GOLDEN HOUR:
THE HANDBOOK OF ADVANCED
PEDIATRIC LIFE SUPPORT

GOLDEN HOUR:
THE HANDBOOK OF ADVANCED
PEDIATRIC LIFE SUPPORT

GOLDEN HOUR:
THE HANDBOOK OF ADVANCED PEDIATRIC LIFE SUPPORT

Third Edition

David G. Nichols, MD, MBA
Mary Wallace Stanton Professor and Vice Dean, Education
The Johns Hopkins University School of Medicine;
Professor, Anesthesiology, Critical Care Medicine, and Pediatrics
The Johns Hopkins Hospital
Baltimore, Maryland

Myron Yaster, MD
Richard J. Traystman Distinguished Professor
Anesthesiology, Critical Care Medicine, and Pediatrics
The Johns Hopkins University School of Medicine
and The Johns Hopkins Hospital
Baltimore, Maryland

Charles L. Schleien, MD, MBA
Executive Vice Chairman, Pediatrics Department
Professor of Pediatrics and Anesthesiology
Columbia University;
Department of Pediatrics
Morgan Stanley Children's Hospital of New York-Presbyterian
New York, New York

Charles N. Paidas, MD, MBA
Professor, Surgery and Pediatrics
Chief, Pediatric Surgery
Associate Dean, Graduate Medical Education
Executive Associate Dean, Clinical and Extramural Affairs
USF Health, University of South Florida College of Medicine
Tampa, Florida

Medical Illustrations by:
Timothy H. Phelps, MS, FAMI
Associate Professor and Medical Illustrator
Department of Art as Applied to Medicine
The Johns Hopkins University
Baltimore, Maryland

ELSEVIER
MOSBY

ELSEVIER
MOSBY

1600 John F. Kennedy Blvd.
Ste 1800
Philadelphia, PA 19103-2899

GOLDEN HOUR: THE HANDBOOK OF ADVANCED   ISBN: 978-0-323-02486-0
PEDIATRIC LIFE SUPPORT, THIRD EDITION

Notices

Knowledge and best practice in this field are constantly changing. As new research and experience broaden our understanding, changes in research methods, professional practices, or medical treatment may become necessary.

Practitioners and researchers must always rely on their own experience and knowledge in evaluating and using any information, methods, compounds, or experiments described herein. In using such information or methods they should be mindful of their own safety and the safety of others, including parties for whom they have a professional responsibility.

With respect to any drug or pharmaceutical product identified, readers are advised to check the most current information provided (i) on procedures featured or (ii) by the manufacturer of each product to be administered, to verify the recommended dose or formula, the method and duration of administration, and contraindications. It is the responsibility of practitioners, relying on their own experience and knowledge of their patients, to make diagnoses, to determine dosages and the best treatment for each individual patient, and to take all appropriate safety precautions.

To the fullest extent of the law, neither the Publisher nor the authors, contributors, or editors assume any liability for any injury and/or damage to persons or property as a matter of products liability, negligence or otherwise, or from any use or operation of any methods, products, instructions, or ideas contained in the material herein.

Previous editions copyrighted 1996, 1991

Library of Congress Cataloging-in-Publication Data
Golden hour : the handbook of advanced pediatric life support / [edited by] David G. Nichols … [et al.] ; medical illustrations by Timothy H. Phelps—3rd ed.
    p. ; cm.
    Handbook of advanced pediatric life support
    Includes bibliographical references and index.
    ISBN 978-0-323-02486-0 (pbk. : alk. paper) 1. Pediatric emergencies. 2. Life support systems (Critical care) I. Nichols, David G. (David Gregory), 1951- II. Title: Handbook of advanced pediatric life support.
    [DNLM: 1. Child—Handbooks. 2. Emergencies—Handbooks. 3. Infant—Handbooks. 4. Critical Care—Handbooks. 5. Life Support Care—Handbooks. 6. Wounds and Injuries— Handbooks. WS 39]
RJ370.G65   2011
618.92'0025—dc22

                                                                    2010039987

Acquisitions Editor: James Merritt   *Project Managers:* Louise King, Antony Prince
Developmental Editor: Barbara Cicalese   *Designer:* Steven Stave
Publishing Services Manager: Anne Altepeter   *Medical Illustrations:* Timothy H. Phelps, MS,
Team Manager: Radhika Pallamparthy   FAMI

Working together to grow
libraries in developing countries
www.elsevier.com | www.bookaid.org | www.sabre.org

ELSEVIER   BOOK AID International   Sabre Foundation

Printed in the United States of America

Last digit is the print number:
9 8 7 6 5 4 3 2 1

#66513014|

The unexpected passing of one of our editors, Dorothy G. Lappe, RN, has saddened the journey of this third edition of *Golden Hour*. Dottie was the glue for both this and the previous editions. It is with great pride that we dedicate this to her loving memory. We owe all who contributed to this edition of *Golden Hour* a huge debt of gratitude, but we are especially thankful for Dottie's inspiration and wisdom.

Contributors

Michael C. Ain, MD
Associate Professor
Orthopaedics and Neurosurgery
The Johns Hopkins Hospital
Baltimore, Maryland

Katherine Biagas, MD, FCCM, FAAP
Associate Professor, Clinical Pediatrics
College of Physicians and Surgeons, Columbia University;
Pediatric Critical Care
Morgan Stanley Children's Hospital of New York-Presbyterian
New York, New York

G. Patricia Cantwell, MD, FCCM
Professor and Chief
Pediatric Critical Care Medicine
Miller School of Medicine;
Holtz Children's Hospital
Miami, Florida

George P. Chrousos, MD, MACE, MACP, FRCP (London)
Professor and Chairman
First Department of Pediatrics
University of Athens;
Director, Department of Pediatrics and Division of Endocrinology,
    Metabolism, and Diabetes, Aghia Sophia Children's Hospital
Athens, Greece

Paul M. Colombani, MD, MBA, FACS, FAAP
Chief and Robert Garrett Professor
Pediatric Surgery
The Johns Hopkins University School of Medicine;
Pediatric Surgeon-in-Charge
The Johns Hopkins Hospital
Baltimore, Maryland

Robert A. Cowles, MD
Assistant Professor, Surgery, Division of Pediatric Surgery
Columbia University;
Assistant Attending Surgeon, Pediatric Surgery
Morgan Stanley Children's Hospital of New York-Presbyterian
New York, New York

Gustavo Del Toro, MD
Associate Professor, Department of Pediatrics
Director, Pediatric Hematopoietic Cell Transplantation Service
Mount Sinai School of Medicine
New York, New York

Jayant K. Deshpande, MD, MPH
Professor, Anesthesiology and Pediatrics
Vanderbilt University Medical Center;
Anesthesiologist-in-Chief
Monroe Carell Jr. Children's Hospital at Vanderbilt
Nashville, Tennessee

Jennifer G. Duncan, MD
Assistant Professor, Department of Pediatrics
Washington University School of Medicine;
Pediatric Critical Care
St. Louis Children's Hospital
St. Louis, Missouri

R. Blaine Easley, MD
Assistant Professor
Pediatrics and Anesthesiology/Critical Care Medicine
The Johns Hopkins Hospital;
Director, Respiratory Care
Kennedy Kreiger Rehabilitation
Baltimore, Maryland

Anne C. Fischer, MD, PhD
Assistant Professor, Surgery
University of Texas Southwestern Medical School;
Staff Surgeon, Dallas Children's Medical Center
Dallas, Texas

Lisa M. Grimaldi, MD
Assistant Clinical Professor, Pediatrics
University of Arizona College of Medicine;
Pediatric Cardiac Intensive Care
Eller Congenital Heart Center
St. Joseph's Hospital and Medical Center
Phoenix, Arizona
Assistant Clinical Professor, Pediatrics
Creighton University School of Medicine
Omaha, Nebraska

Anne-Marie Guerguerian MD, PhD
Assistant Professor, Pediatrics
University of Toronto;
Assistant Professor, Critical Care Medicine
Hospital of Sick Children;
Scientist, Neuroscience and Mental Health
Research Institute of the Hospital for Sick Children
Toronto, Ontario, Canada

Steven Haun, MD
Pediatric Intensivist
Children's Respiratory & Critical Care Specialists, P.A.;
Attending Staff
Children's Hospitals & Clinics of Minnesota
St. Paul, Minnesota

Maria Oliva-Hemker, MD
Stermer Family Professor of Pediatric Inflammatory Bowel Disease
Division of Pediatric Gastroenterology and Nutrition
The Johns Hopkins University School of Medicine
Baltimore, Maryland

Jeff C. Hoehner, MD, PhD
Assistant Professor, Pediatric Surgery
Duke University
Durham, North Carolina

Allan J. Hordof, MD
Professor, Clinical Pediatrics
Columbia University;
Pediatric Cardiology Attending
Morgan Stanley Children's Hospital of New York-Presbyterian
New York, New York

Elizabeth Hunt, MD
Assistant Professor
Anesthesiology and Critical Care Medicine
The Johns Hopkins Hospital
Baltimore, Maryland

Joshua E. Hyman, MD, FAAP
Associate Professor, Clinical Orthopaedic Surgery
Columbia University College of Physicians and Surgeons;
Attending Physician, Pediatric Orthopaedic Surgery
Morgan Stanley Children's Hospital of New York-Presbyterian
New York, New York

Karen Michiko Kling, MD, FACS
Assistant Professor
University of California—San Diego School of Medicine;
Division of Pediatric Surgery
Rady Children's Hospital
San Diego, California

John Kuluz, MD
Staff Physician, Pediatrics
Baptist Children's Hospital
Miami, Florida

Christopher T. Lancaster, MD
Attending Anesthesiologist
Nationwide Children's Hospital
Columbus, Ohio

Eric L. Lazar, MD, MS, FACS, FAAP
Director, Children's Surgical Services
Goryeb Children's Hospital at Morristown Memorial
Morristown, New Jersey

Enrico M. Ligniti, MSCP, PharmD
Clinical Manager, Pediatric Critical Care Medicine
Columbia University Medical Center;
Clinical Manager, Department of Pharmacy Services
Morgan Stanley Children's Hospital of New York-Presbyterian
New York, New York

Steven J. Lobritto, MD
Associate Clinical Professor, Pediatrics and Medicine
Columbia University;
Associate Clinical Professor, Pediatrics and Medicine
Morgan Stanley Children's Hospital of New York-Presbyterian
New York, New York

Lynn D. Martin, MD, MBA
Professor, Anesthesiology and Pain Medicine, Pediatrics
University of Washington School of Medicine;
Director, Anesthesiology and Pain Medicine
Seattle Children's Hospital
Seattle, Washington

Michael A. Nares, MD
Assistant Professor, Clinical Pediatrics
Miller School of Medicine
University of Miami;
Director, Pediatric Critical Care Fellowship
Holtz Children's Hospital
Miami, Florida

David G. Nichols, MD, MBA
Mary Wallace Stanton Professor and Vice Dean, Education
The Johns Hopkins University School of Medicine;
Professor, Anesthesiology, Critical Care Medicine, and Pediatrics
The Johns Hopkins Hospital
Baltimore, Maryland

George Ofori-Amanfo, MD
Associate Professor
Pediatrics and Critical Care Medicine
Duke University
Durham, North Carolina

Charles N. Paidas, MD, MBA
Professor, Surgery and Pediatrics
Chief, Pediatric Surgery
Associate Dean, Graduate Medical Education
Executive Associate Dean, Clinical and Extramural Affairs
USF Health, University of South Florida College of Medicine
Tampa, Florida

Ronald Pauldine, MD
Clinical Associate Professor, Anesthesiology and Pain Medicine
University of Washington School of Medicine;
Anesthesiology Service
VA Puget Sound Health Care System
Seattle, Washington

Timothy H. Phelps, MS, FAMI
Associate Professor and Medical Illustrator
Department of Art as Applied to Medicine
The Johns Hopkins University
Baltimore, Maryland

Richard J. Redett, MD
Associate Professor, Plastic and Reconstructive Surgery
The Johns Hopkins Hospital
Baltimore, Maryland

Michael X. Repka, MD
Professor, Ophthalmology and Pediatrics
The Johns Hopkins University School of Medicine;
Active Staff, Ophthalmology, The Johns Hopkins Hospital
Baltimore, Maryland

Mark R. Rigby, MD, PhD
Assistant Professor, Pediatrics and Surgery
Emory University School of Medicine;
Attending Physician, Pediatric Critical Care
Children's Healthcare of Atlanta at Egleston
Atlanta, Georgia

Lisa Saiman, MD, MPH
Professor, Clinical Pediatrics, Columbia University;
Attending Pediatrician
Morgan Stanley Children's Hospital of New York-Presbyterian;
Hospital Epidemiologist, Infection Prevention and Control
New York Presbyterian Medical Center
New York, New York

Janet N. Scheel, MD
Assistant Professor, Pediatric Cardiology
The Johns Hopkins University School of Medicine;
Assistant Professor, Pediatric Cardiology, The Johns Hopkins Hospital
Baltimore, Maryland

Charles L. Schleien, MD, MBA
Executive Vice Chairman, Pediatrics Department
Professor, Pediatrics and Anesthesiology, Columbia University;
Department of Pediatrics
Morgan Stanley Children's Hospital of New York-Presbyterian
New York, New York

Jennifer Schuette, MD
Assistant Professor, Pediatrics
George Washington School of Medicine and Health Sciences;
Program Director, Pediatric Critical Care Medicine Fellowship
Attending Physician, Cardiac Intensive Care Unit
Children's National Medical Center
Washington, District of Columbia

Deborah Schwengel, MD
Residency Director and Assistant Professor
Anesthesiology and Critical Care Medicine
The Johns Hopkins Hospital
Baltimore, Maryland

Donald Shaffner, MD
Director, Division of Pediatric Anesthesia and Critical Care Medicine
Associate Professor, Pediatrics
The Johns Hopkins University School of Medicine
Baltimore, Maryland

Arthur Smerling, MD
Associate Clinical Professor
Pediatrics and Anesthesiology
Columbia University;
Department of Pediatrics
Morgan Stanley Children's Hospital of New York-Presbyterian
New York, New York

Charles Stolar, MD
Chief, Division of Pediatric Surgery
Surgeon-in-Chief
Morgan Stanley Children's Hospital of New York-Presbyterian;
Rudolph N. Schullinger Professor, Surgery and Pediatrics
Director, Center for Extracorporeal Membrane Oxygenation
Columbia University Medical Center
New York, New York

Steven Stylianos, MD
Clinical Professor, Surgery and Pediatrics
Florida International University College of Medicine;
Department Chief, Pediatric Surgery
Medical Director, Pediatric Trauma Program
Miami Children's Hospital
Miami, Florida

Robert C. Tasker, MBBS, MD
Senior Lecturer, Paediatrics
School of Clinical Medicine
University of Cambridge
Cambridge, England

Allen R. Walker, MD, MBA
Associate Professor, Pediatrics
Division of Pediatric Emergency Medicine
The Johns Hopkins University School of Medicine;
Medical Director, Pediatric Emergency Department
The Johns Hopkins Children's Center
Baltimore, Maryland

Michael Wilhelm, MD
Assistant Professor, Pediatrics
University of Wisconsin—Madison
Madison, Wisconsin

S. Lee Woods, MD, PhD
Medical Director, Center for Maternal and Child Health
Maryland Department of Health and Mental Hygiene
Baltimore, Maryland

Myron Yaster, MD
Richard J. Traystman Distinguished Professor
Anesthesiology, Critical Care Medicine, and Pediatrics
The Johns Hopkins University School of Medicine
and The Johns Hopkins Hospital
Baltimore, Maryland

Susan Ziegfeld, MSN, CRNP-Pediatric
Lead Nurse Practitioner, Pediatric Surgery/Nursing
The Johns Hopkins Children's Center
Baltimore, Maryland

Aaron L. Zuckerberg, MD
Clinical Assistant Professor, Pediatrics
University of Maryland School of Medicine;
Director
Pediatric Anesthesiology and Children's Diagnostic Center
Sinai Hospital
Baltimore, Maryland

Preface

"Elisha came into the house, and there was the boy, laid out dead on his couch. He went in, prayed to the Lord, and placed himself over the child. He put his mouth on its mouth ... and the body of the child became warm."

II Kings 4:32-34

"He who saves a life saves the world."

The Talmud

It has been almost 20 years since the publication of the first edition of *Golden Hour: The Handbook of Advanced Pediatric Life Support,* and 14 years since the last edition. In that time, a revolution in technology and medical science, practice, and education has occurred, necessitating a completely revised and updated edition to reflect those changes. Some basics remain timeless.

The emergency management of a critically ill or injured child is both an exhilarating and terrifying experience. The initial resuscitation often occurs in a tumultuous, chaotic, and emotionally charged atmosphere in which there is little time to think or deliberate on management options. Success often depends on a team approach utilizing well-rehearsed, systematic, evidence-based assessment and management protocols that must be implemented within the first, or *golden*, hour of presentation.

This third edition, like its predecessors, is designed for *front line responders*, namely emergency medical technicians, paramedics, nurses, pediatricians, emergency medicine physicians, surgeons, anesthesiologists, and intensivists. Our emphasis has been and continues to be *how to do it*. Throughout this handbook, the editors and authors have utilized the principles of evidence-based medicine and a culture of safety and quality improvement to impart their battle-tested wisdom to the reader. We believe this is crucial; wisdom is judgment based on knowledge gained through experience. It is quite different than mere intelligence. Wisdom requires experience. It is our profound hope that this edition of *Golden Hour* will facilitate the attainment of wisdom in the readers to improve their management of the critically ill and injured child.

We are thankful that several of the original authors of the first edition have continued to provide their knowledge, expertise, wisdom, and support for this third edition. In addition, we have assembled a new cadre of experts and have tried to maintain the feel and look of the previous editions. Every one of the original chapters in the handbook has been comprehensively updated. Moreover, this third edition includes new chapters dealing with asthma, acute renal failure, endocrine and gastrointestinal emergencies, liver failure, hematologic and oncologic emergencies, general surgical emergencies, hypothermia and hyperthermia, and terrorism and mass casualty events. Images have been added and some revised by our gifted medical illustrator, Tim Phelps. In addition, the editorial board has totally revised treatment protocols and algorithms and tested them in the simulation laboratories, emergency departments, and intensive care units of our hospitals.

Medical and surgical procedures have been redrawn, treatment tables updated, and protocols expanded. They are designed to be clear, uncluttered, and as user friendly as possible.

We are forever grateful to all who have advised, lectured, and participated in our procedure laboratory during our biannual courses at The Johns Hopkins Hospital and in the simulation laboratories. Children from around the globe have benefited from the previous editions of this handbook.

The editors are indebted to all expert contributors. In addition, it is without exaggeration that we remain indebted to all emergency medical technicians, hospital personnel, nurses, and physicians who once again have utilized and critiqued management algorithms in this book.

David G. Nichols, MD, MBA

Charles N. Paidas, MD, MBA

Charles L. Schleien, MD, MBA

Myron Yaster, MD

Acknowledgment

Special thanks to Maura Probst, who worked many extra hours during the past few months to get the third edition of *Golden Hour* to production.

Contents

Chapter 1

Initial Assessment

Deborah A. Schwengel, MD,
Charles N. Paidas, MD, MBA,
and Myron Yaster, MD

I. Overview

    A. The management of a critically ill or injured child requires a systematic, well-rehearsed approach that can be instituted almost reflexively (**Fig. 1-1**).

    B. One must be able to identify the management priorities for stabilization of the patient even before a complete history and physical examination have been obtained.

    C. Definitive therapy may not be possible until resuscitation and stabilization are complete.

    D. Finally, success is only possible if the unique anatomic, physiologic, and pathophysiologic responses of children are understood by the resuscitation team.

II. Primary survey

    A. Definition

    The primary survey involves the first evaluation of the patient's condition, at which time the life-threatening problems are identified. A hierarchy of management priorities for resuscitation and stabilization is established.

    B. Steps in a primary survey

    The primary survey is designed to assess the following items in the order listed:

        1. **A**irway

        2. **B**reathing (ventilation)

        3. **C**irculation (hemorrhage control)

        4. **D**isability (neurologic examination)

        5. **E**xposure (temperature)

        Assessment of children who are able to communicate can be done in 10 seconds by asking the following questions:

        • What is your name?

        • What happened?

        Correct answers to these questions mean that the child has a patent airway, adequate chest wall dynamics for breathing, and intact sensorium to respond appropriately. Thus, when indicated, these questions can facilitate a rapid initial assessment.

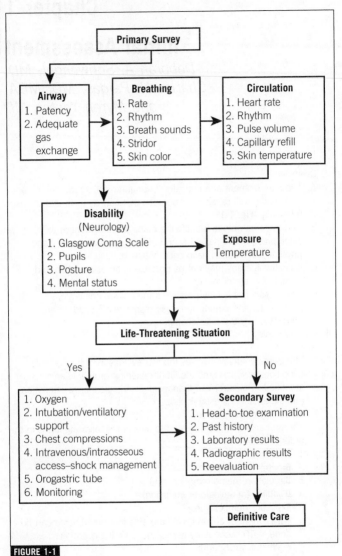

FIGURE 1-1

Algorithm of the initial assessment of a pediatric patient.

C. Airway

The goals of airway management are as follows:

1. Recognition and relief of obstruction
2. Prevention of aspiration of gastric contents
3. Promotion of adequate gas exchange

Further detailed information regarding pediatric airway management is discussed in Chapter 2.

D. Breathing

1. Once the patient's airway is established, the child must be observed for adequate breathing. Air exchange may be deficient from central causes, such as apnea, or from abnormal chest wall dynamics, such as a tension pneumothorax. The cause of the problem should be treated immediately.
2. Assessment of breathing is done as follows:
   a. Physical examination
      (1) Chest rise with inspiration
      (2) Breath sounds
      (3) Skin color (pink nail beds)
   b. Pulse oximetry features
      (1) Noninvasive and continuous
      (2) Late detection of airway obstruction
      (3) Requires perfusion
      (4) Carbon monoxide poisoning—leads to an inaccurate (elevated) reading
      (5) Subject to motion artifact
   c. Capnography (intubated patient)
      (1) Best detection of airway patency and endotracheal tube placement
      (2) Breath-to-breath assessment of breathing, circulation, and carbon dioxide production
      (3) Best assessment of return of spontaneous circulation after cardiac arrest
   d. Arterial blood gas
3. Methods to augment ventilation
   a. Mouth-to-mouth, mouth-to-nose breathing
   b. Mask-bag ventilation
   c. Endotracheal intubation
   d. Cricothyrotomy (needle or surgical)

Emergency breathing techniques are further described in Chapter 2.

E. Circulation

1. The adequacy of circulation is assessed by noting the quality, rate, and regularity of the pulse, centrally and peripherally. Capillary refill and blood pressure are determined. Note that blood pressure is one of the least sensitive measures of adequate circulation in children. Compromised circulation may

TABLE 1-1

APPROXIMATE RANGES OF VITAL SIGNS IN INFANTS AND CHILDREN

Age	Blood Pressure (mm Hg)	Heart Rate (beats/min)
Premature infant	Systolic 40-60	100-160
Full-term newborn	70/50	100-180
1-6 mo	80/50	110-180
6-12 mo	90/65	110-170
12-24 mo	95/65	90-150
2-6 yr	100/60	70-140
6-12 yr	110/60	60-130
12-16 yr	110/65	60-110
16-18 yr	120/65	60-100
Adult	125/75	60-100

Approximate ranges for BP—mean pressure ± 20% = 95% confidence limit. Values for females are approximately 5% lower.

TABLE 1-2

APPROXIMATE BODY WEIGHTS BY AGE

Age	Weight (kg)
Birth	3.5
6 mo	7
12 mo	10
24 mo	12
36 mo	15
5 yr	20
10 yr	30
12 yr	40
14 yr	50

exist despite a normal blood pressure in children. Normal hemodynamic values for children are given in **Table 1-1.**

2. Circulatory support during the primary survey may require the following:
   a. Control of active hemorrhage (see Chapter 6)
      (1) Estimate blood loss (see Table 6-6).
      (2) Estimate blood volume (see Table 6-7).
      (3) Replace volume losses.
   b. Intravenous fluid, crystalloid/blood
   c. External cardiac massage (see Chapter 5)
   d. Defibrillation
   e. Estimated weights. Drug and fluid dosage calculations require estimates of body weight. See **Table 1-2** for estimates of body weight based on age.

F. Disability
   1. A rapid screening neurologic evaluation is performed as part of the primary survey. This includes assessment of pupillary

response, level of consciousness, and notation of any localized findings.

2. A detailed explanation of neurologic assessment is included in Chapters 15 and 16.

G. Exposure
   1. Passive heat loss
      a. A complete physical examination requires undressing the patient.
      b. Because of their large surface–to–body mass ratio, children cool rapidly, particularly when homeostatic mechanisms may be disrupted by disease states.
   2. Hypothermia and hyperthermia are discussed in Chapter 28.

III. Secondary survey
   A. Definition
      The secondary survey includes a detailed physical examination. Other components of the secondary survey include the following:
      1. History of the illness or trauma event
      2. Brief past history
      3. Indicated laboratory and radiographic studies, which may lead to a specific diagnosis or problem list
   B. Head
      1. The face is examined for the following:
         a. Evidence of maxillofacial trauma
            (1) Palpation of bony prominences
            (2) Presence of bloody or cerebral spinal fluid discharge from the nose, mouth, or ears
         b. Dehydration
            (1) Sunken eyes and/or fontanel
            (2) Dry mouth mucosa
         c. Poisoning and metabolic problems
            (1) Odor from mouth
            (2) Discoloration of mucosa
      2. The eyes are examined for pupillary size and reaction, fundoscopic appearance, and vision, if possible (see Chapter 25).
      3. The scalp is carefully examined for laceration or hematoma. Specific signs of basilar skull fractures include Battle sign (ecchymoses behind the ear) and raccoon eyes (ecchymoses around both eyes; see Chapter 15).
   C. Neck
      1. The neck is palpated for obvious signs of fractures and midline position of the trachea.
      2. Cervical spine injury is presumed until it can be excluded. Therefore, flexion, extension, and rotation of the neck are avoided and a cervical collar is applied until neck injury has been excluded.

D. Chest
  1. The chest is inspected for adequacy of respiratory excursion, asymmetry of respiration, and/or presence of a flail segment.
  2. The chest is then carefully palpated, and the lung fields and heart are auscultated.
  3. Thoracic trauma is discussed in Chapter 21, asthma in Chapter 4, and respiratory failure in Chapter 3.
  4. A chest radiograph and electrocardiogram should be obtained if chest trauma has occurred.
E. Abdomen
  1. Initial examination of the abdomen includes inspection for ease of abdominal wall movement with respiration, gentle palpation for localized guarding or mass, and auscultation for bowel sounds.
  2. The flanks are observed for hematoma and palpated.
  3. Serial examinations are often needed to establish a correct diagnosis.
  4. In females of childbearing age, pregnancy and pregnancy-related problems must be investigated.
  5. Abdominal trauma is discussed in Chapter 22.
F. Pelvis
  1. The bony prominences of the pelvis are palpated for tenderness or instability, and examined for ecchymoses.
  2. The perineum is examined for laceration, hematoma, active bleeding, or discharge (inflammatory). Child abuse is discussed in Chapter 31.
G. Rectum
  A rectal examination is indicated if pelvic fracture, bowel pathology, or child abuse is suspected.
H. Extremities
  1. The extremities are examined for signs of abrasion, contusion, hematoma formation, or deformity. Soft tissue injuries are discussed in Chapter 26.
  2. Bony instability is noted and a neurovascular examination is performed on all extremities.
  3. Orthopedic injuries are discussed in Chapter 24.
I. Neurologic examination
  1. This includes motor, sensory, cranial nerve, and level of consciousness in an in-depth examination.
  2. The tympanic membranes and the nose are examined for signs of basilar skull fracture.
  3. The fundi are examined.
  4. A coma score may aid in subsequent examination, and the modified Glasgow Coma Scale score is recommended here (see Chapter 15).
  5. The possibility of spinal cord trauma is noted (e.g., flaccidity, hypotension without tachycardia, absent reflexes).

   6. The patient's current pain levels are assessed and a pain
      history is obtained. Develop a plan to treat the pain (see
      Chapter 20).
   7. Neurologic assessment is further discussed in Chapters 15 and
      16.
J. Bony structures of the back
   1. The patient with suspected spinal cord trauma is immobilized
      on a backboard and with a cervical collar (see Chapter 15).
   2. If there is no obvious spinal cord injury and paralysis, the
      patient should be turned gently to examine the back for
      evidence of trauma.
K. Skin
   The skin should be examined simultaneously during all previous
   steps.
   1. Bruises. The color and size may be suggestive of trauma or
      coagulopathy.
   2. Rash. Hemorrhagic, stellate, rapidly expanding rashes may
      suggest life-threatening conditions (e.g., septic shock,
      meningococcemia, anaphylaxis, drug-induced blood dyscrasia).
L. Other care
   1. History. A thorough and concise review of the presentation and
      history needs to be performed. This can be most easily
      accomplished remembering the mnemonic **AMPLE: A,** allergies;
      M, medications; **P,** past illnesses; **L,** last meal; and **E,** events
      preceding the injury or illness.
   2. Radiographic and laboratory studies
   3. Continuous monitoring and reevaluation
   4. Request for appropriate consultants
   5. Definitive care. The person who performs the initial evaluation
      and stabilization needs to remain the responsible physician and
      function as the child's advocate until responsibility for the
      child's total care is undertaken by another.

Chapter 2

Airway Management

Christopher T. Lancaster, MD,
and Myron Yaster, MD

I. Goals of airway management
   A. **Recognition and relief** of anatomic obstruction
   B. **Prevention** of aspiration of gastric contents
   C. **Promotion** of adequate gas exchange
II. Anatomy of the pediatric airway
   Understanding the anatomic differences among infants, children, and adults is crucial in airway management (**Fig. 2-1**).
   A. Nose
      1. Infants to 3 months of age are obligate nose breathers.
      2. Anatomic (choanal atresia) or upper respiratory infection obstruction will cause respiratory distress.
      3. The abundant lymphoid tissue bleeds easily.
   B. Tongue
      1. The tongue is relatively large in relation to the mandible in children younger than 2 years.
      2. Visualization of the larynx is difficult.
      3. The tongue is the most common cause of upper airway obstruction in unconscious patients of any age.
   C. Larynx
      1. Position—higher (superior, rostral) in the neck than adults: Located at the second to fourth cervical vertebrae (C2-C4) in infants, and at the fourth to fifth cervical vertebrae (C4-C5) in adults (see Fig. 2-1)
         a. Exaggerated in patients with mandibular hypoplasia (e.g., Pierre-Robin syndrome)
      2. Vocal cords: 40% ligament, 60% arytenoid cartilage in infants; ratios reversed in adults
   D. Epiglottis
      1. The infant's epiglottis is omega-shaped, floppy, and has a 45-degree angle of entry into the pharyngeal wall. Better visualization of the larynx is made by lifting the epiglottis directly with a straight blade.
      2. The adult's epiglottis is stiff, flat, and parallel to the tracheal wall. Visualization of the larynx is made indirectly by placing the curved (MacIntosh) laryngoscope blade in the vallecula (see Fig. 2-1).

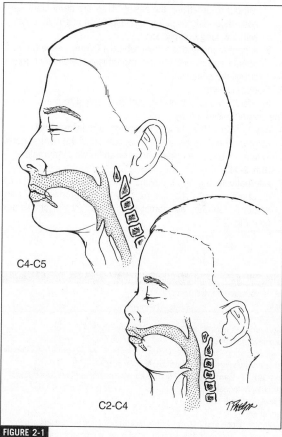

C4-C5

C2-C4

T.Phelps

FIGURE 2-1

Comparison of the adult and infant airways.

E. Subglottis (cricoid cartilage)
   1. The cricoid is the only complete ring of cartilage and is nonexpandable. It is the narrowest part of the airway in children younger than 8 to 10 years and is ellipsoid in shape.
   2. To avoid cuff trauma to this structure, noncuffed tubes have historically been used in children younger than 8 to 10 years. However, newer polyurethane, high-volume, low-pressure cuffed tubes can be used in younger children and infants

without traumatizing the airway. They are particularly useful for patients at risk for pulmonary aspiration of gastric contents or with low lung compliance.

   3. A tight-fitting endotracheal tube (ETT) may cause tracheal edema and stenosis that compromises the airway (croup or subglottic stenosis).

F. Tracheal length

   In infants, the length of the trachea is only 4 to 5 cm.

III. The compromised airway

A. Airway obstruction, or loss of protective reflexes, most commonly occurs because of depression of the central nervous system or because of peripheral or anatomic abnormalities (**Box 2-1**).

B. Alternatively, the upper airway, defined as the nasopharynx, oropharynx, and hypopharynx, may be compromised by normal anatomic features, or anomalies, of the infant's or child's airway (see Fig. 2-1).

BOX 2-1   Major Causes of Upper Airway Obstruction

Central nervous system dysfunction
- Shock
- Head trauma
- Drug overdose (alcohol, sedative/hypnotics, opioids)
- Hypoxemia, hypercarbia
- Metabolic derangements (↑ or ↓ glucose, sodium, potassium levels; hepatic or uremic encephalopathy; metabolic acidosis; sepsis)
- Increased ICP leading to vocal cord paralysis (hydrocephalus, obstructed ventriculoperitoneal shunts)

Peripheral anatomic causes

Congenital anomalies
- Mandibular hypoplasia—Pierre Robin syndrome, Treacher Collins syndrome
- Macroglossia—Beckwith-Wiedemann syndrome, glycogen storage diseases, hypothyroidism, Down syndrome
- Tracheal, laryngeal lesions—subglottic stenosis, web, cyst, laryngocele, tumor, laryngomalacia, laryngotracheoesophageal cleft, tracheomalacia, trachea-esophageal fistula, juvenile papillomatosis

Infection
- Supraglottic—epiglottis, retropharyngeal abscess, Ludwig angina, peritonsillar abscess, juvenile papillomatosis
- Subglottic—laryngotracheobronchitis (croup), staphylococcal tracheitis

Trauma—external trauma, postintubation croup, post-tracheostomy

Foreign body aspiration

Burns
- Thermal (fire, steam); chemical (lye, acid)

Anaphylaxis, laryngospasm

ICP, Intracranial pressure.

IV. Assessment and history
  A. Important questions to ask when obtaining a history in a patient with noisy breathing and distress:
   1. Does it occur with feeding (laryngotracheoesophageal cleft or fistula) or only when the child is stressed (e.g., subglottic stenosis, laryngeal web, or laryngomalacia)?
   2. Is it positional? Specifically, does the prone position provide relief (e.g., supraglottic process, laryngomalacia, or enlarged tongue)?
   3. Is it an acute process associated with infection and fever (e.g., croup, epiglottitis, or retropharyngeal abscess), with a possible foreign body aspiration, or following any external or internal (postintubation) trauma?
   4. Is this a chronic process associated with other problems, such as prematurity (subglottic stenosis), hydrocephalus (vocal cord paralysis), or neuromuscular disease (aspiration pneumonia)?
   5. Does the child snore or breathe noisily (adenoidal hypertrophy, obstructive sleep apnea)?
   6. Is the voice hoarse (e.g., laryngitis, vocal cord paralysis, papillomatosis, granuloma)?
   7. Will the patient eat or drink or swallow the normal oral secretions? Dysphagia is associated with a supraglottic pathology (epiglottitis or retropharyngeal abscess).
   8. Is there a history of a congenital syndrome (e.g., Pierre Robin syndrome, see Box 2-1)?
  B. Physical examination
  Observation and physical examination progress simultaneously while taking a history (see Chapter 1). Signs and symptoms of upper airway obstruction include the following:
   1. Paradoxical chest movements
     a. Chest collapses inward on inspiration; abdomen protrudes outwardly.
     b. When exaggerated, the sternum cups inward; this mimics pectus excavatum.
   2. Use of accessory muscles
     a. Retractions—suprasternal (sternocleidomastoid muscle), intercostals, and subcostal (abdominal muscles)
     b. Nasal flaring
   3. Stridor
     a. Inspiratory stridor suggests obstruction above the larynx.
     b. Inspiratory **and** expiratory stridor suggest obstruction below the larynx.
   4. Cough
     a. Brassy, "dog barking in the night," croupy cough suggests pathology below the larynx and is unusual in epiglottitis.

    5. Nonspecific signs of respiratory distress include the following:
       a. Decreased air movement
       b. Cyanosis, pallor
       c. Somnolence—sign of imminent respiratory arrest (severe hypercarbia, hypoxemia)
    6. Anatomic findings suggesting difficult intubation include the following:
       a. Size of mouth and mouth opening
       b. Size of tongue and its relationship to other pharyngeal structures; the Mallampati classification helps predict the potential for difficult intubation (**Fig. 2-2**).
       c. Loose or missing teeth

  C. Radiographic studies

    Usually unnecessary, the radiographic examination may help confirm a diagnosis suspected by history and physical examination. Specific tests include the following:
    1. Lateral neck film—retropharyngeal abscess, foreign body, macroglossia, enlarged tonsils (sleep apnea)
    2. Anteroposterior view of the chest—croup, foreign body, pneumonia, asthma
    3. Fluoroscopy of the chest—foreign body, paralyzed diaphragm
    4. Barium swallow—tracheoesophageal fistula, vascular ring

V. Airway equipment

  The most common cause of upper airway obstruction in the unconscious patient is neck flexion. This causes the tongue to rest against the roof of the mouth, cutting off air flow.

  A. Oropharyngeal airway
    1. Indications
       a. Relief of airway obstruction by the tongue in unconscious patients (**Fig. 2-3,** *A*)
       b. Bite block when securing an ETT
    2. Size
       a. Length is estimated by placing the airway next to the face, with the flange at the level of the teeth.
       b. The tip should reach the angle of the jaw.
    3. Complications
       a. When placed incorrectly, this device may actually obstruct the airway by pushing the tongue backward into the hypopharynx.

  B. Nasopharyngeal airway (nasal trumpet)
    1. Indication
       a. Relief of nasopharyngeal (NP) obstruction and obstruction by the tongue (see Fig. 2-3, *B*).
       b. The nasal trumpet is well tolerated in conscious or semiconscious patients, and rarely provokes vomiting or laryngospasm.

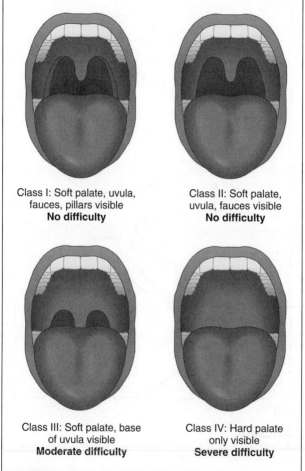

Class I: Soft palate, uvula,
fauces, pillars visible
No difficulty

Class II: Soft palate,
uvula, fauces visible
No difficulty

Class III: Soft palate, base
of uvula visible
Moderate difficulty

Class IV: Hard palate
only visible
Severe difficulty

FIGURE 2-2

Mallampati classification.

2. Insertion
   a. A vasoconstrictive spray, such as 0.25% phenylephrine
      (Neo-Synephrine), shrinks the nasal mucosa and reduces
      the incidence of bleeding.
   b. A local anesthetic lubricant (2% lidocaine jelly or ointment)
      facilitates painless insertion.

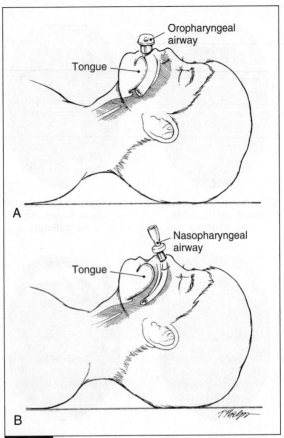

FIGURE 2-3

A, Oropharyngeal and **B,** nasopharyngeal airways relieve obstruction of the hypopharynx by the tongue.

3. Size
   a. The length is estimated by measuring the distance from the tip of the nose to the angle of the jaw; the nares can be progressively dilated by slowly increasing size of the NP airway.
   b. Available sizes are 12 to 36 Fr.
4. Complications
   a. Epistaxis
   b. Avulsion, fracture of the adenoids or nasal conchae

TABLE 2-1			
OXYGEN DELIVERY EQUIPMENT			
Device	**FIo$_2$**	**Patient Size**	**Comments**
Nasal cannula	0.22-0.4	Neonate, infant, child, adult	Least restrictive; best tolerated; FIo$_2$ unknown; entrains room air; does not require humidification; flows 0.5-6 L/min
Simple face mask	0.22-0.5	Infant, child, adult	Entrains room air; requires humidification; flow 4-6 L/min
Nonrebreathing face mask	0.22-1	Child, adult	Reservoir provides 100% FIo$_2$; requires humidification; flows 4-8 liter/min
Oxygen hood	0.22-1	Neonate, infant <10 kg	Requires humidification; flows >10 L/min to flush out CO$_2$

CO$_2$, Carbon dioxide; *FIo$_2$,* fraction of inspired oxygen.

5. Contraindications
   a. Bleeding diathesis
   b. Cerebrospinal fluid leak (especially with basilar skull fractures, raccoon eyes, and Battle sign) because of the possibility of infection or passage of the nasal trumpet into the intracranial vault
   c. Deformity of the nose impeding passage of the tube (never force passage of the tube through the airway)

C. Suction
   1. Indication: Suction of emesis, blood, particulate matter, or oral secretions
   2. Technique: Suction should be set at the highest vacuum rate possible.
   3. Equipment: Rigid, wide-bore catheters (Yankauer) or 14 to 18 Fr soft tracheal suction catheters

VI. Oxygen (O$_2$) therapy equipment
   A. O$_2$ is the first and most important drug to be used in any pediatric crisis situation. There is **never** a resuscitation situation in children in which 100% delivered O$_2$ is contraindicated!
   B. Commonly used O$_2$ therapy equipment is shown in **Figure 2-4** and described in **Table 2-1.**

VII. Manual ventilation equipment
   The airway is opened with the triple jaw maneuver, which relieves obstruction by the tongue (**Figs. 2-5** and **2-6**). Once a patent airway has been established, determine if the patient has adequate ventilation. If not, manual ventilation by bag, mask, and 100% O$_2$ is started.
   A. Resuscitation (ventilation) face mask
      1. A face mask consists of a rubber or plastic body, connecting port, and rim (rigid or malleable) that allows a tight face seal during ventilation.

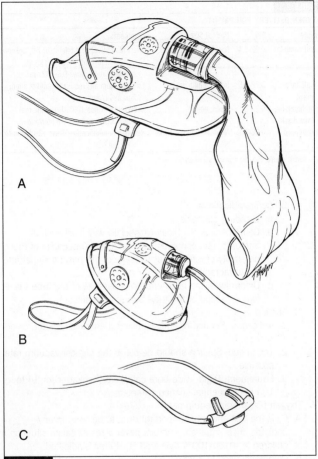

FIGURE 2-4

Oxygen delivery equipment. **A,** Nonrebreathing face mask with reservoir.
B, Simple face mask. **C,** Nasal cannula.

    2. Equipment types
       a. Soft—with or without a cushioned edge to mold to the
         shape of the face
       b. Rigid—low profile, hard edge, minimal dead space
       c. Opaque (black) or clear—clear masks allow early
         identification of emesis or excess secretions in the pharynx.
   B. Manual resuscitation bags or positive pressure O_2 delivery
     systems

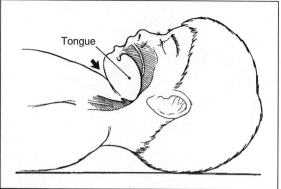

FIGURE 2-5

The tongue obstructs the hypopharynx.

1. Indication: The bag provides a rapid means of delivering positive pressure breaths when connected to a resuscitation face mask.
2. Self-inflating bags (**Fig. 2-7**)
   a. These bags entrain room air, unless a reservoir is attached for 100% O_2.
   b. Spring-loaded disk valves will not open during spontaneous ventilation.
   c. Patients must be manually ventilated.
   d. These bags reinflate automatically after each breath.
3. Anesthesia bags (**Fig. 2-8**)
   a. These require a minimum of 3 L/min flow and do not refill spontaneously.
   b. Patients can breathe spontaneously or be manually ventilated.
   c. Adequacy of ventilation is easy to assess.
   d. 100% O_2 can be delivered without a reservoir.

VIII. Bag and mask ventilation
   A. Overview
      When a patient's breathing is inadequate, the temptation is to intubate the trachea immediately. This is rarely necessary. Ventilation and oxygenation by bag and mask (or rarely mouth to mouth) technique are essential and should routinely precede intubation.
   B. Technique
      1. Infants and small children
         a. The mask is held in the left hand and should be pressed against the nasal bridge with the thumb at the same time that the index finger exerts downward pressure on the base of the mask over the chin.

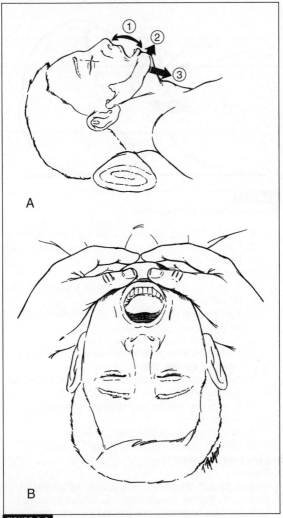

FIGURE 2-6

Triple jaw maneuver. **A, B,** Mouth open (1); mandible displaced anteriorly (2) and downward (3).

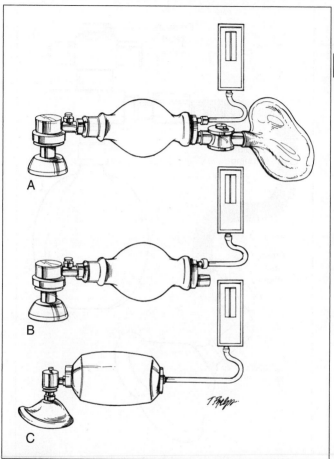

FIGURE 2-7

Self-inflating bags. **A,** Ambu bag with reservoir for delivery of 100% oxygen. **B,** Ambu bag without reservoir entrains room air. **C,** PMR bag without oxygen supply valve or oxygen accumulator delivers 45% to 50% oxygen.

    b. These two fingers encircle the mask and make a C. They provide the mask seal that allows the delivery of positive pressure ventilation.

    c. The middle finger lies directly under the chin, across the mandible, lifting it up.

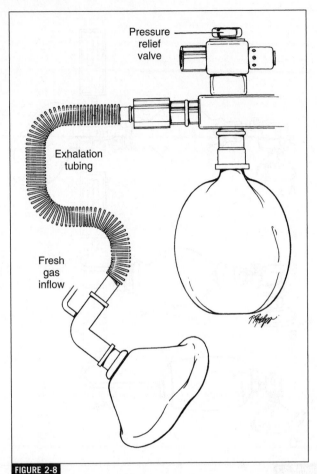

FIGURE 2-8
Anesthesia bag—Mapleson D. This delivers 100% oxygen.

  d. The ring and little fingers float to prevent external
   compression of the airway in the soft tissues of the
   submental area of the neck (**Fig. 2-9**).
 2. Adults and older children
  This is done as with infants and small children, except that the
  ring finger grips the mandible and the little finger engages the
  angle of the jaw, lifting the mandible forward. The wrist is
  cocked to tilt the head backward.

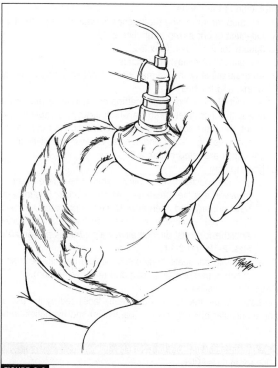

FIGURE 2-9

Bag and mask ventilation. The thumb and index finger produce the seal and the middle finger lies on the mandible to lift the jaw upward.

C. Adjuvants to make ventilation easier
  1. Airways
     An oropharyngeal or nasopharyngeal airway used in conjunction with the face mask helps relieve airway obstruction (usually caused by the tongue; see Fig. 2-3).
  2. Continuous positive airway pressure (CPAP)
     a. CPAP helps in overcoming airway obstruction by dilating the upper airway. This is helpful for spontaneously breathing patients with upper airway obstruction (e.g., large tonsils or croup).
     b. Positive pressure should not exceed 10 mm Hg to avert the risk of vomiting and aspiration caused by air forced into the stomach.

IX. Intubation of the trachea

The method for intubating the trachea is dependent on the following:

A. **Judgment** of one's own intubation skills

B. **Options** for intubation (**Box 2-2**)

C. The patient's **hemodynamic status**

D. An **assessment** of the normalcy of the patient's upper airway, larynx, and trachea

Although there is no single method of anatomic evaluation of the airway that absolutely predicts which airway is simple and which is not, the most commonly used classification is the Mallampati system (see Fig. 2-2). Conditions associated with difficult intubation are listed in **Box 2-3.**

E. Backup plan

1. The unexpected difficult airway should be a rare event; however, it is life-threatening when it occurs. It is imperative to have primary and alternative strategies prepared and available.

2. A reasonable decision tree based on the American Society of Anesthesiologists' difficult airway algorithm is presented in **Figs. 2-10** and **2-11.**

3. Maintain adequate oxygenation while a definitive course of action is pursued (e.g., bag and mask ventilation).

X. Drugs for intubation

Intubation of the trachea can be greatly facilitated by the use of neuromuscular blocking agents (paralytics) and hypnotics-amnestics.

BOX 2-2 Options and Indications for Emergency Intubation

Awake intubation (no sedation)
- Difficult airway: congenital anomalies, trauma, burns
- Hemodynamically unstable or hypotensive patient
- Unconscious patient
- Newborn

Rapid sequence induction (crash)—rapid pharmacologic paralysis, sedation, and cricoid pressure (see Figs. 2-10 and 2-11)
- Bowel obstruction, peritonitis, peritoneal dialysis, ascites
- History of gastroesophageal reflux (history of gastroesophageal fistula repair)
- Pregnancy (later than second trimester)
- Increased intracranial pressure
- Undocumented fasting period or documented fast of <8 hr for solid food
- Multiple trauma, pain

General anesthesia—requires operating room, anesthesiologist, and surgeon for possible bronchoscopy and tracheostomy
- Airway obstruction (acute supraglottitis)
- Foreign body aspiration

Sedation and paralysis
- Elective intubation (prior to gastric lavage, radiographic procedures, cardioversion)
- Emergent intubation in hemodynamically stable patient

BOX 2-3   Syndromes Associated with Difficult Intubation

- Micrognathia—cri-du-chat (also narrow larynx), DiGeorge (also hypocalcemic tetany), Pierre Robin, Treacher Collins, Noonan, Turner, trisomy 13 and trisomy 18 syndromes
- Macroglossia—Beckwith-Wiedemann, trisomy 21 (Down), Hurler, and Hunter (mucopolysaccharidoses) syndromes; also short neck, hypothyroidism, glycogen storage disease (Pompe disease), Scheie (prognathism, short neck) syndromes
- Midface hypoplasia—craniofacial dysostosis (maxilla and/or mandible), Apert, Crouzon, Goldenhar (oculoauriculovertebral), median cleft face (cleft lip, nose, palate) syndromes; cherubism (fibrous dysplasia of mandible); hemifacial microsomia
- Short neck, rigid neck—ankylosing spondylitis; rheumatoid arthritis; Hurler, Hunter, Morquio, Klippel-Feil syndromes
- Temporomandibular joint disease—collagen vascular disease (rheumatoid arthritis, polyarteritis nodosa, dermatomyositis, systemic lupus erythematosus); trismus (following trauma, local infection); infection (Ludwig angina, retropharyngeal abscess); arthrogryposis multiplex
- Airway edema, fibrosis—angioedema (anaphylaxis, hereditary), pregnancy, epidermolysis bullosa, Stevens-Johnson syndrome
- Any patient in a halo traction device

A. Sedative-hypnotics and analgesics
  1. **Awake patients should not receive paralytic drugs!**
  2. The drug and dose used to produce unconsciousness is dependent on the patient's clinical condition and hemodynamic status.
  3. It must be emphasized that there are no correct dosages of these drugs.
     a. Some patients may require enormous amounts of drug and others very little.
     b. The only way to use these drugs is by titration to effect.
     c. It is always better to use a lower dosage and to titrate upward as needed.
     d. Suggested doses are listed in **Table 2-2.** A treatment algorithm is presented in **Figure 2-12.**
B. Neuromuscular blocking agents
  These are listed in **Table 2-3.** A treatment algorithm is given in **Figure 2-13.** Paralytic drugs are classified by the following:
  1. Mechanism
     a. Depolarizing muscle relaxants (succinylcholine)
     b. Nondepolarizing muscle relaxants (pancuronium, vecuronium, rocuronium, cisatracurium)
  2. Duration of action
     a. Short (succinylcholine)
     b. Intermediate (rocuronium, vecuronium, cisatracurium)
     c. Long (pancuronium, doxacurium)

Text continued on p. 31.

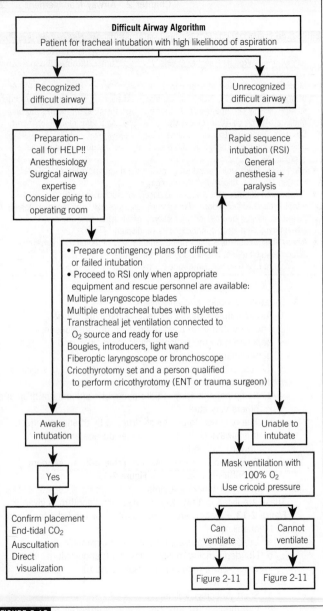

FIGURE 2-10

Algorithm for treatment of the difficult airway (part 1).

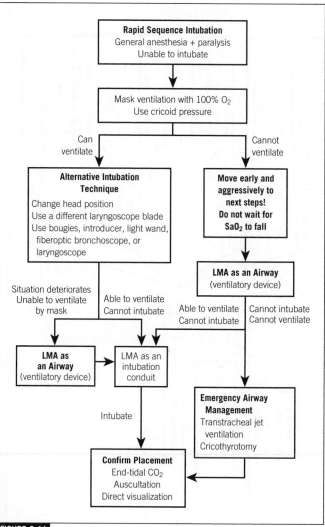

FIGURE 2-11

Algorithm for treatment of the difficult airway (part 2).

ENT, Ear, nose, and throat; *LMA,* laryngeal mask airway; *SaO₂,* oxygen saturation.

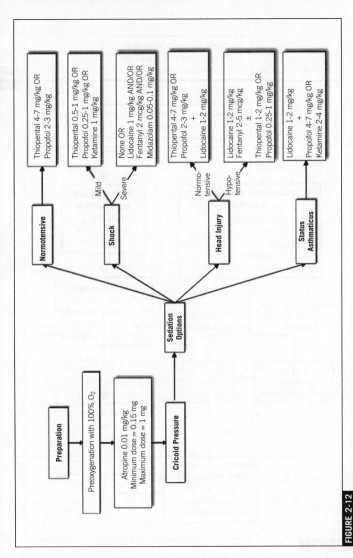

FIGURE 2-12

Treatment algorithm for sedative choices for intubation.

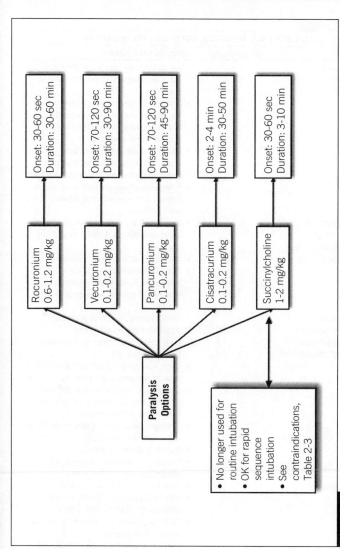

FIGURE 2-13

Treatment algorithm for selection of neuromuscular blocking agents for intubation.

TABLE 2-2

INTRAVENOUS SEDATIVES, HYPNOTICS, AND OPIOIDS FOR INTUBATION

Drug	Dosage (mg/kg)	Indications and Comments
Propofol • Normovolemia • Hypovolemia	 2-3 0.5-1	• Rapidly (<30 sec) produces general anesthesia, loss of consciousness, amnesia; no analgesic properties • ↓ Intracranial pressure (ICP); ↓ cerebral blood flow (CBF); ↓ cerebral oxygen consumption (C_{MRO_2}); anticonvulsant at intubating doses, proconvulsant at lower doses • Myocardial depression; hypotension in hypovolemia; apnea, respiratory depression; painful on injection, particularly into small veins • Prolonged continuous infusions in the intensive care unit associated with fatal, refractory acidosis and heart failure
Thiopental or thiamylal • Normovolemia • Hypovolemia	 4-7 0.25-1	• Rapidly (<30 sec) produces general anesthesia, loss of consciousness, amnesia; no analgesic properties • ↓ICP; ↓CBF; ↓C_{MRO_2}; potent anticonvulsant • Myocardial depression; hypotension in hypovolemia; apnea, respiratory depression; intra-arterial injections → gangrene because pH >11
Ketamine • Normovolemia • Hypovolemia • Intramuscular (IM)	 1-2 0.5 3-7	• Potent analgesic (2-5× more potent than morphine); amnestic; hallucinogen • Rapid loss of consciousness (<30 sec) when given intravenous (IV) • Shock: increases blood pressure and heart rate by releasing endogenous catecholamines • Bronchodilator, ideal for asthmatics; ↑ oral secretions, requires antisialogogue (atropine); blunts airway protective reflexes • Emergence delirium and nightmares, which may be prevented with concomitant benzodiazepine • Contraindicated in patients with ↑ICP • Useful in congenital heart disease except aortic stenosis and severe cardiomyopathy
Etomidate	0.3	• Rapid loss of consciousness (<1 min) • Almost no hemodynamic effects; use in shock, patients with congenital heart disease • Blunts steroidogenesis and may worsen outcome in septic shock patients • Painful on IV injection, pretreat with fentanyl (2 mcg/kg) • Myoclonic jerks common; anticonvulsant; ↓ICP, ↓CBF, ↓C_{MRO_2}

TABLE 2-2

INTRAVENOUS SEDATIVES, HYPNOTICS, AND OPIOIDS FOR INTUBATION—cont'd

Drug	Dosage (mg/kg)	Indications and Comments
Midazolam		• Sedative-anxiolytic; general anesthetic at higher doses; amnestic, no analgesic properties; anticonvulsant
• Normovolemia		
IV	0.05-0.1	
IM	0.1-0.15	• Minimal hemodynamic effects in healthy children
Rectally	0.5-1	• Hypotension in newborns with cardiac disease
• Hypovolemia	0.025-0.05	• Apnea following rapid IV administration
		• $\downarrow$ICP, $\downarrow$CBF, $\downarrow$CMRO$_2$
Fentanyl	0.002-0.01	• Potent analgesic blunts response to intubation; mildly sedating
		• Hemodynamically most stable of all opioids
		• Chest wall rigidity at high dose (>5 mcg/kg), reversed with naloxone or paralytic
Lidocaine	1-2	• Analgesic, decreases the cardiovascular responses to intubation when administered IV or topically (4% solution)
		• $\downarrow$ICP spikes associated with intubation and respiratory toilet
Scopolamine	0.02	• Amnestic, antisialogogue
		• Can be administered IV or IM
		• Mild tachycardia; no blood pressure effects

TABLE 2-3

NEUROMUSCULAR BLOCKING AGENTS

Drug	Contraindications	Side Effects, Comments
Rocuronium Dose: 0.6-1.2 mg/kg Onset: 30-60 sec Duration: 40-60 min	None	1. Minimal vagolytic effect 2. 80% hepatic excretion 3. Reversible in ≈30 min 4. Only nondepolarizing muscle relaxant approved for rapid sequence intubation **5. Precipitates with thiopental and other drugs; flush IV before and after administration.**
Vecuronium Dose: 0.1-0.2 mg/kg Onset: 70-120 sec Duration: 30-90 min	None	1. No effect on heart rate or blood pressure 2. <25% renal elimination; primarily metabolized in liver 3. Reversible in ≈30-45 min after IV dose **4. Faster onset and longer duration in infants**

Continued

TABLE 2-3		
NEUROMUSCULAR BLOCKING AGENTS—cont'd		
Drug	Contraindications	Side Effects, Comments
Pancuronium Dose: 0.1-0.2 mg/kg Onset: 70-150 sec Duration: 45-90 min	Renal failure; tricyclic antidepressant use	1. Vagolytic: ↑ heart rate and blood pressure 2. 60%-90% renal elimination 3. Reversible in ≈45-60 min after IV dose 4. Interaction with tricyclic antidepressants → ventricular arrhythmias 5. No histamine-releasing properties

Succinylcholine
Dose
  IV: 1.5-2 mg/kg
  IM: 3-4 mg/kg
Onset
  IV: 30-60 sec
  IM: 180 sec
Duration
  IV: 3-10 min
  IM: 5-20 min
 	
Defasciculation—in children >4 yr, defasciculation with a nondepolarizing muscle relaxant is commonly suggested; use 10% of intubating dose of nondepolarizing agent.
	Progressive muscular dystrophies; myasthenia gravis; Guillain-Barré syndrome; demyelinating disease; crush, burn, electrical injuries; spinal cord injuries after 24 hours; open globe injury; malignant hyperthermia; myotonia congenita; ↑ intracranial pressure
	
	Black box FDA warning: No longer to be used for routine intubation in children because of increased risk of lethal hyperkalemia in undiagnosed muscular dystrophy
		1. Dysrhythmias: Sinus arrest, bradycardia, nodal and ventricular arrhythmias; bradyarrhythmias prevented by pretreatment with atropine
		2. Fasciculation: ↑ intra-abdominal, intrathoracic, and intracranial pressure
		3. Muscle pain: 10% of patients, ↑ pain may be minimized with prior defasciculation using 0.01 mg/kg pancuronium
		4. Potassium efflux (↑ serum K$^+$ = 0.5 mEq/L in all patients); K$^+$ = 10 mEq/L in myasthenia, Guillain-Barré syndrome, spinal cord injury (starts 24 hr after injury and lasts for 6 mo), crush or electrical injury, muscular dystrophy
		5. Contraction of extraocular muscles
		6. Muscle rigidity—myotonic dystrophy, malignant hyperthermia
		7. Nonreversible; Requires plasma cholinesterase for biodegradation

Cisatracurium Dose: 0.1-0.2 mg/kg Onset: 2-4 min Duration: 30-50 min	Asthma, hypotension; need for rapid onset	1. Histamine release 2. Onset in ~2 min 3. Hofmann elimination and ester hydrolysis; makes it ideal for patients with kidney or liver failure 4. Reversible in 30-45 min after IV administration

TABLE 2-3

NEUROMUSCULAR BLOCKING AGENTS—cont'd

Drug	Contraindications	Side Effects, Comments
Doxacurium Dose: 0.03-0.07 mg/kg Onset: 240-420 sec Duration: 60-120 min	Asthma, hypotension	1. Histamine release 2. Very long-acting 3. 40%-60% renal excretion
Neostigmine Dose: 0.07 mg/kg; max, 3 mg Onset: 180-600 sec Duration: 75 min *plus either* Atropine Dose: 0.01-0.02 mg/kg Onset: 15-30 sec Duration: 90 min *or* Glycopyrrolate Dose: 0.005-0.01 mg/kg Onset: 15-30 sec Duration: 90 min	None	1. Used to antagonize nondepolarizing neuromuscular blockade 2. Muscarinic effects: Bradycardia, salivation, bladder contraction; bronchospasm; must always pretreat with atropine or glycopyrrolate

FDA, U.S. Food and Drug Administration; *IM*, intramuscular; *IV*, intravenous.

C. Antagonism of neuromuscular blockade
   1. Nondepolarizing muscle relaxants act by competitive inhibition of the neuromuscular junction and can be antagonized (reversed) with acetylcholinesterase inhibitors (e.g., neostigmine).
   2. These reversal agents cause profound bradycardia. Pretreatment with either IV atropine, 0.01 to 0.02 mg/kg, or glycopyrrolate, 0.005 to 0.01 mg/kg, is mandatory.
D. Inability to antagonize neuromuscular blockade
   Circumstances that prevent reversal of neuromuscular blockade include the following:
   1. Intense neuromuscular blockade (not enough time has elapsed from last dose of paralytic drug)
   2. Respiratory acidosis
   3. Drug interactions (aminoglycosides, magnesium, corticosteroids)
   4. Organ failure (liver, kidney)
   5. Hypothermia
   6. Plasma cholinesterase deficiency (leads to prolonged succinylcholine or mivacurium effect)
   7. Underlying myopathy or neuropathy

TABLE 2-4

INTUBATION EQUIPMENT SIZES

Age (yr)	Laryngoscope Blade (size)	Endotracheal Tube Internal Diameter (mm)	Oral Endotracheal Tube Length (cm)	Suction Catheter Size (Fr)
Premature	0	2.5-3	7-9	5
Newborn	0	3-3.5	9-10	6
1	1	4	12	8
2	2	4.5	13	10
4	2	5	14	10
6	2	5.5, uncuffed; 5, cuffed	15	10
8	2-3	6, uncuffed; 5, cuffed	18	10
>10	3-4	7-8 cuffed	21	14

X. Intubation equipment
  A. Laryngoscope
    1. Handles
      a. Different handle shapes and sizes are available.
      b. Pick one that fits most securely in your hand.
    2. Blades (**Table 2-4, Box 2-4, Fig. 2-14**)
      a. Miller, Wis-Hipple (straight); sizes 0 to 4—infants to adults
      b. MacIntosh (curved); sizes 1 to 4—children to adults
    3. Light failure
      a. The electrical contact between the handle and blade and between the bulb and its socket commonly corrode and prevent the flow of electricity. This can usually be scraped clean.
      b. Be prepared for equipment failure and have extra handles and blades available.
  B. Endotracheal tubes
    1. Uncuffed ETTs
      a. Patients younger than 8 to 10 years have historically been intubated with uncuffed ETTs to reduce the risk of subglottic edema and stenosis.
      b. An uncuffed tube of appropriate size will provide a reasonable seal at the cricoid ring, the narrowest part of the airway.
    2. Cuffed ETTs
      a. Newer polyurethane, high-volume, low-pressure, cuffed ETTs can be safely used in younger children and infants without traumatizing the airway. They are particularly useful in patients at risk for pulmonary aspiration or with low lung compliance.
      b. When using a cuffed ETT, do not inflate the cuff above 25 mm Hg pressure; higher pressures may cause mucosal ischemia or necrosis.

> **BOX 2-4**
>
> **INTUBATION EQUIPMENT CHECKLIST**
>
> Suction—rigid Yankauer tonsil sucker or large-bore, disposable, soft, tracheal suction catheters
>
> Oxygen delivery equipment
> - Bag-valve ventilation device (Ambu bag, Laerdal bag, vital signs disposable bag)
> - Anesthesia ventilation bag (Mapleson C, D)
>
> Airway
> - Oropharyngeal airways, various sizes
> - Nasopharyngeal airways, various sizes
>
> Face masks—various sizes (Rendell-Baker, vital signs)
>
> Laryngoscope blades
> - Miller straight blades; sizes 0, 1, 1.5, 2, 3, 4
> - MacIntosh curved blades: sizes 2, 3, 4
>
> Endotracheal tubes
> - Uncuffed, 2.5-7 mm ID
> - Cuffed 3-9 mm ID
>
> Stylet and lubricant
>
> Tongue depressor
>
> Adhesive tape and skin protector—tincture of benzoin, Mastisol
>
> Monitoring equipment
> - Pulse oximeter
> - Electrocardiographic equipment
> - Blood pressure cuff
>
> Drugs
> - Atropine
> - Muscle relaxant
> - Sedative-hypnotic
>
> Endotracheal tube confirmation equipment
> - Expired (end-tidal) carbon dioxide
> - Self-inflating bulb
> - Auscultation

ID, Internal diameter.

3. Size (see Table 2-4 and Box 2-4)
   a. The internal diameter (ID) of the ETT can be estimated by using this formula:

$$ID = (16 + age [years])/4$$

   b. Always have additional tubes available, one size smaller and one size larger than the calculated size.
4. Distance (length at lips, in centimeters)
   a. The distance between the ETT marker at the lips and the midtrachea approximately equals three times the ETT ID (in millimeters; e.g., a 5-mm tube is taped at the 15-cm marker at the lip).
   b. In newborns weighing less than 3.5 kg, the ETT distance at the lip is 6 + weight in kilograms.

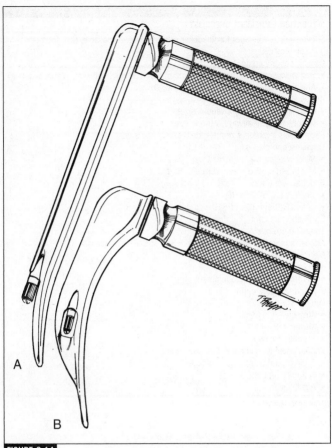

FIGURE 2-14
Laryngoscope blades. **A,** Straight (Miller). **B,** Curved (MacIntosh).

   C. Stylet
      1. Elongated metal or plastic rod that alters the natural curve of
         an ETT and facilitates intubation
      2. Indication
         a. Used when difficult intubation is anticipated
         b. Rapid sequence intubation (RSI)
      3. Technique
         a. Lubricate the stylet before inserting it into the ETT to
           facilitate its removal after intubation.

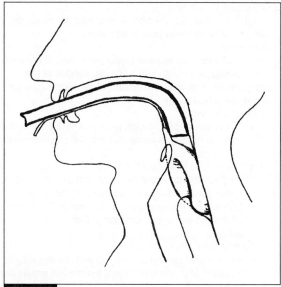

FIGURE 2-15

Insertion technique of the laryngeal mask airway.

        b. The stylet must never extend beyond the distal end of the
           ETT and must never be used to force entry into the trachea.
    4. Complications
        a. Submucosal dissection
        b. Lacerations, hemorrhage, hematomas
        c. Tracheal perforation
        d. Pneumothorax
        e. Pneumomediastinum
  D. Alternative airway devices
    1. Laryngeal mask airways (**Fig. 2-15;** see Fig. 2-11)
    2. Lighted stylet (light wand)
    3. Fiberoptic bronchoscope or laryngoscope (GlideScope)
    4. Tracheostomy equipment
XI. Techniques for intubation
  A. Preoxygenation
    Ventilation with 100% O_2 should always precede intubation to
    avoid hypoxemia.
  B. Monitoring
    Electrocardiography, pulse oximetry, and noninvasive blood
    pressure are the minimum requirements, except during
    cardiorespiratory arrest, when immediate intubation is necessary.

C. Equipment preparation

Box 2-4 is a checklist of essential equipment for intubation; these items must be reviewed prior to intubation.

D. Positioning

Successful intubation requires proper positioning of the head and neck, opening the mouth widely, proper insertion of the laryngoscope, with clear visualization of the vocal cords, and proper placement of the ETT.

1. Head and neck
   a. The proper position for the head and neck maximizes the alignment of the laryngeal axis with the oropharyngeal axis and mouth.
   b. The head is tilted backward, extending the atlanto-occipital joint with the hand and by elevating the occiput with a folded towel underneath the head (sniffing position).
   c. Extension of the head without elevation of the occiput rotates the larynx anteriorly and makes visualization difficult.

2. Cervical spine injury
   a. Patients with cervical spine injury and atlanto-occipital instability (e.g., achondroplasia, trisomy 21) require special consideration.
   b. An assistant straddles the patient and applies a gentle traction force in the cephalad direction to the patient's mastoid processes, keeping the mastoid process in line. This should counter any extension or flexion of the cervical spine during laryngoscopy (see Chapter 15).

3. Opening the mouth
   a. The mouth is opened widely by depressing the lower teeth and mandible with the right thumb while pushing against the upper teeth with the right middle finger (scissor maneuver).
   b. This minimizes trauma to the teeth, lips, and gums.

4. Cricoid pressure
   a. Compression of the cricoid ring with the thumb and index finger occludes the esophagus and prevents passive regurgitation (**Fig. 2-16**). It may also help visualize the larynx.
   b. In RSI, cricoid pressure is maintained until ETT placement is confirmed.

5. Laryngoscopy
   a. Blade insertion
      (1) The laryngoscope blade is gripped firmly in the left hand and inserted from the right side of the mouth, gently lifting and sweeping the tongue to the left (**Fig. 2-17**).
      (2) The visualized larynx is shown in **Figure 2-18.**

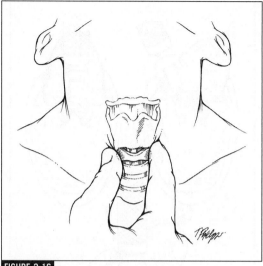

FIGURE 2-16

Cricoid pressure to prevent passive regurgitation during intubation.

   b. Curved blade advancement
     (1) The curved blade is advanced slowly along the base
        of the tongue until the epiglottis is visualized
        (**Fig. 2-19,** *A*).
     (2) The tip of the blade is inserted into the space between
        the base of the tongue and the epiglottis (the vallecula).
     (3) The operator's wrist is then fixed in position and further
        exposure is gained by lifting the laryngoscope vertically
        forward, without using leverage on maxillary structures.
     (4) The epiglottis is elevated and the glottis visualized.
        (a) Pressure on the cricothyroid cartilages may improve
            visualization of the glottis.
        (b) Never pull backward, flex the wrist, or lean on the
            patient's upper teeth with the laryngoscope blade.
     (5) The curved blade is the preferred blade for children
        older than 2 years.
   c. Straight blade advancement
     (1) The straight blade is advanced below the epiglottis
        along the posterior wall (Fig. 2-19, *B*).
     (2) The laryngoscope is then lifted and retracted slowly
        while elevating the soft tissue until the glottis appears.
     (3) The ETT is placed as noted earlier.

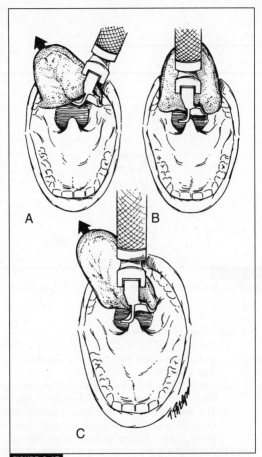

FIGURE 2-17

The laryngoscope is inserted from the right side of the mouth.
The tongue is swept from the right to the left. **A,** Incorrect. The
laryngoscope has not returned to the middle. **B,** Incorrect. The
tongue hangs over the right side of the blade. **C,** Correct. This
is the final position.

(4) The straight blade is the preferred blade for infants and
small children because of their floppy epiglottis.
(5) Inserting the curved or straight blade into the vallecula
may result in failure because the vertical lift of the
blade may not pull up the infant epiglottis.

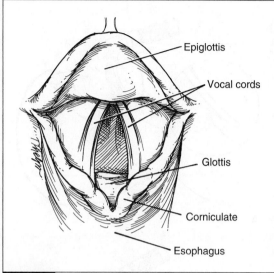

FIGURE 2-18

The larynx.

6. Placement of the ETT. The tube is inserted from the right side, using a stylet if necessary, and the tip is passed between the vocal cords.
   a. Uncuffed ETT
      (1) The distal line markings should be used to gauge the depth of insertion.
          (a) If the ETT has a single distal line marker, that line should be visible at the true vocal cords.
          (b) If the ETT has two or three distal line markers, the second or third line markers should be visible above the true vocal cords.
   b. Cuffed ETT
      (1) Stop advancing the ETT as soon as the cuff is below the vocal cords.
      (2) Continued advancement may result in endobronchial intubation.
7. ETT position confirmation
   a. Following intubation, the position of the ETT must be confirmed prior to securing the tube with waterproof adhesive tape.
   b. Auscultation in the axilla and over the stomach is not a reliable method to confirm proper positioning of the ETT.

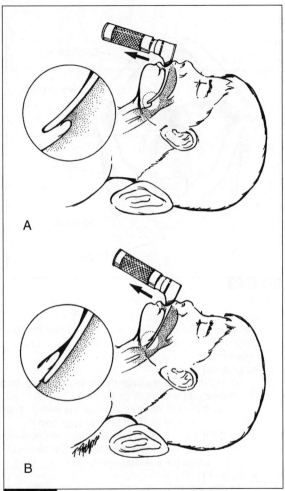

FIGURE 2-19

Sagittal view of laryngoscopy. **A,** Curved blade is placed in the vallecula.
B, The tip of the straight blade is placed under the epiglottis.

   c. **The presence of expired (end-tidal) CO_2 is the gold standard
   for confirmation of correct tube position.** However, there
   must be pulmonary circulation for this test to be positive.

   d. In an arrest situation, CO_2 may not be present in the ETT if
   chest compressions are inadequate, even though the tube
   is correctly positioned in the trachea.

XII. Complications of intubation
  A. Complications during laryngoscopy or intubation
    1. Corneal abrasion
    2. Dental and soft tissue trauma (laceration, abrasion, tooth loss)
    3. Cardiac arrhythmia
    4. Autonomic instability
      a. Hypertension, tachycardia
      b. Hypotension, bradycardia
      c. Vagally mediated reflexes (apnea, laryngospasm, bronchospasm, vomiting)
    5. Pulmonary aspiration of stomach contents
    6. Esophageal intubation
    7. Endobronchial intubation
    8. Arytenoid cartilage dislocation
  B. Complications with tube in place
    1. Increased resistance to breathing
    2. ETT obstruction (plugging or kinking)
    3. Accidental extubation
    4. Autonomic instability (see earlier)
  C. Complications after intubation
    1. Laryngeal damage or edema (e.g., pharyngitis, laryngitis, laryngeal granuloma or ulceration, laryngeal web, vocal cord paralysis)
    2. Tracheal damage or edema (e.g., tracheal mucosa ischemia, tracheal stenosis)
XIII. Cricothyrotomy
  A. Indications
    1. Occasionally, a patient can neither be ventilated nor intubated and an emergency needle cricothyrotomy is required to establish the airway.
    2. Figures 2-10 and 2-11 depict the algorithms for failed ventilation and/or endotracheal intubation.
  B. Technique
    1. Emergency cricothyrotomy
      a. The neck is extended and the thyroid and cricoid cartilages are identified (**Fig. 2-20**).
      b. The skin is cleansed with antiseptic.
      c. A 14-gauge, 5-cm over-the-needle catheter is attached to a 5-mL syringe.
      d. The needle is directed at a 45-degree angle caudally in the midline of the cricothyroid membrane.
      e. The syringe is aspirated while advancing the needle until air is obtained.
      f. The catheter is advanced over the needle and an ETT adapter from a 3-mm (pediatric) ETT is inserted into the hub of the catheter.

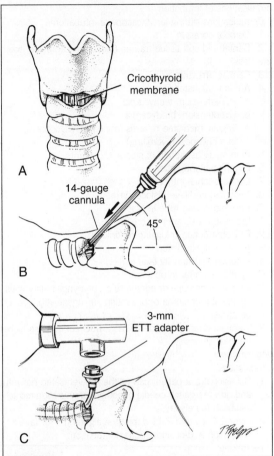

FIGURE 2-20

Cricothyrotomy. **A,** Anatomic view. **B,** Insertion of 14-gauge
intravenous cannula. **C,** Bag attached to a 3-mm endotracheal tube
adaptor connected to the intravenous cannula.

     g. The catheter is secured and the ETT adaptor is connected
       to a positive pressure ventilation bag to allow ventilation
       with 100% O_2.

  2. Alternatively, a Seldinger wire technique can be used (**Fig.
    2-21**).

     a. Following needle puncture of the cricothyroid membrane, a
       wire is passed through the needle into the trachea.

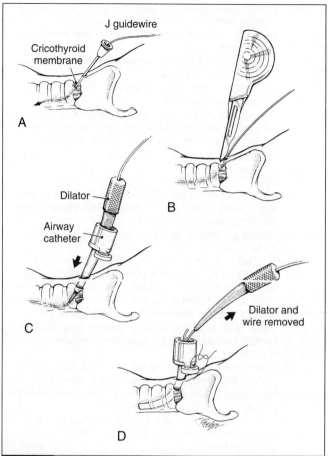

FIGURE 2-21

Seldinger wire technique for cricothyrotomy. **A,** Following needle puncture of the cricothyroid membrane, a wire is placed through the needle into the trachea. **B,** A scalpel is used to cut down through the skin and muscle to the trachea. **C,** A dilator tracheostomy tube is inserted over the wire into the trachea. **D,** The wire and dilator are removed and the tracheostomy tube is secured in place.

  b. A scalpel is used to cut down through the skin and muscle to the trachea.

  c. A dilator tracheostomy tube is inserted over the wire into the trachea.

  d. The wire and dilator are removed and the tracheostomy tube is sutured in place.

  e. The chest is then observed and auscultated to assess the adequacy of ventilation.

 This is a temporary measure only, and alternative methods for securing the airway should be undertaken. Complications of needle cricothyrotomy include hemorrhage, aspiration, asphyxia, and perforation of the trachea.

XIV. Laryngeal mask airway

 A. Overview

  1. A laryngeal mask airway (LMA) can rapidly provide a clear and secure airway without the skill required for laryngoscopy and tracheal intubation (see Fig. 2-15).

  2. Patients can breathe spontaneously or be ventilated with positive pressure.

  3. The LMA is inserted blindly (i.e., without laryngoscopy).

  4. It can be used in anticipated or unexpected difficult airway situations and for cardiopulmonary resuscitation. It facilitates continuous ventilation during and between intubation attempts and can be used to facilitate fiberoptic intubations.

  5. Classic LMAs and other, specially designed *intubating* LMAs facilitate intubations over fiberoptic bronchoscopes.

 B. Insertion technique

  1. With the neck flexed and the head extended, a deflated and lubricated LMA is held like a pencil and inserted along the hard palate, using the index finger to press the mask into the posterior pharyngeal wall and downward.

  2. When positioned, the cuff is inflated, the glottic and LMA apertures are in line with each other, and the mask forms a seal around the larynx.

  3. The LMA does not prevent regurgitation and should not be used in full stomach conditions.

 C. Alternative insertion technique

  1. The LMA is inflated to the maximum and then deflated until the first crease is seen.

  2. With the neck flexed and the head extended, the lubricated LMA is inserted upside down along the hard palate; when resistance is felt at the posterior pharyngeal wall, the LMA is turned 180 degrees and advanced downward.

  3. When positioned, the cuff is inflated, the glottic and the LMA apertures are in line with each other, and the mask forms a seal around the larynx.

TABLE 2-5

LARYNGEAL MASK AIRWAY

Mask Size	Patient Weight (kg)	Internal Diameter (mm)	Length (cm)	Maximum Cuff Volume (air) (mL)
1	<5 (neonates, infants)	5.25	10	4
1.5	5-10 (infants)			7
2	10-20 (infants, toddlers)	7	11.5	10
2.5	20-30 (children)	8.4	12.5	14
3	31-70 (children, small adults)	10	19	20
4	50-70 (adolescents, small adults)	12	19	30
5	>70 (large adults)	—	—	40
6	>100 (very large adults)	—	—	50

D. Sizing

Weight-appropriate sizing for the LMA is listed in **Table 2-5.**

E. Fiberoptic intubation and bronchoscopy

The LMA can also be used as a guide for fiberoptic intubation and bronchoscopy (**Table 2-6**).

XV. Lighted stylet

A. Overview

1. A lighted stylet is a useful adjunct for the management of a difficult pediatric airway.

2. It is a malleable stylet with a high-intensity light at the tip.

B. Technique

1. The stylet is prebent to 90 degrees and well lubricated, and then inserted within an ETT.

2. It is introduced into the mouth and follows the curvature of the tongue.

a. When positioned in the trachea, a sharp, well-defined bright circle of light is observed, transilluminating the neck directly in the midline at the level of the cricothyroid membrane.

b. When in the esophagus, the light is diffuse or not seen at all.

TABLE 2-6

LARYNGEAL MASK AIRWAY: ENDOTRACHEAL AND FIBEROPTIC PLACEMENT ASSIST GUIDE

Mask Size	Largest Endotracheal Tube (ID, mm)	Maximum Fiberoptic Bronchoscope (OD, mm)	Bronchoscope Type
1	3.5, uncuffed	2.7	Olympus PF-27M Olympus ENF-P2 Olympus BF-N20 Pentax FB-10H Pentax FI-10P
1.5	4, uncuffed	3	Olympus PF-27M Olympus ENF-P2 Olympus BF-N20 Pentax FB-10H Pentax FI-10P
2	4.5, uncuffed	3.5	Olympus ENF-P3 Olympus BF-3C20 Pentax FNL-15S
2.5	5, uncuffed	4	Olympus LF-1
3	6, cuffed	5	Olympus BF-2TR Olympus BF-P20D Pentax FB-19H Pentax FB-19H3
4	6, cuffed	5	Olympus BF-2TR Olympus BF-P20D Pentax FB-19H Pentax FB-19H3
5	7, cuffed	5	Olympus BF-2TR Olympus BF-P20D Pentax FB-19H Pentax FB-19H3
6	7, cuffed	5.5	Olympus BF-2TR Olympus BF-P20D Pentax FB-19H Pentax FB-19H3

ID, Internal diameter; *OD*, outer diameter.

Chapter 3
Respiratory Failure

R. Blaine Easley, MD,
David G. Nichols, MD, MBA,
and Charles L. Schleien, MD, MBA

3

I. Overview
   A. Definition
      Respiratory failure is defined as any clinical condition that results in impaired oxygenation and/or ventilation (removal of carbon dioxide [CO_2] from the blood).
   B. Classification by cause
      Respiratory failure can be divided into two broad categories, lung failure and respiratory pump (or bellows) failure (**Table 3-1**).
      1. Lung failure arises from various diseases affecting the airways, alveoli, alveolar capillary membranes, or pulmonary circulation and leads to varying degrees of hypoxemia, hypercapnia, and respiratory acidosis (**Tables 3-2** and **3-3**).
      2. Pump failure may result from any disease resulting in dysfunction of the pathway from the respiratory center of the brain to the upper spinal cord, phrenic nerves and other motor neurons or other diaphragmatic dysfunction, and chest wall as well as other structures of the chest, including bones and skin. It leads primarily to hypercapnia (see Table 3-3).
      3. Apnea has many causes in children that differ from those seen in adults (**Table 3-4**).
   C. Evaluation
      1. Physical examination is the most important tool in the diagnosis of acute respiratory failure. Most patients have the typical picture of respiratory distress (**Box 3-1**). However, a small group of patients with respiratory pump failure may exhibit only hypoventilation (i.e., bradypnea and/or apnea) and few signs of distress. Patients should also be assessed for signs of chronic respiratory insufficiency (e.g., barrel chest, severe scoliosis, clubbing).
      2. Pulse oximetry provides continuous information regarding a patient's oxygen saturation (SaO_2). An SaO_2 <90% corresponds to a partial pressure of arterial oxygen (PaO_2) lower than 60 mm Hg. An SaO_2 >90% does not preclude respiratory

---

TABLE 3-1

MOST COMMON CAUSES OF RESPIRATORY FAILURE IN CHILDREN

Lung Failure	Pump Failure	Miscellaneous
Asthma	Drug overdose	Hypothermia
Bronchiolitis	CNS disease	Metabolic alkalosis
Chronic lung disease	Neuromuscular disease	Starvation
ARDS	Phrenic nerve disease (usually post-surgical)	
Upper airway obstruction	Chest wall abnormalities (e.g., flail chest, scoliosis, extensive burns)	

ARDS, Acute respiratory distress syndrome; *CNS*, central nervous system.

TABLE 3-2

CAUSES AND TREATMENT OF HYPOXEMIA

Physiologic Classification	Clinical Entities	Treatment
Low inspired O_2 concentration	Disconnection from O_2 High altitude	Secure supplemental O_2 source
Hypoventilation	Drug overdose Sleep apnea Brain stem injury	Assisted ventilation (e.g., BiPAP) Antidote to opiate or benzodiazepine overdose (e.g., naloxone, flumazenil)
$\dot{V}/\dot{Q}$ mismatch	Atelectasis Pneumonia, bronchiolitis ARDS Pulmonary embolism Asthma Primary pulmonary hypertension	Chest physiotherapy ↑ Lung volume with end-expiratory pressure (PEEP, BiPAP) Bronchoscopy to remove airway plug
Shunt ($\dot{V}/\dot{Q} = 0$)	Cyanotic congenital heart disease Pulmonary hypertension	Prevent agitation Surgical correction of congenital heart defect Inhaled NO and/or other specific pulmonary vasodilators ECMO
Impaired O_2 delivery to tissues	Shock Anemia + mild lung disease	Blood transfusion Inotropes Supplemental O_2 and PEEP

BiPAP, Bilevel positive airway pressure; *ECMO*, extracorporeal membrane oxygenation; *NO*, nitric oxide; *O_2*, oxygen; *PEEP*, positive end-expiratory pressure.

failure; significant hypercarbia ($Paco_2$ >45 mm Hg) is possible with normal Sao_2. Sao_2 <90% implies the following:

a. Supplemental oxygen (O_2) and possibly assisted ventilation are needed.

b. Causes of respiratory failure should be sought.

c. The patient must be monitored closely for further decompensation.

d. Causes of false pulse oximetry readings include low cardiac output with severe vasoconstriction, abnormal hemoglobins

TABLE 3-3

CAUSES AND TREATMENT OF HYPERCARBIA

Physiologic Classification	Clinical Entity	Treatment
↓ CO_2 ELIMINATION		
↑↑ $\dot{V}/\dot{Q}$ ratio (e.g., ↑ dead space ventilation)	Pulmonary embolism Asthma, bronchiolitis Shock Apparatus attached to the airway—low fresh gas flow	Assisted ventilation Bronchodilators; steroids ↑ Pulmonary blood flow (↑ intravascular volume, inotropes, remove obstruction)
↓↓ Minute ventilation	All causes of respiratory pump failure	Assisted ventilation Specific treatment: • Opiate, benzodiazepine antagonists • Anticholinesterase for myasthenia gravis • Plasmapheresis, IV immunoglobulin, Guillain-Barré syndrome
↑ CO_2 PRODUCTION		
↑↑ Metabolic rate	Hyperthermia Sepsis Hypertonic dextrose Malignant hyperthermia Neuroleptic malignant syndrome Nutrition (high carbohydrate load)	Assisted ventilation—increased minute ventilation Specific treatment: • Cooling, antipyretics • Dantrolene for malignant hyperthermia

CO_2, Carbon dioxide.

TABLE 3-4

CAUSES OF APNEA

System Affected/Disorder	Cause
Central nervous system	Seizure, head injury, meningitis-encephalitis, Chiari syndrome, posterior fossa mass, acute or chronic hydrocephalus with shunt malfunction, central apneic syndromes.
Circulation	Arrhythmia, congestive heart failure
Infection	Sepsis, meningitis
Gastrointestinal disease	Gastroesophageal reflux disease
Metabolic disease	Poisons, medications, hypoglycemia, hypothermia, inborn errors of metabolism

       (e.g., carboxyhemoglobin, methemoglobin), IV dye (methylene blue), and certain nail polishes.
   3. Laboratory tests should include the arterial blood gas (**Table 3-5;** see Box 3-1) and chest radiograph, which may only show minor abnormalities and must be interpreted in the context of the physical examination.

II. Upper airway obstruction
   Commonly seen in children, upper airway obstruction is the most common cause of cardiac arrest in children. It results in

---

BOX 3-1

PHYSICAL EXAMINATION AND ARTERIAL BLOOD GAS IN ACUTE RESPIRATORY FAILURE

SIGNS AND SYMPTOMS

Tachypnea
Respiratory pattern—irregular or regular, nasal flaring, retractions
Grunting
Body position
- Sniffing position with upper airway obstruction
- Splinting of chest with pneumonia; pain; flail chest
Chest wall shape
- ↑ anteroposterior diameter—asthma, cystic fibrosis
- Scoliosis
- Asymmetry, abnormal shape—neuromuscular disease, skeletal abnormalities, pneumothorax, paralyzed diaphragm
Growth parameters, neurodevelopment
Diminished breath sounds: Adventitial sounds—wheezing, stridor, rales, friction rub, absent sounds
Cyanosis, clubbing
Lethargy, depressed level of consciousness
Pulsus paradoxus >10 mm Hg

BLOOD GASES

PaO_2 <60 mm Hg (FIO_2 >0.6)
$PaCO_2$ >50 mm Hg
pH <7.3

FIO$_2$, Fraction of inspired oxygen; *PaCO$_2$*, partial pressure of arterial carbon dioxide; *PaO$_2$*, partial pressure of arterial oxygen.

TABLE 3-5

NORMAL ARTERIAL BLOOD GAS VALUES IN ADULTS AND CHILDREN*

Parameter	Age			
	Newborn (24 hr)	Infant (1-24 mo)	Child (7-9 yr)	Adult
pH	7.37 ± 0.06	7.40 ± 0.06	7.39 ± 0.02	7.40 ± 0.03
$PaCO_2$ (mm Hg)	33 ± 6	34 ± 8	37 ± 3	39 ± 5
PaO_2 (mm Hg)	70 ± 8	90 ± 7	96 ± 9	100 ± 10
$[HCO_3^-]$ (mEq/L)	20 ± 3	20 ± 4	22 ± 2	24 ± 2

PaCO$_2$, Partial pressure of arterial carbon dioxide; *PaO$_2$*, partial pressure of arterial oxygen.
*Mean ± 2 standard deviation.

hypoventilation, can lead to hypoxemia, and may lead to cardiopulmonary collapse with respiratory and/or cardiac arrest. Successful management is dependent on the following:
- Rapid, accurate diagnosis
- Appreciation of the severity of the obstruction
- Skilled medical team that can intervene appropriately
A. Pathophysiology
   The laws of physics (Poiseuille's and Bernoulli's laws) that govern the flow of gas through narrow tubes explain the susceptibility of

TABLE 3-6

POISEUILLE'S LAW

Flow	Equation for Resistance
Laminar flow	$\text{Resistance} = \dfrac{8 \times \text{length} \times \text{viscosity}}{\pi r^4}$
Turbulent flow	$\text{Resistance} = \dfrac{K \times \text{density}}{\pi r^5}$

K, Constant; *r*, radius.

infants and small children to acute upper airway obstruction. The clinical presentation with respiratory distress, retractions, and stridor is frequently more dramatic in small children than in adults.

1. Poiseuille's law indicates that air flow is turbulent through a narrowed trachea (**Table 3-6**).
    a. Resistance increases further because it is now inversely proportional to the fifth power of the radius of the lumen.
    b. Gas exchange is dramatically reduced with only minor degrees of narrowing of an infant's trachea.
    c. Thus, the child cannot tolerate lesions with the same degree of narrowing that usually does not produce symptoms in the adult.
2. Bernoulli's principle states that as the velocity of a gas flowing through the narrowing of a collapsible tube increases, the distending pressure that holds the tube open will decrease, thereby causing collapse of the tube.
    a. Stridor in a crying infant with laryngotracheomalacia is an example of the Bernoulli principle.
    b. Stridor and respiratory distress worsen as airflow velocity increases with increased agitation.

B. Assessment
    1. Signs and symptoms
        a. Stridor
        b. Retractions
        c. Dysphagia
        d. Paradoxical chest wall motion during inspiration (chest collapses inward rather than expanding outwardly)
        e. Dyspnea
        f. Coughing
    2. Late signs of impending respiratory failure
        a. Cyanosis
        b. Depressed consciousness
    3. General approach
        a. Determine the severity of obstruction.
            (1) Stridor, retractions, air entry, color, consciousness

(2) Assess need for endotracheal intubation prior to precise diagnosis.
   b. Determine the cause of obstruction.
      (1) History: Prodrome, rate of progression, sore throat, drooling, abnormal or absent voice, fever
      (2) Radiology (neck, chest radiographs): Perform only if stable
      (3) Endoscopy: Only by otolaryngologist
      (4) Other laboratory tests (complete blood cell count, cultures)
   c. Carefully monitor for respiratory deterioration: SaO_2, electrocardiogram, frequent observation.
   d. Initiate supportive and specific therapy (see later). For life-threatening upper airway obstruction, do the following:
      (1) Direct high-flow, humidified O_2 to the child's face ("blow-by O_2").
      (2) Avoid disturbing the child (e.g., needle sticks), which increases functional obstruction.
      (3) Summon help from anesthesiologist and/or otolaryngologist
      (4) If patient is becoming obtunded or hypoxemic, apply continuous positive airway pressure (CPAP) or positive pressure ventilation with 100% O_2 by bag and mask. Then follow difficult airway algorithm. (See Chapter 2, Figs. 2-10 and 2-11.)
 C. Differential diagnosis
    The differential diagnosis of acute upper airway obstruction is outlined in **Table 3-7.**
III. Laryngotracheobronchitis (LTB)
   LTB is divided into three categories (**Table 3-8**):
   • Viral croup
   • Spasmodic croup
   • Bacterial tracheitis
   All these must be distinguished from epiglottitis and retropharyngeal abscess.

TABLE 3-7

DIFFERENTIAL DIAGNOSIS OF UPPER AIRWAY OBSTRUCTION

Viral laryngotracheobronchitis*	Foreign body aspiration
Spasmodic croup	Corrosive ingestion
Epiglottitis	Neck trauma
Retropharyngeal abscess	Angioedema
Bacterial tracheitis	Diphtheria
Peritonsillar abscess	Infectious mononucleosis

*NOTE: Recurrent croup may indicate an anatomic airway abnormality, such as subglottic stenosis or hemangioma.

TABLE 3-8

DIAGNOSTIC FEATURES OF INFECTIOUS CAUSES OF STRIDOR

	Cause			
Parameter	Viral Croup	Retropharyngeal Abscess	Bacterial Tracheitis	Epiglottitis
HISTORY				
Age	2 mo-3 yr	Children, adults	6 mo-12 yr	>18 yr; now rare in children
Prodrome	None or URI	Pharyngitis, trauma	URI	None
Onset	Gradual	Slow	Variable	Fulminant
Dysphagia	Rare	Common	Rare	Common
SIGNS				
Fever	Low grade	Variable	High, toxic	High, toxic
Stridor	Common	Unusual	Common	Usual
Drooling	Rare	Common	Rare	Common
Posture	Lying down	Variable	Variable	Sitting
TESTS				
White blood cell count (cells/μL)	<10,000	>10,000	>10,000	>10,000
Neck radiograph	Subglottic narrowing	Widened retropharynx	Subglottic irregularity	Swollen supraglottis

URI, Upper respiratory infection.

A. Classification
  1. Viral croup
     a. Causes: Parainfluenza virus A, respiratory syncytial virus (RSV), and adenovirus are most common.
     b. Clinical features
        (1) Seasonal illness, mostly in winter
        (2) Age: Usually 6 months to 3 years
        (3) Symptoms: Prodromal infection, barking cough, inspiratory stridor, respiratory distress
        (4) Pathophysiology: Swelling of the tracheal mucosa in the subglottic region
     c. Radiology: Trachea has a gradual progressive narrowing of its lumen, reaching narrowest point just below the vocal cords (steeple sign)
     d. Clinical course
        (1) Therapy: None required in most patients
        (2) Hospitalization: Required in up to 10% of children
        (3) Artificial airway: Required in minority (5% to 10%) of hospitalized children
  2. Spasmodic croup
     a. Cause: An allergic reaction to viral antigens rather than a true infection

      b. Clinical course: Recurrent episodes of acute stridor with or without a febrile upper respiratory infection prodrome.

      c. Onset: Usually acute and at night with a mild course

      d. Resolution: Typically occurs with emesis or exposure to cold air or mist

      e. Age: 6 months to 5 years

  3. Bacterial tracheitis

      a. Cause: An uncommon infection usually caused by a secondary *Staphylococcus aureus* infection superimposed on viral LTB

      b. Pathology: Infraglottic inflammation with extensive exudate and edema within the trachea and bronchi

      c. Clinical course

        (1) Usual prodromal viral infection or illness

        (2) Affected children usually become acutely ill and develop respiratory distress, stridor, and toxic appearance.

      d. Diagnosis: Frequently made after endoscopic examination of the airway, which is performed because of worsening respiratory distress or the clinical suspicion of epiglottitis

      e. Tracheostomy may be required for adequate pulmonary toilet.

B. Management (**Table 3-9**)

  1. Avoid agitation and pain. Severity can usually be judged clinically (**Table 3-10**).

      a. No radiographs needed if symptoms are severe.

  2. Humidifier, mist O_2

  3. Fever control, hydration if necessary

  4. Corticosteroids

      a. Mild symptoms: A single dose of oral corticosteroids can be considered, although efficacy has not been proven.

      b. Moderate to severe symptoms

        (1) Efficacy

          (a) Shortened duration of symptoms

          (b) Reduced need for endotracheal intubation or inhaled epinephrine

          (c) Hastened improvement over first 24 hours

          (d) Shortened duration of hospitalization

          (e) Decreased frequency of readmission

        (2) Mechanism: Generally unknown

          (a) May reduce airway inflammation and edema by vasoconstriction of mucosa

      c. Dexamethasone: 0.15 to 0.6 mg/kg intravenously (IV), orally (PO), or intramuscularly (IM) × one dose

TABLE 3-9

HOSPITAL THERAPY OF VIRAL LARYNGOTRACHEOBRONCHITIS

Croup Score*	Clinical Severity	Management
≤4	Mild	Outpatient mist O_2 therapy; consider oral corticosteroids
5-6	Mild to moderate	Outpatient if child: 1. Improves in ED after mist O_2 *and* 2. Is >6 mo old *and* 3. Has reliable caregivers 4. Give oral corticosteroids. Consider inpatient if: 1. Improves, but <6 mo old *or* 2. If socially indicated (e.g., poor follow-up or no transportation)
7-8	Moderate	Consider outpatient if child: 1. Meets above criteria *and* 2. Received corticosteroids, a single nebulized epinephrine treatment, and improves in ED after 3 to 4 hr of observation *or* 3. Received corticosteroids, more than one nebulized epinephrine treatment, and improves in ED after 12 hr of observation *and* 4. Is without stridor at rest 5. Consider additional corticosteroid therapy. Admit if child: 1. Is improved, but fails above criteria 2. Needs O_2 therapy for desaturation 3. Consider systemic corticosteroids. 4. Consider ICU access.
≥9	Severe	Admit to ICU: 1. Do not disturb child. 2. Give O_2 therapy continuously. 3. Give nebulized epinephrine. 4. Give systemic corticosteroids. 5. Consider heliox. 6. Consider noninvasive ventilation. 7. Prepare for intubation.

ED, Emergency department; *ICU*, intensive care unit; O_2, oxygen.
*See Table 3-10.

TABLE 3-10

ESTIMATION OF SEVERITY OF RESPIRATORY DISTRESS IN CROUP

	Degree of Severity—Croup Score			
Sign	**0**	**1**	**2**	**3**
Stridor	None	Only with agitation	Mild at rest	Severe at rest
Retraction	None	Mild	Moderate at rest	Severe
Air entry	Normal	Mild	Moderate ↓	Marked ↓
Color	Normal	Normal	Normal	Cyanotic
Level of consciousness	Normal	Restless	Restless when disturbed	Lethargic when undisturbed

        (1) A single dose can be effective in reducing the severity of moderate to severe disease.

        (2) The oral route has been shown to be as efficacious as others.

        (3) Intramuscular route is an alternative but should be avoided, along with other forms of agitation.

    d. Prednisone: 1 to 2 mg/kg PO × one dose

    e. Nebulized budesonide: 0.25 to 2 mg in 4 mL normal saline; indicated if child vomits or unable to take oral steroids.

    f. Patients with moderate or severe symptoms who improve following steroid administration should be observed for up to 4 hours in the emergency department (ED).

        (1) Discharge only when no stridor is observed. If symptoms are improved, but not resolved, steroid dosage should be repeated at 12 hours and consideration given for nebulized epinephrine or IV steroids.

5. Nebulized epinephrine

    a. Mechanism of action: The α-adrenergic properties of epinephrine produce topical mucosal vasoconstriction and thereby reduce mucosal edema.

    b. Dose: 0.05 mL/kg of 2.25% racemic solution (or 0.5 mL/kg of 1:1000 epinephrine) diluted with 3 mL normal saline. Maximum dose: 0.5 mL (of 2.25% solution) or 5 mL (of 1:1000 epinephrine).

    c. Interval: May be used as frequently as every 30 minutes; if no improvement after three doses or 90 minutes, consider endotracheal intubation.

    d. Following nebulized epinephrine treatments, recommend admission because of the potential for rebound worsening of airway obstruction.

        (1) However, the experience and evidence of symptomatic benefit from steroids, with and without multiple epinephrine nebulizations, supports more recent recommendations for potential discharge to home from the ED as an alternative to admission,

        (2) This should be recommended only after a prolonged observation period (up to 12 hours; see Table 3-10).

6. Antibiotics: Antibiotic therapy is not indicated in the treatment of viral LTB.

7. Helium-O_2 mixture

    a. Mechanism of action: Low-density gas

        (1) Reduces the work of breathing by decreasing the resistance to turbulent gas flow through a narrowed airway (Poiseuille's law).

BOX 3-2

INDICATIONS FOR INTUBATION OF A PATIENT WITH VIRAL LARYNGOTRACHEOBRONCHITIS*

Increasing severity of retractions
Decreasing air entry
Worsening stridor
Decreasing stridor but increasing expiratory wheeze
Cyanosis
Depressed sensorium
Worsening hypoxia and/or hypercarbia

*Even with medical interventions (e.g., steroids, inhaled epinephrine).

(2) Only used in an intensive care unit (ICU) with continuous pulse oximetry monitoring
(3) Hypoxemia may occur with helium-O_2 mixtures, because the inspired helium concentration must be >60% (i.e., inspired O_2 concentration <40%) for this therapy to be effective.
8. Noninvasive positive pressure ventilation
   a. Types: CPAP or bilevel positive airway pressure (BiPAP)
   b. Mechanism of action: Assists in stenting open the upper airway
      (1) May be integrated with heliox therapy to assist in air movement
      (2) Should only be instituted in a setting in which endotracheal intubation can be performed safely
9. Endotracheal intubation (**Box 3-2**)
   a. Use when LTB is refractory to medical intervention.
   b. Use smaller endotracheal tube (ETT) than usual for age.
   c. Tracheotomy offers no advantage; only use in an emergency when intubation impossible.
   d. Extubation: Use leak test.
IV. Chronic lung disease of the newborn
   A. Definition
      1. Chronic lung disease of the newborn (CLD) occurs in infants who have suffered acute lung disease in the neonatal period.
         a. Risk factors
            (1) Prematurity
            (2) Exposure to mechanical ventilation
            (3) Past or present need for supplemental O_2
   B. Pathophysiology
      1. Involves damage to airways and alveolar-capillary units, which may result in hypoxia, hypercapnia, increased airway resistance, and cor pulmonale.

TABLE 3-11

BLOOD GAS VALUES IN CHRONIC LUNG DISEASE:
ACUTE AND CHRONIC RESPIRATORY FAILURE

Parameter	Value
PaO_2	<60 mm Hg (with FIO_2 ≥0.6)
$PaCO_2$	20 mm Hg over baseline (may have baseline ≥50 mm Hg; very high levels)
pH	<7.30
$[HCO_3^-]$	>24 mEq/liter

FIO_2, Fraction of inspired oxygen; $PaCO_2$, partial pressure of arterial carbon dioxide; PaO_2, partial pressure of arterial oxygen.

---

2. Infection, fluid overload, bronchospasm, mucus plugging, or tracheobronchial collapse may add acute respiratory failure to the existing chronic respiratory condition.

C. Management
   1. Diagnosis of acute respiratory failure in the CLD patient depends on recognition of the usual signs and symptoms of respiratory distress.
      a. A parental history is helpful in determining if the patient's condition is different from the usual baseline state.
      b. Arterial blood gas levels (**Table 3-11**) reflect acute and chronic respiratory failure with a partially compensated respiratory acidosis.
   2. The status of the patient's airway determines the order of steps used in the management of acute respiratory decompensation in CLD (**Fig. 3-1**).
      a. Some patients with severe CLD will present with a tracheostomy, which allows ready access to the airway for suctioning and institution of controlled ventilation.
      b. Patients without a tracheostomy may receive bronchodilator and diuretic therapy before proceeding to emergency intubation unless they exhibit evidence of impending respiratory arrest.
   3. Typical CLD patient presenting in acute distress
      a. History of extreme low birth weight (<1000 g) and/or prolonged neonatal hospitalization
      b. Relatively mild acute respiratory disease triggers decompensation
      c. Short duration of new or increased O_2 ventilator support (~72 hours)
      d. O_2 requirement—usually persists

V. Bronchiolitis
   A. Definition
      1. Acute lower airway disease
      2. Signs and symptoms: Rhinorrhea, cough, low-grade fever, wheezing, and tachypnea
      3. Cause: RSV

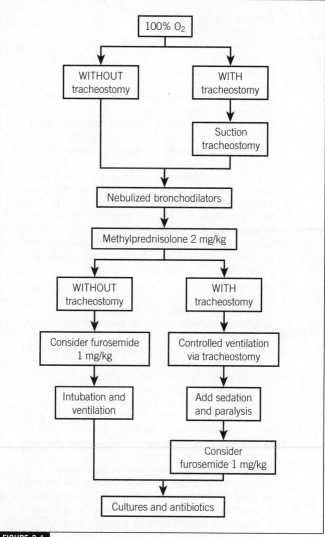

FIGURE 3-1

Management algorithm for chronic lung disease patients with acute respiratory failure.

      4. Age: Infants
      5. High-risk patients
        a. Congenital heart disease
        b. Chronic lung disease
        c. Prematurity
        d. Immunodeficiency

B. Pathophysiology
  1. Lower airway obstruction secondary to mucosal inflammation and mucus plugging
  2. Leads to hyperinflation and increased work of breathing
  3. Intrapulmonary shunting caused by bronchiolar obstruction with decreased ventilation to lung units, resulting in hypoxemia
  4. Although patients also have increased dead space ventilation, they are able to maintain normocapnia by breathing faster.
  5. Fatigue occurs when the infant has been forced to increase work of breathing for prolonged periods, which leads to hypercapnia and worsening hypoxia.
  6. Central apnea with complete absence of respiratory effort—may develop suddenly and after only minor symptoms in young infants.

C. Management
  1. Close observation and monitoring
    a. For infants with respiratory distress
    b. Infants in high-risk categories, even if their distress is relatively mild.
  2. High incidence of nosocomial spread of RSV bronchiolitis
    a. Infected patients should be isolated or cohorted.
    b. Strict contact isolation: Gloves, gowns
  3. Supplemental O_2
  4. Maintenance IV fluids after correcting dehydration
  5. Corticosteroids and bronchodilators may be tried in patients with a prior history of reactive airway disease.
  6. In patients with central apnea, CPAP has been used to support patients.
    a. Use only in a highly monitored setting in which endotracheal intubation is a readily available alternative.
    b. CPAP or BiPAP can assist in helping stimulate the infant to breathe as well as to promote oxygenation and prevent atelectasis. Starting pressure is usually 5 cm H_2O (CPAP), 8/4 cm H_2O (BiPAP) and can be administered via nasal prongs or a nasal mask.

VI. Acute respiratory distress syndrome
  A. Definition
    Acute respiratory distress syndrome (ARDS) is a syndrome of parenchymal lung injury characterized by acute onset, hypoxia

with decreased pulmonary compliance, diffuse infiltrates on chest radiograph, and absence of left ventricular failure.

B. Causes
1. Shock
2. Sepsis
3. Pneumonia
4. Near-drowning
5. Aspiration

C. Pathophysiology
1. ARDS represents the final common pathway following a variety of pulmonary or extrapulmonary insults.
2. The fundamental pathophysiologic abnormality appears to be disruption and increased permeability of the alveolar capillary membrane.
3. An unbalanced inflammatory response from activated granulocytes and O_2 free radicals results in cytokine release, macrophage infiltration, and further disruption of the alveolar-capillary membrane.
4. The final result is an inflammatory cascade of lung injury and respiratory failure.

D. Management
1. Supplemental O_2 by mask; prepare for probable endotracheal intubation.
2. Fluid resuscitation to restore normovolemia (if necessary)
3. Broad-spectrum antibiotics after blood culture and sputum culture
4. Intubation criteria: Inability to maintain PaO_2 higher than 60 mm Hg with fraction of inspired oxygen (FIO_2) of 0.6 or higher
5. Following intubation
   a. Start mechanical ventilation with positive end-expiratory pressure (PEEP) of 5 to 10 cm H_2O to prevent alveolar collapse.
   b. Increase PEEP to maintain PaO_2 higher than 60 mm Hg with FIO_2 of 0.6.
   c. Note that PEEP higher than 14 cm H_2O may be associated with hypotension and increased risk of barotrauma.
6. Consider measuring central venous pressure to titrate supplemental fluid and inotropic drug administration.
7. Consider bronchoalveolar lavage (BAL) if infectious pneumonia cannot be diagnosed by routine tracheal cultures. Open lung biopsy may be considered in immuno-suppressed patients if BAL cultures are negative.
8. Early, low dose, prolonged glucocorticoid treatment may be of benefit in ARDS as suggested by recent meta-analysis of

controlled trials and cohort studies (Tang BM, Crit Care Med 2009;37;1594). Early (within 72 hours of diagnosis) methylprednisolone 1 mg/kg/day for 14-21 days followed by slow tapering has been associated with decreased mortality, multiple organ dysfunction, and length of ICU stay without an increase in complications.

9. $PaCO_2$ of any value usually is tolerated as long as pH is higher than 7.2.

10. Endogenous nitric oxide (NO) works as a potent vasodilator.
    a. When inhaled, exogenous NO is a potent pulmonary vasodilator, without systemic effects.
    b. Inhaled NO therapy in ARDS is thought to improve oxygenation transiently by improving blood flow to ventilated regions (improved $\dot{V}/\dot{Q}$ ratio).
    c. Dosing: 5 to 40 parts per million and weaned to minimize toxicity of methemoglobinemia
    d. Research in children is ongoing, but no long-term benefit in ARDS has been demonstrated.

11. Consider prone positioning.
    a. Research in children has demonstrated transient improvements in oxygenation with no long-term benefit on duration of mechanical ventilation or hospitalization, as well as no effect on morbidity and mortality.
    b. Mechanism: Improved ventilation and perfusion matching, with increased uniformity

12. Consider referral for extracorporeal membrane oxygenation if a potentially reversible cause is suspected.

VII. Mechanical ventilatory support
   A. Goals of therapy
      In the setting of respiratory failure or compromise to maintain adequate gas exchange (i.e., delivery of O_2 to and removal of CO_2 from the body)
   B. Methods of mechanical ventilatory support
      1. Noninvasive: Patient is able to maintain and protect own airway and has intrinsic ventilatory drive. Delivery can be via nasal prongs, nasal mask, or face mask.
         a. CPAP: Delivers a set airway pressure with flow to the patient; usually start with 5 cm H_2O.
         b. BiPAP: Delivers air flow to maintain set inspiratory and expiratory airway pressures.
            (1) Some devices can also provide a ventilatory rate for controlled breaths.
            (2) Usually, start with low settings—4 to 5 cm H_2O expiratory pressure and 8 to 10 cm H_2O inspiratory pressure.

              (3) Increase pressures in stepwise fashion (e.g., 5/10,
                  6/12 cm H_2O).
   2. Invasive
       a. The patient has an artificial airway, either an ETT or
          tracheostomy.
       b. The ventilator can be adjusted to support ventilation and
          oxygenation fully.
       c. In addition, this mode can be safely weaned as the need
          for mechanical ventilation resolves.
       d. Conventional ventilation methods
           (1) Pressure-limited: Peak inflating pressure (PIP) set per
               delivered breath; tidal volume (VT) variable (dependent
               on compliance)
           (2) Volume-limited: Delivered VT set; variable PIP.
       e. Alternative method
           (1) High-frequency oscillatory ventilation: Method of
               ventilation for patients with severe lung disease who
               have failed conventional ventilatory measures
   C. Initial mechanical ventilator settings
       1. Pressure-limited: A difference in pressure is prescribed (**Table
          3-12**).
           a. FIO_2: Start at 1.0 and adjust down to maintain targeted SaO_2
              (>93% to 95%) and PaO_2 (>60 mm Hg) in patients without
              intracardiac shunt.
           b. PIP: Start with 15 cm H_2O for infants and 20 to 25 cm H_2O
              for older children, and adjust up or down as needed to
              produce adequate (but not excessive) chest wall
              movement. Avoid PIP >30 cm H_2O.
           c. Inspiratory time (IT): Start with 0.5 second in infants, 0.75
              second in children, and 1 second in adolescents. Normally,
              adjust to give an inspiration-to-expiration ratio (I:E) of 1:2.
           d. Respiratory rate:
               (1) Infant: 24 to 28/min
               (2) Child: 18 to 22/min
               (3) Adolescent: 12 to 16/min

TABLE 3-12

EFFECTS OF CONVENTIONAL VENTILATOR CHANGES ON BLOOD GAS PARAMETERS

Ventilatory Setting	Effects on Blood Gas Values	
	$PacO_2$	PaO_2
↑ PEEP	↓ or ↑	↑
↑ Respiratory rate	↓	↑ (minimal)
↑ PIP	↓	↑
↑ I:E	Variable	↑

I:E, Inspiration-to-expiration ratio; *Paco₂,* partial pressure of arterial carbon dioxide; *Pao₂,* partial pressure of arterial oxygen; *PEEP,* positive end-expiratory pressure; *PIP,* peak inflating pressure.

Adjust respiratory rate and PIP to maintain targeted $Paco_2$ or end-tidal CO_2.

   e. PEEP: Start with 5 cm H_2O and increase to recruit collapsed alveoli as indicated by improved oxygenation, increased lung compliance, and increased lung aeration (chest radiograph or computed tomography scan).

   f. Mode

     (1) Select synchronized intermittent mandatory ventilation (SIMV), if available.

     (2) This permits patient to initiate breaths and breathe faster than the set respiratory rate.

     (3) If pressure support (PS) is available, PS can be added to SIMV, allowing independent breaths of the patient to be supported.

     (4) Start with a PS = 10 cm H_2O.

   g. Evaluation

     (1) Once mechanical ventilation has been initiated, obtain a blood gas measurement, chest radiograph, and look for expiratory V_TS of ~6 mL/kg.

     (2) Lower exhaled V_TS may indicate a leak around the ETT.

  2. Volume-limited: A V_T is prescribed.

   a. Fio_2, I_T, respiratory rate, PEEP; mode as earlier.

   b. V_T: ~6 mL/kg. Chest wall should move with each breath. If no chest wall movement, increase by 1 or 2 mL/kg every other breath.

VIII. Tracheostomy complications

  A. Mucus plugging

   1. Diagnosis: Observe for signs of airway obstruction.

   2. Treatment

    a. Assume that there is plugging and suction trachea.

    b. Change tracheostomy tube if obstruction encountered that cannot be removed with suctioning.

  B. Mechanical problems

   1. Cause: Weight of tube on mucosa and skin

   2. Results in the following:

    a. Erosion

    b. Skin laceration

    c. Granulation tissue growth

    d. Bleeding (especially caused by aggressive suctioning)

  C. Leaks in ventilated patients

   1. Usually associated with uncuffed tracheostomy tubes

   2. If possible, change to a larger tracheostomy tube or a tube with a cuff.

   3. If volume ventilation:

    a. Attempt to increase V_T to compensate for leak.

       b. Change to a pressure-limited modality.
         (1) Adjust pressure limit to desired PIP.
         (2) Increase to high VT setting.
         (3) When pressure limit is reached, pressure will plateau at that level and remainder of VT is not delivered to patient.

IX. Transfusion-related acute lung injury

  A. Pathophysiology

    1. May be immune-mediated such that antibodies in blood products activate neutrophils and lead to cytokine release.

    2. Results in neutrophil-mediated endothelial injury, capillary leak, and acute lung injury

  B. Treatment

    1. Same as for ARDS

  C. Prevention

    1. Avoidance of blood products from individuals with known leukocyte antibodies

    2. Leukoreduction of blood components

    3. Shortening storage time of cellular components to reduce cytokine levels

    4. Cellular components washed before transfusion

Chapter 4

Acute Asthma

Charles L. Schleien, MD, MBA,
David G. Nichols, MD, MBA,
and R. Blaine Easley, MD

I. Definitions
   A. Asthma is a chronic inflammatory disease of the airways marked by intermittent acute cough, wheezing, shortness of breath secondary to bronchoconstriction, airway hyperreactivity, and airway edema.
   B. Status asthmaticus (SA) is an acute asthma attack that is resistant to multiple doses of β-agonist therapy.
   C. Near-fatal asthma is an acute asthma attack that progresses to respiratory arrest.

II. Cause
    The precise cause of asthma is unknown, but contributing factors have been identified.
    A. Innate immunity
       1. Downregulation of the Th1 response and upregulation of the Th2 response lead to an increased incidence of allergic disease and asthma.
       2. These changes in innate immunity may be related to the overuse of antibiotics or the infection pattern in early life.
    B. Genetics
       1. There is a hereditary component to asthma, but it is likely that multiple polymorphisms are involved.
    C. Environmental factors
       1. Exposure to respiratory viruses (e.g., respiratory syncytial virus), tobacco smoke, dust, mites, air pollution, and furry animals have been associated with asthma.

III. Pathophysiology
     A. Cholinergic (parasympathetic) stimulation
        This results in bronchial smooth muscle constriction and increased mucus production.
     B. β-adrenergic (sympathetic) stimulation
        This results in smooth muscle relaxation, improved ciliary movement, decreased bronchial edema, and diminished vascular permeability.

TABLE 4-1

IMPAIRMENT FROM CHRONIC ASTHMA

	Degree of Impairment		
Parameter	Mild	Moderate	Severe
Symptoms	>2 days/week, but not daily	Daily	All day
SABA	Use <2 times/wk	Use once daily	Use ≥bid
PEF	>80%	60%-80%	<60%

Modified from the National Heart, Lung, and Blood Institute: Expert panel report 3: Guidelines for the diagnosis and management of asthma, August 28, 2007 (http://www.nhlbi.nih.gov/guidelines/asthma/asthgdln.pdf National Asthma Guidelines).

PEF, Peak expiratory flow; *SABA,* short-acting β-agonist.

C. Cellular mediators of inflammation

These mediators (e.g., histamine, leukotrienes) may aggravate bronchoconstriction, increase mucus secretion, and reduce mucociliary clearance.

IV. Epidemiology

Details are available from the American Lung Association (http://www.lungusa.org).

A. Most common serious chronic disease of childhood

B. Peak prevalence occurs between the ages of 5 and 17 years.

C. SA is the third leading cause of hospital admission for children younger than 15 years.

V. Impairment and risk

A. Severity

1. The severity of the underlying chronic asthma condition correlates with the severity on presentation to the emergency department (ED) and subsequent risk of decompensation.

2. **Table 4-1** indicates the patient's baseline degree of impairment.

3. The major risk factors associated with severe or life-threatening acute asthma include the following:

a. History of mechanical ventilation

b. History of previous intensive care unit (ICU) admission

c. Increasing inhaled β-agonist use

d. Poor compliance

B. Counseling

Children and families with moderate to severe impairment and/or major risk factors should receive specific counseling.

1. Receive care from a pediatric pulmonologist or someone with experience in managing severe asthma.

2. Learn how to measure peak expiratory flow (PEF) regularly and understand the signs of worsening asthma.

3. Seek medical attention early in the presence of worsening condition or PEF lower than 80% of baseline.

TABLE 4-2

CLASSIFICATION OF ACUTE ASTHMA SEVERITY IN THE EMERGENCY DEPARTMENT

	Severity		
Parameter	Moderate	Severe	Life-Threatening
Signs, symptoms	Dyspnea with activity	Dyspnea at rest	Dyspnea: Unable to speak
Peak expiratory flow (PEF)* (% of baseline)	40%-70%	25%-40%	<25%
Response to SABA	Relief (≤3 doses)	Partial relief	No relief
Disposition	Discharge home (with 5-day course of oral steroids) Careful follow-up Improved asthma education	Admit to hospital	Admit to intensive care unit (ICU)

Modified from the National Heart, Lung, and Blood Institute: Expert panel report 3: guidelines for the diagnosis and management of asthma, August 28, 2007 (http://www.nhlbi.nih.gov/guidelines/asthma/asthgdln.pdf National Asthma Guidelines).

SABA, Short-acting β-agonist.

*If PEF is unavailable or the patient cannot cooperate with the measurement, the modified CAS (see Table 4-3) has proved useful for determining whether a patient requires admission to the ICU or intubation and assisted ventilation.

---

    4. Comply with the chronic medication regimen, especially the use of inhaled steroids.

VI. Presentation to the emergency department

  A. Clinical examination

    1. Patients present to the ED with symptoms ranging from mild to severe and even near-arrest.

    2. **Table 4-2** lists these symptoms and the corresponding PEF measurements that correlate with severity, and on which therapy is based.

    3. If the patient has used PEF at home and knows his or her personal best PEF, the results of a PEF test in the ED should be used to guide therapy.

  B. Chest radiograph criteria

    1. Most patients with known asthma who improve promptly in the ED do not require a chest radiograph.

    2. Obtain chest radiograph if the following occur:

      a. Patient fails to improve and requires admission to the hospital

      b. Patient is strongly suspected of pneumonia (fever, rales) or another complicating diagnosis (e.g., foreign body aspiration)

VII. Management

  A. Initial ED phase

    See **Figure 4-1**.

    1. Measure oxygen saturation (SaO_2); administer O_2 by nasal prongs or face mask.

    2. Measure PEF rates if patient knows his or her personal best and can cooperate with the test (Table 4-2). If not, assess clinical asthma score (CAS; **Table 4-3**).

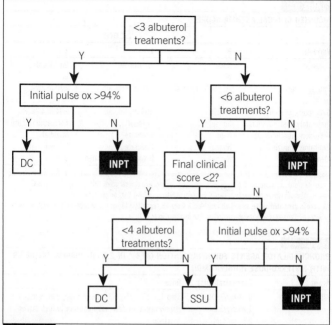

FIGURE 4-1

Clinical decision model to predict successful discharge of SA patients from the emergency department. *(From Gorelick M, Scribano PV, Stevens MW, et al. Predicting need for hospitalization in acute pediatric asthma. Pediatr Emerg Care 2008;24:735.) Clinical score,* Clinical asthma score (see Table 4-3); *DC,* discharge; *pulse ox,* pulse oximeter SaO$_2$; *INPT,* inpatient; *SA,* status asthmaticus; *SSU,* short stay unit.

3. Administer short-acting β-agonist (SABA) if patient is wheezing and PEF more than 25% (of personal best) or CAS lower than 5 (**Table 4-4**).
4. Administer prednisone, 1 to 2 mg/kg orally twice daily (maximum, 60 mg/day), for 3 to 10 days or until PEF is higher than 70% of personal best. Use inhaled steroids concurrently or after oral steroids.
5. If PEF is less than 25% or CAS is higher than 5, proceed to impending respiratory failure sequence (see later).

B. Therapies that are not recommended
   1. Aminophylline: Increased risk of vomiting
   2. Sedation: Risk of respiratory depression; if used, must be prepared to ventilate the patient immediately
   3. Mucolytics: No evidence of improved outcomes

TABLE 4-3

MODIFIED CLINICAL ASTHMA SCORE*

Variable	Score		
	0	1	2
Cyanosis	None	In room air	On 40% O_2
or	*or*	*or*	*or*
Pao_2 (mm Hg)	70-100 in room air	<70 in room air	<70 in 40% Fio_2
or	*or*	*or*	*or*
Sao_2 (pulse oximetry, %)	95-100	<94 in room air	<94 in 40% Fio_2
Inspiratory breath sounds	Normal	Unequal	Decreased or absent
Accessory muscle usage	None	Moderate	Maximal
Expiratory wheezing	None	Moderate	Marked
Mental status	Normal	Depressed or agitated	Coma

Modified from Downes JJ, Wood DW, Harwood I, et al. Intravenous isoproterenol infusion in children with severe hypercapnia due to status asthmaticus. Effects on ventilation, circulation, and clinical score. Crit Care Med 1973;1:63.

Fio_2, Fraction of inspired oxygen; Pao_2, partial pressure of arterial oxygen; Sao_2, oxygen saturation.

*A score is generated as the sum of all variables. A score ≥5 suggests a higher risk of impending respiratory failure. A score ≥7 correlates with respiratory failure. The maximal score is 10.

TABLE 4-4

BRONCHODILATOR AGENTS FOR NEBULIZATION (NEB)* IN 2.5 mL NORMAL SALINE OR WITH METERED-DOSE INHALER (MDI)†

Agent	Concentration(s)	Dose
Albuterol Neb	0.63 mg/3 mL	Step 1: 0.15 mg/kg ×3 (min, 2.5 mg; max, 5 mg)
	1.25 mg/3 mL	Improvement → decrease frequency to 0.15 mg/kg q1-4h
	2.5 mg/3 mL	
	5 mg/mL	No improvement → 0.5 mg/kg/hr continuous Neb
Albuterol MDI	90 mcg/puff	Step 1: 4-8 puffs q20 min ×3
		Improvement → decrease frequency to 4-8 puffs q1-4h
		No improvement → 0.5 mg/kg/h continuous Neb
Levalbuterol Neb	0.31 mg/3 mL	Step 1: 0.075 mg/kg ×3 (min, 1.25 mg; max, 2.5 mg)
	0.63 mg/3 mL	Improvement → decrease frequency to 0.075-0.15 mg/ kg q1-4h
	1.25 mg/0.5 mL	
	1.25 mg/3 mL	No data on continuous levalbuterol Neb
Levalbuterol MDI	45 mcg/puff	Same as albuterol MDI
Ipratropium bromide	500 mcg/2.5 mL	250 to 500 mcg q4-6h

*Nebulizers driven with 5-10 L/min O_2.

†Use valve-holding chamber (VHC) for all children. Use mask and VHC in children <4 yr.

C. Impending respiratory failure

If CAS is higher than 5 or the patient cannot cooperate with nebulization treatment (or nebulization equipment is not immediately available), use subcutaneous (SC) injection:
- Epinephrine (1:1000), 0.01 mL/kg SC (maximum, 0.3 mL), every 20 minutes (up to three doses)

  or
- Terbutaline, 0.01 mg/kg SC (maximum, 0.4 mg), every 20 minutes (up to three doses)

1. Monitor heart rate (HR), blood pressure (BP), and Sao_2. Start intravenous (IV) line.
2. Convert to continuously inhaled SABA if patient can cooperate.
3. Methylprednisolone, 2 mg/kg IV once, then 1 mg/kg IV every 6 hours
4. Ipratropium bromide (IB; see Table 4-4)
   a. Anticholinergic inhaled bronchodilator
   b. Minimal systemic absorption: No systemic effects
   c. Onset: 50% effect in 3 minutes; peak effect in 90 minutes
   d. For mild to moderate acute asthma: No additional benefit when IB is added to SABA
   e. For severe acute asthma: Conflicting data on incremental benefit of IB over SABA alone. It is our practice to add IB to SABA for severe acute asthma.

D. Adjunctive therapies for severe asthma and impending respiratory failure
   1. Magnesium sulfate, 25 to 75 mg/kg (maximum 2 g) IV over 20 minutes; may repeat the dose up to four times
   2. Terbutaline infusion: Terbutaline, 10 mcg/kg IV load over 30 minutes, then 0.1 to 4 mcg/kg/min

E. Impending respiratory failure
   1. Diagnosis: Various symptoms, signs, or laboratory data may indicate the need for ventilatory support in acute asthma.
      a. CAS higher than 7
      b. Sao_2 less than 90% or fraction of inspired oxygen (Fio_2) more than 40%
      c. Decreased level of consciousness
      d. Arterial blood gas (ABG): Partial pressure of arterial carbon dioxide ($Paco_2$) higher than 40 to 60 mm Hg
         Even a $Paco_2$ of approximately 40 mm Hg is inappropriately elevated in a patient with severe asthma, and such a patient requires meticulous observation in the ICU. However, not every patient with acute asthma and $Paco_2$ of 40 mm Hg requires assisted ventilation. Clinical judgment is required.
         Decreasing level of consciousness, increasing O_2 requirement, and rapidly rising $Paco_2$ favor the decision to institute assisted ventilation.
      e. Chest radiograph: Rule out pneumothorax or major atelectasis.
   2. Monitoring: In addition to noninvasive monitoring (e.g., HR, BP, Sao_2), an arterial line should be placed for continuous BP and frequent ABG monitoring.
   3. Management: Bilevel positive airway pressure (BiPAP)
      a. BiPAP devices maintain continuous gas—O_2 or air—flow with intermittent positive pressure ventilation by mask.

Positive pressure is triggered by patient inspiratory effort. A mandatory backup frequency (breaths/minute) may also be added.

   b. Mask options—nasal or full face: Some physicians advocate a nasal mask in the hope of limiting gastric insufflation and vomiting. Nasal masks require patient cooperation to keep the mouth closed. Some younger children are too agitated to establish synchronous breathing with BiPAP.
   c. Inspiratory and expiratory positive airway pressures (IPAP, EPAP) in SA with impending respiratory failure:
      (1) IPAP range: 8 to 14 cm H_2O
      (2) EPAP range: 4 to 5 cm H_2O; may be increased in the presence of hypoxemia or major areas of atelectasis on chest radiograph
   d. Maintain continuous nebulization of SABA during BiPAP.
4. Outcomes
   a. Most patients improve within 3 to 6 hours after initiation of BiPAP as measured by decreased respiratory rate and improved blood gas values.
   b. The benefit may result from respiratory muscle unloading and airway recruitment.
   c. Avoidance of tracheal stimulation during intubation is another major benefit.
F. Frank respiratory failure
   1. Diagnosis
      a. CAS higher than 8
      b. Unresponsive
      c. Bradypnea
      d. SaO_2 lower than 90% on FIO_2 of 60% or greater
      e. $PaCO_2$ higher than 80 mm Hg or higher than 60 mm Hg and rising rapidly
   2. Management
      Once frank respiratory failure has been diagnosed (usually after bronchodilator therapy and BiPAP have failed), endotracheal intubation and mechanical ventilation are necessary.
      a. The following extreme risks of endotracheal intubation during refractory SA should be anticipated:
         (1) Worsening bronchospasm
         (2) Vomiting and aspiration
         (3) Pneumothorax
         (4) Hypotension
      b. The management plan must take these risks into account:
         (1) Rapid fluid bolus of normal saline, 10 to 20 mL/kg, in anticipation of hypotension during positive pressure ventilation and administration of general anesthesia

(2) Rapid sequence induction of general anesthesia (see Chapter 2)

(a) Preoxygenation (ventilation with FIO_2 of 100%) and strict application of cricoid pressure

(b) Anesthetic: Ketamine, 1 mg/kg IV

(c) Anticholinergic: Atropine 0.01, mg/kg IV

(d) Muscle relaxant: Succinylcholine, 1 to 2 mg/kg IV, or rocuronium, 1 mg/kg IV

(e) Verify patient has no contraindications to succinylcholine (see Chapter 2).

(f) Low tidal volume ventilation strategy

(g) Ventilatory mode: Pressure support, pressure control

(3) Low tidal volume ventilation strategy

(a) Low tidal volume: 6 mL/kg

(b) Limit peak inflating pressure—less than 30 cm H_2O

(c) Positive end-expiratory pressure: 0 to 5 cm H_2O

(d) Frequency: 5 to 10 breaths/minute (if patient breathing spontaneously with pressure support ventilation)

(e) FIO_2: As needed to maintain SaO_2 higher than 90%

(4) Continuous administration of general anesthesia: Certain general anesthetics produce significant bronchodilation and are therefore useful adjuncts in life-threatening asthma.

(a) Ketamine infusion, 1 mg/kg/hr IV, *or*

(b) Isoflurane, 0.5% to 1.5% inhaled

It is advisable to add a benzodiazepine (lorazepam or diazepam) to ensure amnesia (during low-dose isoflurane) or to prevent hallucinations with ketamine. Only individuals with experience and competency in the use of general anesthetics should attempt to manage life-threatening asthma with general anesthesia.

3. Adverse events

a. Hypotension

(1) Causes: Hypovolemia, inhaled anesthetic effect, increased intrathoracic pressure limiting venous return

(2) Management

(a) If small cardiac silhouette (teardrop) and poor perfusion (cool mottled extremities)—normal saline, 20 mL/kg, *or*

(b) Dopamine, 5 to 10 mcg/kg/min, or phenylephrine, 1 to 10 mcg/kg/min

TABLE 4-5

PHENOTYPIC DESCRIPTION OF NEAR-FATAL ASTHMA (NFA)

	Onset	
Feature	**Sudden (Asphyxic or Hyperacute Asthma)**	**Gradual**
Onset	Hours (usually <2 hr)	Days-weeks
Past history	Asthma, partially responsive	Asthma, poorly controlled
Trigger	Massive allergen exposure (food, NSAIDs); emotional upset	Underusage of inhaled and oral steroids; depression, denial
Frequency of NFA events	20%	80%
Airway findings	No mucus plugging; submucosal neutrophilic infiltrate	Dense mucus plugging; submucosal eosinophilic infiltrate
Pathophysiologic features	Blunted perception of dyspnea	PEF highly variable with diurnal variation (early morning drop in PEF)
Recovery	Rapid	Slow

NSAIDS, Nonsteroidal anti-inflammatory drugs; *PEF,* peak expiratory flow.

  b. Steroid myopathy
    (1) Definition: Steroid myopathy is a myopathy or polyneuropathy that may present with weakness, including quadriparesis, and last for months.
    (2) Causes: Prolonged use (days) of steroids and nondepolarizing muscle relaxants
    (3) Management: Nondepolarizing muscle relaxants should be avoided or used sparingly if there is no other alternative to ventilate the patient.
VIII. Near-fatal asthma
  A. Phenotypes
    See **Table 4-5.**
  B. Management
    1. Acute ED and hospital management (see Section VII)
    2. Emergency management in the field
      a. Respiratory effort and breath sounds present: O_2 by face mask
      b. Breath sounds absent: Bag or mask ventilation with 100% O_2
      c. Epinephrine (1:1000), 0.01 mL/kg SC (maximum, 0.3 mL)
      d. Intubation: If bag-mask ventilation is not effective, transport to ED will be delayed (>20 minutes), or patient requires cardiopulmonary resuscitation
  IX. Disposition from the ED
    See Figure 4-1.
  X. Long-term management
    Schedule follow-up visits, preferably with a pediatric pulmonologist, every 2 to 6 weeks until asthma is under control (i.e., no symptoms, infrequent use of β-agonist inhaler).

Chapter 5

Cardiopulmonary Resuscitation

Elizabeth Hunt, MD,
Donald H. Shaffner, MD,
John Kuluz, MD,
and Charles L. Schleien, MD, MBA

I. Overview

The American Heart Association (AHA) has established guidelines for basic and advanced cardiopulmonary resuscitation (CPR) for infants and children. These guidelines establish a hierarchy of tasks—airway, breathing, and circulation (the ABCs)—that should be followed in the resuscitation of any critically ill infant or child. **Figure 5-1** compares techniques for infants and children.

II. Assessment and initial response

A. Airway and breathing

1. Basic CPR is instituted once inadequate breathing and circulation have been confirmed.

2. The rescuer immediately ensures that the airway is open, looks for chest excursions, and listens for breathing.

3. If absent, one should give two rescue breaths by bag–valve–mask (BVM) ventilation and call for help. (This chapter is focused on the health care provider, and thus we will not discuss mouth-to-mouth ventilation.) Other than Figure 5-1, which addresses CPR in the out-patient setting, this chapter is focused on in-hospital resuscitation.

B. Circulation

1. If an Ambu bag is not immediately available, proceed to assessment of circulation while a team member is getting the Ambu bag.

2. It is important not to delay compressions if they are needed.

3. Although the ABC steps appear to be sequential, in a hospital setting with multiple health care providers, they may be done simultaneously.

   a. Carotid or brachial pulses are then checked, if absent, or if the heart rate is <60 beats/min with signs of poor perfusion.

   b. Compressions then should be started immediately.

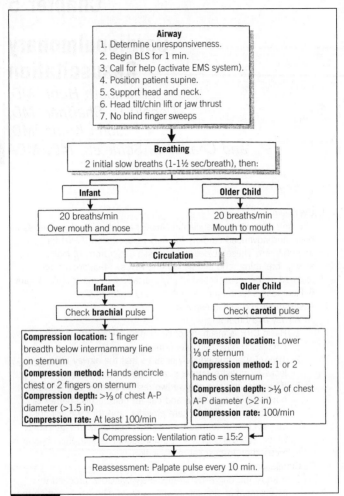

FIGURE 5-1

Comparison of basic CPR techniques for infants and children. *A-P,* Anterior-posterior; *BLS,* basic life support; *EMS,* emergency medical services.

4. For children of any age, an automated external defibrillator (AED) or manual defibrillator should be placed on the patient as soon as it is available.
5. If no care providers trained in pediatric advanced life support (PALS) are readily available, the team should activate the AED

as soon as possible, with the goal of defibrillating a child with a shockable rhythm (ventricular fibrillation [V Fib] or pulseless ventricular tachycardia [V Tach]) in less than 3 minutes from the onset of cardiopulmonary arrest.

6. The same time goal is used if a PALS provider is available, but this individual will use the manual mode of defibrillation if the child is in a shockable rhythm.

7. In the meantime, emergency equipment should be brought to the bedside.
   a. Backboard
   b. Step stool
   c. Code cart
   d. Emergency drug box

III. Organization
   A. Factors to consider
      1. Effective resuscitation requires meticulous organization.
      2. Roles should be clearly assigned and rehearsed during mock arrests.
      3. The responder most experienced in resuscitation assumes overall command and coordinates the effort (or may supervise a trainee acting as leader, but is still responsible for the quality of the event).
      4. An individual skilled in airway management provides positive pressure ventilation with 100% oxygen (O_2) via a mask or an endotracheal tube (ETT) (see Chapter 2).
      5. If positive pressure ventilation is being delivered by a face mask, another provider applies cricoid pressure until ETT placement is confirmed and acts as the airway assistant.
         a. However, it is not essential to provide cricoid pressure if not enough people are available.
         b. If the provider is not able to move the chest with positive pressure ventilation when cricoid pressure is applied, it should be immediately released.
      6. A fourth person administers chest compressions and one or two others should be ready to take over compressions every 2 minutes to ensure that the compressions are of good quality throughout the event.
      7. One responder is focused on obtaining rapid vascular access, administering rescue medications, and assisting with other procedures per the PALS algorithms.
      8. Another responder prepares medications.
      9. A record keeper is needed to document all events, medications, and vital signs during the resuscitation.
      10. Excess personnel may hamper effective resuscitation.

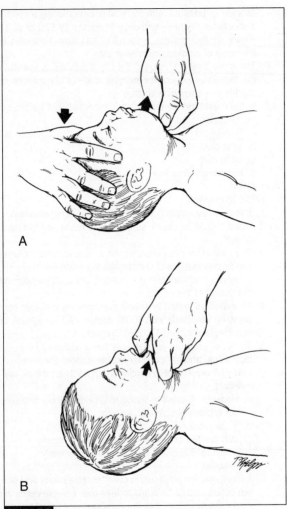

FIGURE 5-2
A, Head tilt, neck lift. **B,** Chin lift.

IV. Airway management for basic CPR
  A. Positioning
  Proper head, neck, and jaw positioning is designed to relieve
  airway obstruction, usually caused by the tongue.
    1. Head tilt, lift (**Fig. 5-2,** *A*)

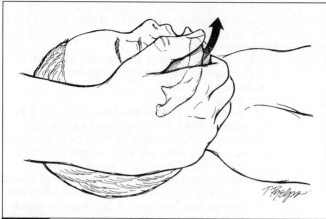

FIGURE 5-3

Jaw thrust. The mouth is opened with the thumb and the mandible is elevated with the middle fingers.

5

       a. If there is no suspicion of neck trauma, the rescuer's hand is placed on the victim's forehead while applying firm backward pressure to tip the head backward.

       b. Simultaneously, the other hand is placed under the neck to lift and support it upward.

       c. If neck injury is suspected, avoid head tilt and maintain in-line traction.

   2. Chin lift method (see Fig. 5-2, *B*)

       a. The fingertips of one hand are placed under the mandible.

       b. This brings the chin forward, which supports the jaw and tilts the head back.

   3. Jaw thrust (**Fig. 5-3**)

       a. This technique provides additional forward movement of the jaw when the rescuer grabs the angles of the mandible and lifts with both hands, displacing the mandible forward and tilting the head backwards.

       b. It is used if neck trauma is suspected and is also very effective in other scenarios.

       c. In-line traction should be maintained throughout resuscitation.

 B. Foreign body obstruction

   1. Evaluation

       a. Symptoms: Stridor and cyanosis

       b. History: The child playing with small objects prior to the choking spell

       c. Age: Uncommon in infants but possible, particularly if in close proximity to an older child, who might feed the infant the foreign body

  2. Management: Infants

       a. If the child is still **breathing and acyanotic,** no attempt is made to dislodge the foreign body. O_2 is applied by face mask during transport.

       b. Not breathing or cyanotic

          (1) The infant is positioned prone over the forearm of the rescuer with the infant's head lower than the trunk.

          (2) While providing support to the baby's head, five back blows are delivered rapidly with the heel of the hand between the infant's shoulder blades (**Fig. 5-4,** *A*).

          (3) With persistent obstruction, the infant is turned supine.

          (4) The infant's back is placed on the rescuer's thigh with the head lower than the trunk, and five chest thrusts are delivered in rapid succession.

          (5) Chest thrusts are given in the same manner as chest compressions (see Fig. 5-4, *B*).

       c. Blind finger sweeps are never indicated.

  3. Management: Children

       a. Manual thrusts (Heimlich maneuvers) are performed by standing behind the victim and wrapping one's hands around the waist (**Fig. 5-5**).

       b. The rescuer grasps one fist with the other hand and places the thumb side of the fist against the victim's abdomen, between the waist and rib cage.

       c. In this position, the rescuer then presses the fist five times into the victim's abdomen, with a quick inward and upward thrust.

       d. The unconscious victim is placed in the supine position.

          (1) The rescuer faces the patient kneeling astride the patient's hips.

          (2) With hands on top of each other, the heel of the bottom hand is thrust midway between umbilicus and xiphoid process in an inward and upward direction.

V. Airway management in advanced CPR

  A. Critical step in escalating from basic to advanced life support

    1. This occurs when 100% O_2 can be delivered by positive pressure ventilation.

  B. Technique

    1. Initially 100% O_2 is delivered with the BVM technique while cricoid pressure is applied to limit the risk of aspiration.

    2. As long as the team is able to move the chest adequately with bilateral breath sounds, and the child has intravenous (IV) or intraosseous (IO) access to deliver medications, then

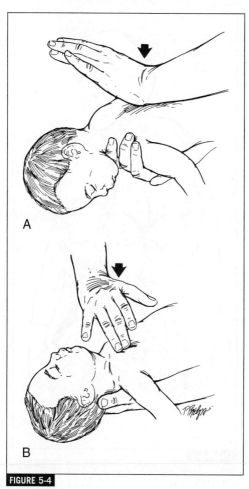

FIGURE 5-4

Relief of foreign body obstruction in infants. **A,** Back blows.
B, Chest thrusts.

intubation does not need to be performed immediately if there
are not enough team members to carry out other essential
tasks (e.g., compressions, early defibrillation).
3. Compressions should not be stopped for intubation attempts
unless necessary.
   a. Pauses should never exceed 10 seconds.

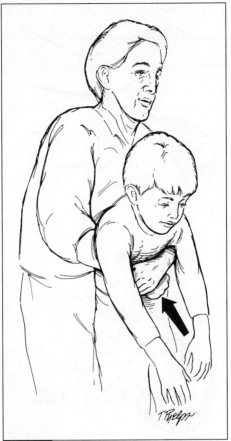

FIGURE 5-5

Relief of foreign body obstruction in children (Heimlich maneuver).

    b. However, as soon as there are adequate personnel present, the airway is secured with endotracheal (ET) intubation to guarantee delivery of 100% O_2, to prevent aspiration, and as a route to deliver certain medications if IV or IO access is not yet available (see Chapter 2).

4. Confirmation of ETT placement should include the use of an end-tidal carbon dioxide ($ETCO_2$) device.

    a. If there is very low or no blood flow through the pulmonary bed, there may be no $ETCO_2$ reading.

  b. This is a poor prognostic sign, particularly if ETT placement
     is confirmed with direct laryngoscopy and $ETCO_2$ is still not
     obtainable after deeper chest compressions and drug
     administration.
 5. Once the patient is intubated, compressions should no longer
    be paused for ventilation.
 6. Ventilations should be delivered at ~10 breaths/min in the
    intubated patient.
 7. Ensure good chest excursions, but avoid hyperventilation,
    because this can impede cardiac output.
VI. Circulation
  A. Assessment
    1. Cardiac arrest is defined as the absence of a pulse in the large
       arteries of an unconscious patient who is not breathing (or has
       agonal breaths).
    2. The brachial pulse is used to assess the presence of a pulse
       in an infant; the carotid pulse is used in the child.
    3. After determining a patient is pulseless, electrocardiographic
       analysis is necessary to determine which PALS algorithm will
       be used for subsequent therapy.
  B. Chest compressions
    1. Infant (**Fig. 5-6**)
      a. Technique: Two techniques may be used to compress the
         chest in infants.
        (1) The technique of choice is to use the hands to
            encircle the chest, providing a firm surface to the back,
            and to compress the chest at midsternum with the
            thumbs.
        (2) Alternatively, two fingers are placed on the sternum
            one fingerbreadth below the intermammary line;
            this may be preferred when only one rescuer is
            present.
          (a) Sternal compression depth: One third to one half
              the depth of the chest
          (b) Compression rate: 100 times/min
          (c) Compression–to–ventilation ratio = 15:2
            (i) Compressions should be paused for ventilation
                until intubated.
            (ii) They then should be continuous—that is, with
                 no need to synchronize ventilations and
                 compressions.
    2. Children 1 year of age to puberty (~12 years old) (**Fig. 5-7**)
      a. Technique: The heel of one hand is placed on the lower
         half of the sternum.
      b. Sternal compression depth: One third to one half the depth
         of the chest

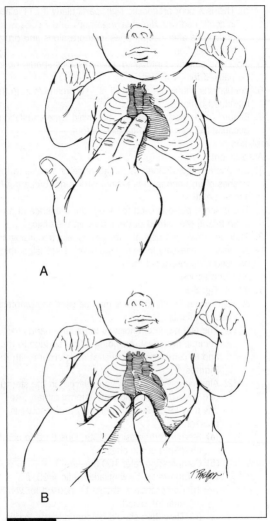

FIGURE 5-6

Chest compressions in the infant. **A,** Two-finger method.
B, Encircling method.

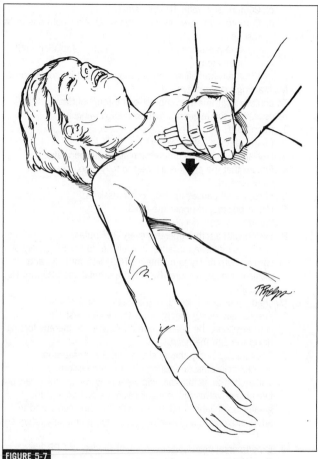

FIGURE 5-7
Chest compressions in the child 1 to 12 years of age. See text for details.

     c. Compression rate: 100 times/min
     d. Compression–to–ventilation ratio = 15:2.
       (1) Compressions should be paused for ventilation until
          intubated.
       (2) After intubation, compressions should be continuous.
  3. Children older than puberty (~13 years of age and older)
     a. Technique: The heels of both hands are placed on the
       lower half of the sternum.
     b. Sternal compression depth: ≥2 inches.

    c. Compression rate: 100 times/min

    d. Compression–to–ventilation ratio = 30:2 for both one or two rescuers.

      (1) Compressions should be paused for ventilation until intubated.

      (2) After intubation, compressions should be continuous.

C. Maintaining high-quality CPR

To achieve high-quality compressions throughout the resuscitation, the operator must do the following:

1. Push hard.
2. Push fast (see details earlier).
3. Use an appropriate compression–to–ventilation ratio.
4. Ensure that the chest is allowed to fully recoil after each compression.
5. Minimize all pauses in chest compressions.
6. Use a backboard under the child.
7. Stand on a step stool.
8. Switch with another operator every 2 minutes.
9. Use a quantitative measure, if available, to assess quality of cardiac output: Try to maintain $ETCO_2$ >15 mm Hg, and diastolic blood pressure (BP) on the arterial line >25 mm Hg, if possible.

D. Mechanism of blood flow during closed-chest CPR

1. The cardiac pump theory states that with chest compressions, the heart is directly squeezed, thereby forcing blood through the heart.
2. The thoracic pump theory states that the increase in intrathoracic pressure during chest compressions is transmitted to all intrathoracic vessels as well as the heart but, because of valves in the jugular venous system and the greater compliance and collapsibility of veins compared to arteries, blood flows forward through the pulmonary artery and aorta.
3. Experimental investigations in infant models of CPR have yielded data supporting both mechanisms.

E. Open-chest CPR

1. Indications

    a. The vast majority of arrest situations call for closed-chest CPR and do *not* call for extension to open-chest CPR.

    b. The only indications for open-chest CPR are those special situations that already require thoracotomy (**Box 5-1**).

2. Technique

    a. This is most easily done in the operating room during surgical procedures involving the thorax.

BOX 5-1

INDICATIONS FOR OPEN-CHEST CPR FOLLOWING CARDIAC ARREST

- Cardiac arrest during or following an intrathoracic procedure with an unhealed chest
- Penetrating trauma (e.g., stab wounds, gunshot wounds, intrathoracic hemorrhage)
- Massive air embolism
- Massive pulmonary embolism
- Ventricular or aortic aneurysms
- Chest or spine deformities (e.g., severe scoliosis) precluding effective closed-chest CPR
- Left atrial myxoma or other intracardiac obstruction
- Aortic stenosis

5

---

      b. When this is done in the emergency department or intensive care setting, it should only be performed by physicians trained in this procedure.

      c. The heart should be placed between the thumb and second and third fingers and care should be taken not only to squeeze the heart adequately, but also to allow refilling of the heart between direct compressions.

    3. Physiology: Open-chest CPR is superior to closed-chest CPR in generating vital organ blood flow.

    4. Risks include all of those associated with opening the chest:

      a. Infection

      b. Ventricular rupture

      c. Residual pneumothorax

      d. Hemothorax

VII. Rhythm assessment

  A. Comparison of approach in adults and children

    1. Child at the age of puberty or older or a child who has a history of cardiac disease is found unresponsive: **Call first**.

      a. Immediately call for help (request a defibrillator), and *then* initiate basic CPR.

      b. Initial cardiac rhythm is most likely to be pulseless V Tach or V Fib, both of which require defibrillation to convert to sinus rhythm.

    2. Child who has not yet reached puberty: **Call fast**.

      a. Perform 1 minute of CPR before calling for help.

    3. In a hospital setting, it is likely that one can do all steps simultaneously.

      a. Activate the hospital-wide resuscitation response.

      b. Ask a team member to get the defibrillator.

      c. Begin immediate compressions.

4. Younger children are more likely to have a primary respiratory arrest that progresses to a cardiac arrest.
   a. They may respond to early assistance with oxygenation, ventilation, and compressions.
   b. They are most likely to have an initial rhythm, such as pulseless electrical activity or asystole that will not respond to defibrillation.
5. For all children: Once basic CPR has been initiated, assess the cardiac rhythm to determine the appropriate treatment options.

B. Defibrillator
   1. All children who are found unresponsive and pulseless should have an AED attached and activated as soon as possible, and patients of any age should be defibrillated with a manual defibrillator by a PALS-trained provider, if available.
   2. CPR should be performed until the defibrillator is attached.
   3. Using the AED
      a. Turn on the AED device.
      b. Attach pads.
      c. Stop compressions.
      d. Perform AED analysis.
      e. AED will direct the rescuer to deliver a shock if indicated.
      f. AED will recommend that CPR be immediately resumed for another 2 minutes and then will recommend pausing compressions for another analysis.
      g. This cycle will continue every 2 minutes.
   4. Use of the manual defibrillator (**Fig. 5-8**)
      a. Turn on the defibrillator.
      b. Attach pads (or prepare the paddles by placing gel on them) and continue chest compressions.
      c. Select the appropriate energy dose (2 J/kg for the first shock, 4 J/kg for the second and subsequent shocks, to a maximum of 200 J for biphasic defibrillators and 360 J for monophasic defibrillators).
      d. Charge the defibrillator while compressions are being performed.
      e. When the defibrillator is fully charged, clear quickly so that no one is physically touching the patient or the bed, and remove the O_2 away from the bed.
      f. Confirm that the patient is in a shockable rhythm.
      g. Deliver the shock (<10 seconds of paused chest compressions).
      h. Immediately resume chest compressions for 2 minutes and then repeat the cycle.

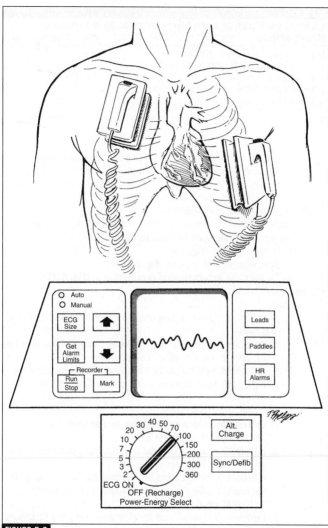

FIGURE 5-8

Defibrillation technique. (1) Energy dose set at 2 J/kg. (2) Choose largest paddles that do not touch each other when placed on chest. (3) Apply gel to paddles. (4) Place one paddle on right upper chest and the second paddle between left nipple and left anterior axillary line. (5) Charge the defibrillator. (6) Clear the bed. (7) Press discharge buttons on paddles simultaneously. (8) Immediately resume compressions (do not check rhythm or pulse first).

BOX 5-2

ROUTES OF MEDICATION DELIVERY: PREFERRED HIERARCHY FOR PEDIATRIC CARDIAC ARRESTS

1. Intravenous (IV) route (central vein)
2. Intravenous (IV) route (peripheral vein)*
3. Intraosseous (IO) route*
4. Endotracheal (ET) route
5. Intracardiac (IC) route

---

*IV and IO routes are equivalent; whichever can be obtained the quickest is the preferred route.

5. For the child between 1 and 8 years of age, use energy attenuator pads, if available, in order to minimize the total energy dose that is delivered when using the AED. If unavailable, use the adult pads.

C. Treatment of specific rhythms
   Other specific rhythms are covered in the 2010 AHA guidelines in the algorithms included in these figures.
   1. Pulseless arrest (**Fig. 5-9**)
   2. Brachycardia with a pulse (**Fig. 5-10**)
   3. Tachycardia with pulse and poor perfusion (**Fig. 5-11**)

VIII. Drugs and fluids
   A. Route
      1. IV or IO routes are the preferred routes for drug administration (**Box 5-2**)
         a. All drugs that are effective via the IV route are also effective IO, with almost no delay in onset time.
         b. A flush solution should be used after drug administration, (~0.25 mL/kg; minimum 5 mL, preferably 10 mL IV or IO).
      2. ET administration of drugs
         a. **Epinephrine, lidocaine, naloxone,** and **atropine** can be administered through the ETT.
         b. If IV or IO access is delayed beyond 2 to 3 minutes, these drugs should be given via the ETT.
         c. Epinephrine dose should be 10 times the IV dose (0.1 mg/kg; use 0.1 mL/kg of 1:1000 solution or 1 mL/kg of 1:10,000 solution).
         d. Lidocaine, naloxone, and atropine given via the ETT should be two to three times the IV dose.
         e. This route is less effective in obtaining a sufficient serum level than the IV and IO routes.
      3. Intracardiac (IC) administration
         a. The IC route is hazardous during CPR due to the risk of coronary artery laceration and should be used only when no other route is available.

B. Resuscitation drugs

See **Table 5-1** for arrest drug dosages, routes of administration, indications, and physiology.

C. Fluid administration

1. Type of fluid: Normal saline (NS), 10 to 20 mL/kg, is given over 2 to 5 minutes.

   a. A rapid 10- to 20-mL/kg volume expansion is justified in almost every pediatric arrest situation unless massive congestive heart failure (e.g., myocarditis, hypoplastic left heart syndrome) caused the arrest.

   b. Place a stopcock in line—in the IV tubing—so that a titrated fluid volume can be administered by syringe bolus.

2. Fluids for hypovolemic arrest (see Chapter 6)

   a. Interstitial fluid loss: If hypovolemia caused the arrest (e.g., trauma, vomiting and diarrhea, sepsis), additional aliquots of lactated Ringer's solution or NS, 20 mL/kg, are given every 5 minutes until adequate perfusion is restored.

   b. Blood loss

      (1) If hypovolemia was caused by blood loss, lactated Ringer's solution should be changed promptly to type O Rh-negative uncrossmatched whole blood or packed red cells.

      (2) Some institutions use O Rh-positive blood as a default, unless the patient is obviously pregnant or a female of childbearing age.

      (3) Type-specific blood can be administered safely (see Chapter 6).

   c. Total fluid volume administration

      (1) There is no arbitrary maximum fluid volume in the face of hypovolemic arrest. Fluid and blood administration is titrated to restore an adequate BP.

      (2) Consider early hemoglobin measurement to diagnose occult hemorrhage.

      (3) Ongoing fluid losses must be subtracted from the administered volume to determine the net fluid volume.

      (4) Pulses, breath sounds, liver size, peripheral edema, capillary refill, and skin color are constantly reassessed.

      (5) Up to 80 mL/kg of fluid can be given before laboratory tests such as hemoglobin and invasive monitoring (i.e., central venous pressure) are needed.

3. Dextrose administration

   a. Routine crystalloid fluid is isotonic and does not contain dextrose; hyperglycemia may aggravate neuronal injury.

   b. However, glucose must be measured to rule out hypoglycemia (Table 5-1 describes treatment regimens).

Text continued on p. 95.

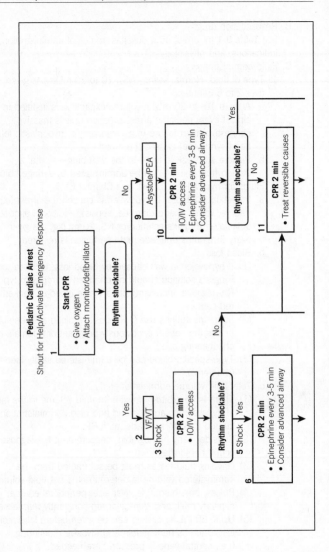

Pediatric Cardiac Arrest
Shout for Help/Activate Emergency Response

1 Start CPR
- Give oxygen
- Attach monitor/defibrillator

Rhythm shockable?

Yes →

2 VF/VT

3 Shock

4 CPR 2 min
- IO/IV access

Rhythm shockable?

Yes →

5 Shock

6 CPR 2 min
- Epinephrine every 3-5 min
- Consider advanced airway

No →

No → **9 Asystole/PEA**

10 CPR 2 min
- IO/IV access
- Epinephrine every 3-5 min
- Consider advanced airway

Rhythm shockable?

Yes →

No →

11 CPR 2 min
- Treat reversible causes

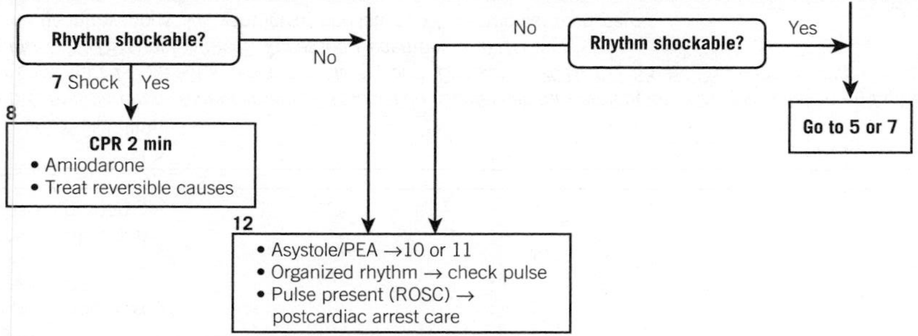
Rhythm shockable?
7 Shock
Yes
No
8
CPR 2 min
• Amiodarone
• Treat reversible causes
No
Rhythm shockable?
Yes
Go to 5 or 7
12
• Asystole/PEA →10 or 11
• Organized rhythm → check pulse
• Pulse present (ROSC) → postcardiac arrest care

Doses/Details

CPR Quality
- Push hard (≥⅓ of anterior-posterior diameter of chest) and fast (at least 100/min) and allow complete chest recoil
- Minimize interruptions in compressions
- Avoid excessive ventilation
- Rotate compressor every 2 minutes
- If no advanced airway, 15:2 compression-ventilation ratio. If advanced airway, 8-10 breaths per minute with continuous chest compressions

Shock Energy for Defibrillation
First shock 2 J/kg, second shock 4 J/kg, subsequent shocks ≥4 J/kg, maximum 10 J/kg or adult dose.

FIGURE 5-9
PALS pulseless arrest algorithm.
(Reprinted with permission from American Heart Association. Guidelines for cardiopulmonary resuscitation and emergency cardiovascular care. Part 14: pediatric advanced life support. Circulation 2010;122:S876-908 (website): http://circ.ahajournals.org/cgi/content/full/122/18_suppl_3/S876. Accessed December 6, 2010.)
BLS, Basic life support; *CPR,* cardiopulmonary resuscitation; *IO,* intraosseous; *IV,* intravenous; *PEA,* pulseless electrical activity; *ROSC,* return of spontaneous circulation; *VF,* ventricular fibrillation; *VT,* ventricular tachycardia.

Continued

Drug Therapy
- **Epinephrine IO/IV Dose:** 0.01 mg/kg (0.1 mL/kg of 1:10 000 concentration). Repeat every 3-5 minutes. If no IO/IV access, may give endotracheal dose: 0.1 mg/kg (0.1mL/kg of 1:1000 concentration).
- **Amiodarone IO/IV Dose:** 5 mg/kg bolus during cardiac arrest. May repeat up to 2 times for refractory VF/pulseless VT.

Advanced Airway
- Endotracheal intubation or supraglottic advanced airway
- Waveform capnography or capnometry to confirm and monitor endotracheal tube placement
- Once advanced airway in place give 1 breath every 6-8 seconds (8-10 breaths per minute)

Return of Spontaneous Circulation (ROSC)
- Pulse and blood pressure
- Spontaneous arterial pressure waves with intra-arterial monitoring

Reversible Causes
- Hypovolemia
- Hypoxia
- Hydrogen ion (acidosis)
- Hypoglycemia
- Hypokalemia/hyperkalemia
- Hypothermia
- Tension pneumothorax
- Tamponade, cardiac
- Toxins
- Thrombosis, pulmonary
- Thrombosis, coronary

FIGURE 5-9

PALS pulseless arrest algorithm.

(Reprinted with permission from American Heart Association. Guidelines for cardiopulmonary resuscitation and emergency cardiovascular care. Part 14: pediatric advanced life support. Circulation 2010;122:S876-908 (website): http://circ.ahajournals. org/cgi/content/full/122/18_suppl_3/S876. Accessed December 6, 2010.)

IO, Intraosseous; IV, intravenous; VF, ventricular fibrillation; VT, ventricular tachycardia.

   4. Maintenance fluids during CPR
      a. Once intravascular volume has been restored, subsequent fluid administration should be reduced to minimize the risk of tissue edema.
      b. Hypovolemia may recur, so constant reassessment is necessary.
IX. Vascular access
   Advanced CPR requires rapid vascular access for the delivery of medications and fluids.
   A. Options: Peripheral IV, IO, and central venous access
      1. Although all three types of vascular access are options for patients of any age, there is generally a different approach for younger versus older children.
      2. IO access is easier in younger children because their bone cortex is softer, but can theoretically be obtained in patients of any age.
      3. Newer IO needles with drill mechanisms make it even easier and more reliable than previously to obtain rapid access in older patients, thus truly extending the use of this lifesaving procedure to older patients.
      4. Central venous access can also be obtained in any age child, but is usually easier and faster to obtain in older children.
   B. Children younger than 8 years
      1. A brief attempt is made to start an IV in the dorsum of the hands or feet or any other readily visible vein, unless a child is in full cardiac arrest.
      2. If full arrest, **immediately** place an IO needle.
      3. The preferred location for first attempt at IO access is in the medial portion of the tibia at the level of the tibial tubercle (**Fig. 5-12**). Long-term access is then achieved with a central vein catheter (e.g., femoral, external, or internal jugular, or subclavian vein) or via a saphenous vein cutdown (**Figs. 5-13** to **5-16**).
   C. Children older than 8 years
      1. Peripheral venous access is generally easier in the older child, but IO needles may be more difficult to place because the bone cortex is thicker.
      2. Success rate of IO placement increases with IO needles with drill mechanisms, so these devices can be used in any aged child.
      3. For traditional IO needles in the older or obese child, consider alternative sites, such as the anterior superior iliac spine or other sites (see later).
      4. If peripheral and IO techniques fail, central line placement or saphenous vein cutdown should be attempted.

Text continued on p. 108.

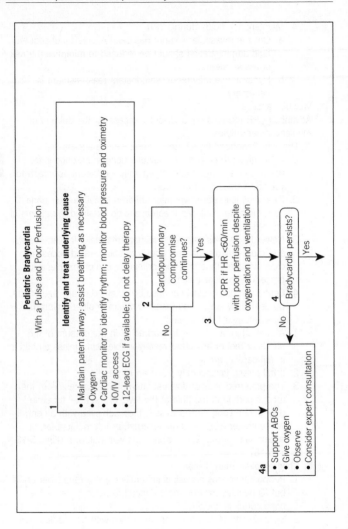

Pediatric Bradycardia
With a Pulse and Poor Perfusion

1

Identify and treat underlying cause

- Maintain patent airway; assist breathing as necessary
- Oxygen
- Cardiac monitor to identify rhythm; monitor blood pressure and oximetry
- IO/IV access
- 12-lead ECG if available; do not delay therapy

2

Cardiopulmonary compromise continues?

No →

Yes ↓

3

CPR if HR <60/min with poor perfusion despite oxygenation and ventilation

4

Bradycardia persists?

No →

Yes →

4a

- Support ABCs
- Give oxygen
- Observe
- Consider expert consultation

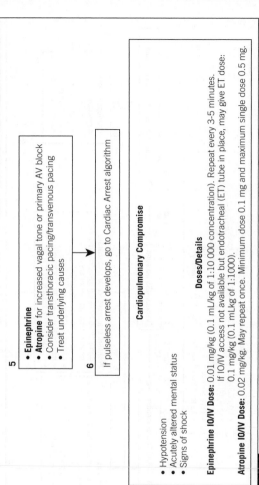

5

- **Epinephrine**
- **Atropine** for increased vagal tone or primary AV block
- Consider transthoracic pacing/transvenous pacing
- Treat underlying causes

6

If pulseless arrest develops, go to Cardiac Arrest algorithm

Cardiopulmonary Compromise

- Hypotension
- Acutely altered mental status
- Signs of shock

Doses/Details

Epinephrine IO/IV Dose: 0.01 mg/kg (0.1 mL/kg of 1:10 000 concentration). Repeat every 3-5 minutes. If IO/IV access not available but endotracheal (ET) tube in place, may give ET dose: 0.1 mg/kg (0.1 mLkg of 1:1000).

Atropine IO/IV Dose: 0.02 mg/kg. May repeat once. Minimum dose 0.1 mg and maximum single dose 0.5 mg.

FIGURE 5-10

PALS bradycardia algorithm.

(Reprinted with permission from American Heart Association. Guidelines for cardiopulmonary resuscitation and emergency cardiovascular care. Part 14: pediatric advanced life support. Circulation 2010;122:S876-908 (website): http://circ. ahajournals.org/cgi/content/full/122/18_suppl_3/S876. Accessed December 6, 2010.)

ABCs, Airway, breathing, circulation; *AV,* atrioventricular; *CPR,* cardiopulmonary resuscitation; *ECG,* electrocardiogram; *HR,* heart rate; *ICP,* intracranial pressure; *IO,* intraosseous; *IV,* intravenous.

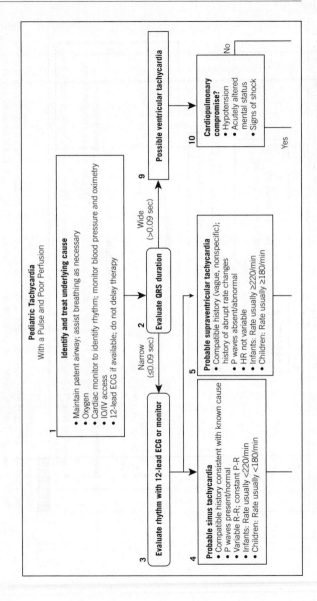

Pediatric Tachycardia
With a Pulse and Poor Perfusion

1
Identify and treat underlying cause
• Maintain patent airway; assist breathing as necessary
• Oxygen
• Cardiac monitor to identify rhythm; monitor blood pressure and oximetry
• IO/IV access
• 12-lead ECG if available; do not delay therapy

2
Evaluate QRS duration

Narrow (≤0.09 sec)

Wide (>0.09 sec)

3
Evaluate rhythm with 12-lead ECG or monitor

9
Possible ventricular tachycardia

4
Probable sinus tachycardia
• Compatible history consistent with known cause
• P waves present/normal
• Variable R-R; constant P-R
• Infants: Rate usually <220/min
• Children: Rate usually <180/min

5
Probable supraventricular tachycardia
• Compatible history (vague, nonspecific; history of abrupt rate changes
• P waves absent/abnormal
• HR not variable
• Infants: Rate usually ≥220/min
• Children: Rate usually ≥180/min

10
Cardiopulmonary compromise?
• Hypotension
• Acutely altered mental status
• Signs of shock

No

Yes

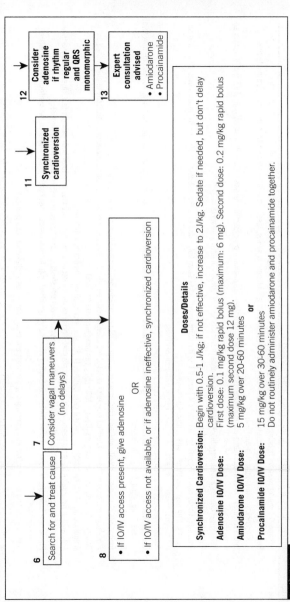

6 Search for and treat cause

7 Consider vagal maneuvers (no delays)

8
- If IO/IV access present, give adenosine

OR

- If IO/IV access not available, or if adenosine ineffective, synchronized cardioversion

11 Synchronized cardioversion

12 Consider adenosine if rhythm regular and QRS monomorphic

13 Expert consultation advised
- Amiodarone
- Procainamide

Doses/Details

Synchronized Cardioversion: Begin with 0.5-1 J/kg; if not effective, increase to 2J/kg. Sedate if needed, but don't delay cardioversion.

Adenosine IO/IV Dose: First dose: 0.1 mg/kg rapid bolus (maximum: 6 mg). Second dose: 0.2 mg/kg rapid bolus (maximum second dose 12 mg).

Amiodarone IO/IV Dose: 5 mg/kg over 20-60 minutes

or

Procainamide IO/IV Dose: 15 mg/kg over 30-60 minutes
Do not routinely administer amiodarone and procainamide together.

FIGURE 5-11

PALS tachycardia algorithm.

(Reprinted with permission from American Heart Association. Guidelines for cardiopulmonary resuscitation and emergency cardiovascular care. Part 14: pediatric advanced life support. Circulation 2010;122:S876-908 (website): http://circ.ahajournals.org/cgi/content/full/122/18_suppl_3/S876. Accessed December 6, 2010.)

ABCs, Airway, breathing, circulation; ECG, electrocardiogram; HR, heart rate; IO, intraosseous; IV, intravenous; QRS, QRS wave complex.

TABLE 5-1

DRUGS AND ELECTRICAL THERAPY FOR PEDIATRIC RESUSCITATION

Arrest Drug	Dosage, Route of Administration, Indications, and Physiology
Adenosine	Dosage: 0.1 mg/kg by rapid IV bolus; if ineffective, 0.2–0.3 mg/kg; max first dose, 6 mg, second, 12 mg Route: IV/IO (because of rapid metabolism, prefer central route; flush with ≥5 mL normal saline; ideally, use stopcock to deliver drug as a fast push, turn stopcock and immediately push flush Indications: SVT in stable children (cardioversion required if BP is unstable); may be used prior to cardioversion if there is no delay (i.e., drug and IV access are available) Physiology: Causes a temporary block through the AV node; interrupts reentry circuits involving AV node
Amiodarone	Dosage: 5 mg/kg; max, 15 mg/kg/day Route: IV, IO (by rapid IV bolus for pulseless V Tach, V Fib; if rhythm reverts, slow down bolus and give the rest over 30–60 min; by infusion over 20–60 min for perfusing supraventricular and ventricular rhythms) Indications: Pulseless V Tach, V Fib, SVT, V Tach with poor perfusion Physiology: Class III antiarrhythmic, increases conduction delay, ↑ V Fib threshold
Atropine	Dosage: 0.02 mg/kg; minimum dose, 0.1 mg (paradoxical bradycardia may occur with smaller doses); max single dose: 0.5 mg, child, 1 g, adolescent; max total dose: 1 mg, child, 2 mg, adolescent Route: IV, IO, SC, ET, IM Indications: Atropine is specifically indicated in sinus or junctional bradycardia and in slow idioventricular rhythms. Physiology: Because of the exaggerated effects of vagal stimulation in children, atropine is used prior to pediatric intubations, particularly in children <2 yr.
Calcium	Dosage: 20 mg/kg calcium chloride (CaCl₂), 100 mg/kg calcium gluconate (CaGluc) Route: CaCl₂, IV, IO, preferably via central vein; CaGluc, IV, IO, give over 5–10 min in perfusing patients. Indications: Hyperkalemia, hypermagnesemia, calcium channel blocker overdose; documented hypocalcemia: ↓ in total body calcium (e.g., hypoparathyroidism, renal failure, pancreatitis), ↓ ionized Ca²⁺ (e.g., following massive blood transfusion, postoperative or post-trauma, critical illness) Physiology: Essential for myocardial excitation-contraction coupling; major effect is to increase myocardial contractility; may increase ventricular automaticity during asystole. Side effects: May vasoconstrict ischemic areas of the heart and brain, worsen intracellular calcium overload.

Cardioversion, defibrillation	Dosage
	<u>V Fib, pulseless V Tach:</u> Asynchronous—first, 2 J/kg; second, 4 J/kg; third, 4 J/kg; first shock should be delivered as rapidly as possible (within 3 min of onset of pulselessness), and immediately followed by 2 min of compressions; if still in shockable rhythm, a second shock should be administered; if not successful, follow drug-shock pattern, shock delivered after drugs circulated for 2 min with CPR
	<u>V Tach with a pulse or SVT:</u> 0.5 J/kg (synchronized) when hemodynamically unstable or if unresponsive to amiodarone or lidocaine, ↑ to 1.0 J/kg on second and subsequent attempts
	Paddle: One paddle on right upper chest quadrant, the other paddle to the left of the left nipple in anterior axillary line
	Placement: One paddle anteriorly or over left precordium, the other posteriorly on the upper back, between the scapulae (ideal for small infants)
	Paddle size: Infant paddles—for infants <1 yr or <10 kg, use largest paddles that do not touch
	Indications: As above; V Fib is unusual in children without congenital heart defect; suspect metabolic abnormalities or intoxication with digitalis or tricyclic antidepressants
	Physiology: V Fib characterized by random depolarization of myocardial cells; defibrillation results in spontaneous depolarization of critical number of myocardial cells. A single pacemaker may then emerge to allow depolarization of the heart.
Epinephrine	Dosage: Initial dose, 10 mcg/kg or 0.1 mL/kg of 1:10,000 solution: ET doses, 100 mcg/kg, 0.1 mL/kg of 1:1000 solution
	Supply: 1:10,000 solution (0.1 mg/mL) premixed resuscitation syringe or 1:1000 solution (1 mg/mL)
	Route: IV, IO, ET
	Indications: Symptomatic bradycardia unresponsive to oxygenation and ventilation, pulseless arrest (asystole, PEA, V Fib, pulseless V Tach)
	Physiology: Epinephrine is an α- and β-agonist. The α-adrenergic effects are responsible for its beneficial effects during CPR, causing a generalized vasoconstriction of the peripheral vasculature and resulting in ↑ in coronary and cerebral blood flow. Epinephrine also causes ↑ inotropy, ↑ chronotropy, ↑ intensity of V Fib thus ↓ defibrillation threshold, ↑ myocardial O₂ requirement.

AV, Atrioventricular; *BP,* blood pressure; *ET,* endotracheal; *IM,* intramuscular; *IO,* intraosseous; *IV,* intravenous; *PEA,* pulseless electrical activity; *SC,* subcutaneous; *SVT,* supraventricular tachycardia; *V Fib,* ventricular fibrillation; *V Tach,* ventricular tachycardia.

Continued

TABLE 5-1

DRUGS AND ELECTRICAL THERAPY FOR PEDIATRIC RESUSCITATION—cont'd

Arrest Drug	Dosage, Route of Administration, Indications, and Physiology
Glucose	Dosage: 2-4 mL/kg of D_{25} (0.25 g/mL of dextrose); neonates: 10 mL/kg of D_{10} (0.10 g/mL of dextrose) Route: IV, IO Indications: Point of care glucose <60 mg%; check glucose early and q30min during resuscitation efforts; empiric glucose is *not* indicated because hyperglycemia may exacerbate ischemic brain injury. Physiology: Children have a smaller liver (thus smaller glycogen stores) and higher metabolic rate than adults. This results in a high risk of hypoglycemia during stressed states, including cardiopulmonary arrest. The glucose level should be checked early and repeatedly.
Lidocaine	Dosage: 1 mg/kg rapid IV push. If repeated doses are needed, initiate an infusion of 20-50 mcg/kg/min. Route: IV, IO, ET Indications: V Fib, V Tach, with or without a pulse Physiology: Class IB antiarrhythmic, ↓ automaticity of pacemaker cells and ↑ V Fib threshold
Sodium bicarbonate	Dosage: 1 mEq/kg (1 mL/kg of 8.4% solution) or bicarbonate (mEq) = 0.3 × body weight (kg) × base deficit; for neonates use dilute solution, 2 mL/kg of 4.2% solution) Route: IV, IO Indications: Bicarbonate should be limited to cardiac arrest associated with the following: (1) hyperkalemia; (2) preexisting metabolic acidosis (e.g., associated with sepsis); (3) after cardiac compressions, defibrillation, support of ventilation, and antiarrhythmics have been given; (4) hypermagnesemia; (5) tricyclic overdose; (6) sodium channel blocker overdose; (7) aspirin overdose Physiology: Bicarbonate is a buffer used to treat metabolic acidosis according to the reaction $$HCO_3^- + H^+ \leftrightarrow H_2CO_3 \leftrightarrow H_2O + CO_2$$ Effective treatment of metabolic acidosis requires the following: (1) effective pulmonary blood flow (i.e., effective chest compressions) so that the metabolic product of the above reaction, CO_2, can be delivered from peripheral tissues to the lungs; and (2) effective ventilation so that accumulated CO_2 can be excreted by the lungs. Unless these two requirements are fulfilled, bicarbonate administration will lead to tissue CO_2 accumulation and hence a combined respiratory and metabolic acidosis in the tissues, including myocardium, which may delay recovery of spontaneous cardiac activity. Potential adverse effects of bicarbonate: (1) hypernatremia; (2) hyperosmolality; (3) shift of O_2 dissociation curve to left, which thereby reduces O_2 unloading in peripheral tissue; (4) myocardial depression (in treating lactic acidosis); (5) intracellular acidosis (especially central nervous system). CO_2 formed by dissociation of bicarbonate rapidly enters neurons, with slower egress of H^+ from cell.

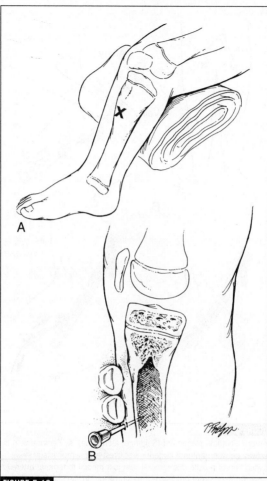

FIGURE 5-12

IO needle placement. **A,** Insert needle 1 to 2 cm below and 1 to
2 cm medial to the tibial tubercle on the medial portion of the tibia.
B, The needle is aimed caudally and laterally.
IO, intraosseous.

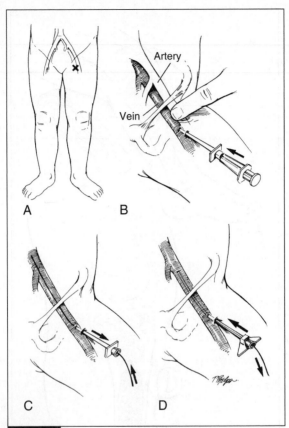

FIGURE 5-13

Femoral vein line placement (Seldinger technique). **A,** Femoral vein is midway between anterior superior iliac crest and symphysis pubis. **B,** Insertion of needle into femoral vein just medial to femoral arterial pulse. **C,** Insertion of guidewire through needle in the vein. Needle is removed once guidewire is in place. **D,** Infusion catheter advanced over guidewire into vein. Guidewire is removed after catheter is in place.

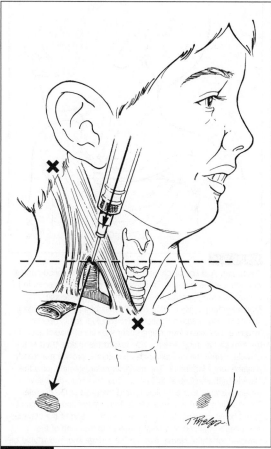

FIGURE 5-14

Internal jugular vein line placement. The head is turned to the opposite side and needle puncture is at the apex of the triangle formed by the heads of the sternocleidomastoid muscle, midway between the sternal notch and the mastoid process. Needle is aimed at the ipsilateral nipple. Use Seldinger technique (Fig. 5-13).

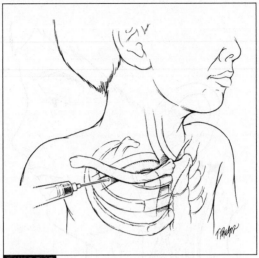

FIGURE 5-15

Subclavian vein line placement. The patient is positioned supine with arms at the side. No Trendelenburg position is needed in the patient receiving positive pressure ventilation (10-degree Trendelenburg position decreases the risk of air embolism in the spontaneously breathing patient). No shoulder roll is needed. Visualize the axillary vein rising under the skin of medial aspect of the arm and arching over the ribs toward the middle third of the clavicle, where the clavicle angles posteriorly, providing a readily palpable bony landmark. The costoclavicular ligament joins the clavicle to the first rib at this point. From this point on, the vein travels posterior to the clavicle toward the head of the clavicle. The insertion point of the needle is 1 cm lateral and 1 cm caudal to the bony angle produced by the posterior bend of the clavicle. The needle is aimed at a point posterior to the head of the clavicle (not at the sternal notch). The syringe and hub should be elevated at a 30-degree angle to the frontal plane of the chest. Then use the Seldinger technique (Fig. 5-13) for line placement.

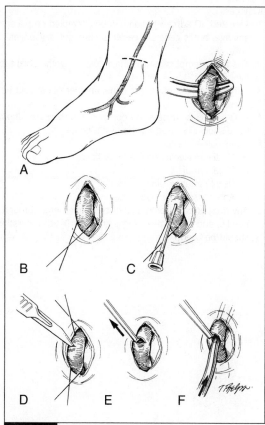

FIGURE 5-16

Saphenous vein cutdown. **A,** 1-cm transverse incision anterior to the medial malleolus; blunt dissection with hemostat. **B,** Control of vein with ligature. **C,** Direct puncture with intravenous catheter or proximal and distal control with ligature, and **D,** incision with no. 11 scalpel blade. **E,** Insertion of right angle vein guide. **F,** Insertion of Silastic catheter underneath vein guide.

D. IO access
   1. As noted, IO administration can be attempted on patients of any age, but is generally easier to carry out in younger children.
   2. The first attempt is usually made just below the tibial tubercle (see Fig. 5-12).
   3. If there is a fracture in that bone, another site should be chosen.
   4. If IO access is successfully obtained and then lost, another bone should be used for the next attempt.
   5. Other potential sites
      a. Medial malleolus on the distal tibia
      b. Distal femur
      c. Distal radius or ulna
      d. Anterior superior iliac spine
   6. Any drug or blood product can be administered through an IO needle, and the same dosages given for IV administration should be used.

Chapter 6

Shock
Mark R. Rigby, MD, PhD,
Katherine Biagas, MD, FCCM, FAAP,
and Charles L. Schleien, MD, MBA

I. Overview
   A. Definition
      1. Shock is a complex syndrome of acute homeostatic derangement in which the body's ability to meet cellular metabolic requirements for oxygen (O_2) and nutrients is severely compromised.
      2. The resultant strain on cellular function may lead to multi-organ dysfunction and failure of cellular metabolism.
      3. Shock is not necessarily low blood pressure (BP) or decreased intravascular blood volume.
   B. Classification (**Table 6-1**)
      1. Hypovolemic shock (root cause is low preload, low circulating volume). Major causes include the following:
         a. Vomiting, diarrhea
         b. Hemorrhage
         c. Third space fluid accumulation associated with peritonitis, surgery, or other inflammatory conditions
      2. Cardiogenic shock (root cause is diminished myocardial ejection, pump failure). Major causes include the following:
         a. Cardiomyopathy
         b. Myocarditis
         c. Congestive heart failure
         d. Congenital heart disease
         e. Cardiac tamponade
         f. Myocardial infarction (anomalous coronary artery)
      3. Distributive shock (root cause is decreased systemic vascular resistance [SVR]). Major causes include the following:
         a. Spinal cord injury
         b. Anaphylaxis
         c. Some types of septic shock
      4. Septic shock (root causes are multifactorial). All cases of septic shock have low preload. The SVR may be low (because of poor vascular tone and increased permeability) or high. Myocardial function is impaired to variable degrees.

TABLE 6-1

CHARACTERISTICS OF MAJOR SHOCK TYPES

Shock Type	Primary Root Cause	HR	CO	SVR	CVP	Pulses/ Perfusion	Initial Therapy
Hypovolemic shock	↓ Intravascular volume	↑	↓	↑	↓	↓/cold	Fluid
Cardiogenic	Poor myocardial contractility	↑	↓	↑	↑	↓/cold	Inotropy
Septic, warm	Vasodilation from inflammation	↑	Usually↑	↓	↓	↑/warm	Fluid, inotropy-pressors
Septic, cold	Vasoconstriction from inflammation	↑	↓	↑	↓	↓/cold	Fluid, inotropy
Distributive	Vasodilation from various causes (e.g., neurogenic)	↑	↑	↓	↓	↑/warm	Fluid, inotropy-pressors
Obstructive	Left ventricular or aortic obstruction	↑	↓	↑	Variable	↓	Fluids, PGE1 only in the newborn

CO, Cardiac output; *CVP*, central venous pressure; *HR*, heart rate; *PGE1*, prostaglandin E1; *SVR*, systemic vascular resistance.

5. Obstructive shock (root cause is obstruction to left ventricular outflow). Major causes include the following:
   a. Critical coarctation of the aorta (newborn)
   b. Hypoplastic left heart syndrome (newborn)
   c. Aortic stenosis (children and adolescents)

II. Pathophysiology
   A. Cardiac function
      1. BP = cardiac output (CO) × SVR.
         a. A reduction in CO (i.e., heart failure) that cannot be compensated for by an increase in SVR will result in a reduction in BP.
         b. Similarly, a reduction in SVR that cannot be compensated for by an increase in CO will also result in a reduction in BP (i.e., septic shock).
      2. CO = stroke volume (SV) × heart rate (HR). Marked reductions in HR or SV result in reduced CO.
         a. Neonates, young infants, and some patients with cardiomyopathies or who have undergone bypass surgery have stiff ventricles and are unable to increase their SV. In these patients, CO is dependent on HR and falls dramatically with decreasing HR.
         b. Ventricular filling is decreased by tachyarrhythmias (>220 beats/min) and/or loss of atrial contraction (loss of P wave), resulting in decreased SV and CO.

III. General principles
   A. Recognizing shock
      1. The signs and symptoms of shock are listed in **Box 6-1.**

BOX 6-1

SIGNS AND SYMPTOMS OF COLD SHOCK

- Abnormal capillary refill time (>3 sec)
- Cold extremities
- Decreased mental status
- Diminished peripheral pulses
- Hypotension
- Ileus
- Oliguria
- Pallor
- Sweating
- Tachycardia

TABLE 6-2

AVERAGE BLOOD PRESSURES AND HEART RATES FOR AGE

Age	Blood Pressure (mm Hg)	Heart Rate (beats/min)
Premature infant	Systolic, 40-60	100-160
Full-term newborn	75/50	100-180
1-6 mo	80/50	110-180
6-12 mo	90/65	110-170
12-24 mo	95/65	90-150
2-6 yr	100/60	70-140
6-12 yr	110/60	60-130
12-16 yr	110/65	60-110
16-18 yr	120/65	60-100
Adult	125/75	60-100

Approximate ranges for BP—mean pressure ± 20% = 95% confidence limit. Values for females are approximately 5% lower.

6

    2. Regardless of cause, tachycardia and/or tachypnea present first and remain the most persistent signs of shock in children.
    3. Normal BPs and HRs by patient age are shown in **Table 6-2**.
  B. Airway and breathing
    1. If airway patent and breathing adequate, 100% O_2 by face mask
    2. If airway or breathing inadequate, bag–valve–mask ventilation followed by endotracheal intubation
  C. Intravenous (IV) access
    1. Place two large-bore IVs.
    2. If IV access cannot be obtained rapidly, place an intraosseous (IO) needle. Once the patient has been resuscitated with fluids, an IV can generally be placed and the IO discontinued (see later).
  D. Laboratory assessment
    1. Obtain dextrostick and hematocrit (Hct) values at the earliest possible moment *without delaying therapy* in any child with shock.
    2. Obtain other laboratory tests after ABCs of resuscitation (airway, breathing, circulation), and depending on the clinical scenario.
  E. Transfer
    After initial stabilization, transfer to a pediatric critical care facility.

IV. Hypovolemic shock
  A. Definition
    1. Result of intravascular volume depletion caused by hemorrhage, trauma, diarrhea, vomiting, renal loss, deprivation, diuresis (diabetes mellitus or insipidus), third-space sequestration
    2. Leads to cellular hypoperfusion, metabolic acidosis, and cell death
    3. Most common cause of shock in children
    4. Reflex tachycardia (baroreceptor reflex) is common. Hypotension is not, so BP is an insensitive index of hypovolemia and, if present, implies profound failure of homeostasis.
  B. Assessment
    1. Assessment of shock severity is based on the physical examination (**Table 6-3**) and measured weight loss. Acute weight loss can be presumed to be the result of extracellular fluid loss.
    2. Fluid deficit: Calculate by multiplying the assessed percentage of dehydration (see Table 6-4) by the child's weight. For example, a 20-kg child who is 10% dehydrated has lost 10% (100 mL/kg) of body weight, or 2000 mL (2 kg) of fluid.
    3. Three types of dehydration (particularly following vomiting and/or diarrhea) are described based on the measured serum sodium level.
      a. Isonatremic (130-150 mEq/L)
      b. Hyponatremic (<130 mEq/L)
      c. Hypernatremic (>150 mEq/L)
      d. Physical examination findings
        (1) In hyponatremic dehydration, all the clinical manifestations appear at lesser degrees of deficit.

TABLE 6-3

CLINICAL ESTIMATION OF HYPONATREMIC OR ISONATREMIC DEHYDRATION

Dehydration (% of body weight)	Clinical Observation
• 5	• ↑ heart rate (10%-15% above baseline)
	• Dry mucous membranes
	• Concentrated urine
	• Lack of tearing
• 10	• Poor skin turgor
	• Oliguria
	• Soft, sunken eyes
	• Sunken anterior fontanel
	• Delayed capillary refill time (>3 sec)
• 15	• ↓ BP, tachycardia, tachypnea
	• Poor tissue perfusion and acidosis
	• Cool extremities
	• Delayed capillary refill time (>5 sec)

BP, Blood pressure.

        (2) In hypernatremic dehydration, the circulating volume is relatively preserved at the expense of cellular water, and less circulatory disturbance is seen for a given amount of fluid deficit.

    e. Laboratory tests: Tests confirming dehydration include the following:

        (1) Urine specific gravity ≥1.030

        (2) Blood urea nitrogen (BUN) ≥20 mg/dL

        (3) Creatinine ≥1 mg/dL

        (4) BUN-to-creatinine ratio ≥20 : 1 (an insensitive marker of dehydration in children)

V. Management of hypovolemic shock

The fluid management of a dehydrated patient requires the restoration of effective circulating volume, replacement of past and ongoing fluid losses, and provision of normal maintenance fluid and electrolyte requirements.

A. Initial management

    1. ABCs: Ensure adequate airway and breathing. Apply 100% O_2.

    2. Reassess BP, HR, peripheral perfusion, and urine output to guide fluid volume replacement. Reassess after administration of every fluid bolus or every 5 to 10 minutes.

    3. Initial fluid resuscitation

        a. Normal saline (NS), 20 mL/kg (recommended) or

        b. 5% albumin, 10 to 20 mL/kg

        The use of colloids, such as albumin, remains controversial. There is no evidence of improved survival with albumin administration compared with NS, nor is there evidence of benefit of other colloids (e.g., hetastarch) over albumin.

        c. Blood (when hypovolemia is caused by hemorrhage): See later (Section VI) for details of blood replacement therapy.

    4. For shock and >15% dehydration

        a. Administer up to 60 mL/kg IV rapidly (within 10 to 15 minutes) in 20 mL/kg aliquots until perfusion and BP improve or until adverse events are noted (i.e., hepatomegaly, rales).

        b. Reassess after every aliquot.

    5. Place Foley catheter into the urinary bladder.

B. Replacement of preexisting fluid deficit

    1. Assume that acute changes in weight from fluid losses (i.e., vomiting, diarrhea) are losses of extracellular fluid.

    2. The weight lost (in kg) equals the fluid deficit to be replaced (in liters).

    3. If the patient is hyponatremic (serum sodium = 120 to 130 mEq/L) or normonatremic (serum sodium = 130 to 150 mEq/L), replace the fluid and sodium deficit over 24 hours.

4. If the patient is *severely hyponatremic* (serum sodium <120 mEq/L and convulsing, give 3% hypertonic saline (i.e., in 5 cc/kg aliquots to increase the serum sodium by ~4 mEq/L with each aliquot) to raise the serum sodium to ~120 mEq/L acutely or until asymptomatic, then raise serum sodium toward the normal range more gradually (over 48 hours).

   a. The choice of fluids depends on the estimated sodium deficit and, more importantly, on monitoring the rate of sodium normalization.

   b. Half (0.45%) or normal (0.9%) saline are the preferred options (depending on condition). (See later and Chapter 8.)

5. If the patient is *severely hypernatremic* (serum sodium >160 mEq/L), replace the fluid deficit over 72 hours.

   a. NS is the preferred IV fluid solution until a predictable rate for sodium normalization has been established, after which 0.45% saline may be used with close monitoring.

   b. See Chapter 8 for more details on the management of hypernatremic dehydration.

C. Replacement of ongoing fluid losses

   1. Measure fluid intake and output (i.e., gastric, enteric, and/or renal) hourly—with Foley catheter, naso-gastric tube or rectal tube if necessary.

   2. Replace enteric losses milliliter for milliliter

   3. Replace excessive renal losses (i.e., 1 mL replacement for 1 mL urine output if urine output exceeds 2-3 mL/kg/hr). Excessive renal losses might be seen in diabetes insipidus or mellitus (with hyperglycemia).

D. Provision of normal maintenance fluid and electrolyte requirements

   1. Maintenance of fluid volume

      a. 4 mL/kg/hr for each of the **first** 10 kg of body weight (100 mL/kg/day)

      plus

      b. 2 mL/kg/hr for each of the **second** 10 kg of body weight (50 mL/kg/day)

      plus

      c. 1 mL/kg/hr for **each additional** kg of body weight (20 mL/kg/day)

      d. Maximum (adult) maintenance fluid volume: 100 mL/hr

   2. Total fluid administration rate in dehydration/shock = maintenance rate + preexisting deficit rate + ongoing loss rate.

   3. Maintenance sodium concentration: Use half-normal (0.45%) or normal (0.9%) saline depending on serum sodium and organ specific (i.e., central nervous system [CNS]) concerns.

4. Maintenance potassium concentration
   a. 20 mEq KCl/L of maintenance fluid will meet potassium maintenance requirements.
   b. Do not add KCl to IV fluids until the patient has voided.
   c. Do not add KCl to maintenance fluids of patients with renal failure, acute crush injuries, or burns.

E. Glucose
   1. Maintenance fluids should contain glucose.
      a. 10% dextrose (D10) for newborns and patients with known or suspected metabolic disease or hypoglycemia
      b. 5% dextrose (D5) for all other normoglycemic patients
   2. Monitoring to prevent hypoglycemia or hyperglycemia is essential.

F. Typical reevaluation of electrolytes, glucose, and renal function during the first 24 hours after shock
   1. Sodium and potassium, q4h
   2. Glucose, q1h until stable, then q4h
   3. Bicarbonate, calcium, and magnesium ×1; repeat if abnormal
   4. Intake and output q1h

G. Typical fluid and electrolyte regimen
   See **Table 6-4.**
   1. First 8 hours
      a. Half of the calculated loss is replaced along with maintenance fluid over the first 8 hours.
      b. Use half-normal (0.45%) or normal (0.9%) saline depending on serum sodium and organ specific (i.e., CNS) concerns. (The maintenance fluid will contain D5 in most cases.)
      c. Add 20 mEq/L of potassium once urine output is established.
      d. Ongoing losses are replaced concurrently (*piggybacked*) with a solution that matches the fluid being lost, either 0.45% saline or Ringer's lactate.
   2. Next 16 hours
      a. The remainder of the calculated deficit is replaced along with maintenance fluid over the next 16 hours. The preferred solution is D5, 0.45% saline, with 20 mEq/L of potassium.
      b. Ongoing losses are replaced as described earlier in Section V.C.
   3. Lack of therapeutic response: If a poor therapeutic response is noted or there is evidence of cardiac or renal disease (e.g., hemolytic-uremic syndrome), a central venous line and vasopressor infusion may be required.

VI. Management of hemorrhagic shock
   A. Classification
      Hemorrhagic shock is a specific form of hypovolemic shock seen most commonly after trauma (particularly of long bones, pelvis, and abdomen). See **Table 6-5** for classification.

TABLE 6-4

SAMPLE CALCULATION OF FLUID REQUIREMENTS

Calculate the fluid requirements for an 18-kg child (was 20 kg last week) who is 10% dehydrated (serum sodium = 132 mEq/L) with persistent diarrheal losses (40 mL/hr).

Deficit	20 kg × 10% (or 100 mL/kg) = 2000 mL
Maintenance	(10 kg × 4 mL/kg/hr) + (10 kg × 2 mL/kg/hr) = 60 mL/hr
Ongoing loss	40 mL/hr*

Timeline	Administered Fluid
0-15 min	20 mL/kg Ringer's lactate
30 min-8 hr	Half-deficit (1000 mL)/8 hr = 125 mL/hr
	125 mL/hr + maintenance fluids (60 mL/hr) + stool replacement (40 mL/hr)
	or 225 mL/hr of D5 0.45% saline + 20 mEq/L potassium
9-24 hr	Half-deficit (1000 mL)/16 hr = 63 mL/hr + maintenance fluids (60 mL/hr) + stool replacement (40 mL/hr)
	or 163 mL/hr of D5 0.45% saline + 20 mEq/L potassium

D5, 5% dextrose.
*Stool replacement will be based on prior-hours stool loss. In this example, stool output is assumed to be constant.

TABLE 6-5

CLASSIFICATION OF HEMORRHAGIC SHOCK

	Class			
Parameter	I	II	III	IV
Estimated blood volume deficit (%)	10-15	20-25	30-35	>40
Heart rate*	Normal or mild tachycardia	Tachycardia	Tachycardia	Tachycardia or bradycardia
Respirations	Normal	Mildly increased	Tachypneic	Tachypneic, apneic
Capillary refill (sec)	<5	5-10	10-15	>20
Blood pressure	Normal	Decreased pulse pressure	Decreased	Severely decreased
Mentation	Normal	Anxious	Confused or lethargic	Unconscious
Urine output	1-3 mL/kg	0.5-1 mL/kg	<0.5 mL/kg	None

*Interpretation of heart rate depends on the patient's age. See Table 6-2 for average heart rates based on age.

B. Specific therapy for hemorrhagic shock by class
   1. Class I
      a. Replace volume loss with NS.
      b. Administer 10 to 20 mL/kg as a bolus, replacing 3 to 5 mL of crystalloid for every 1 mL of circulating blood volume lost.
      c. The rationale for the 3-for-1 rule is that only one third to one fifth of the crystalloid infused remains in the intravascular space.
   2. Class II
      a. Same as class I hemorrhage, except that blood is frequently required as well.

      b. Ongoing blood losses are replaced milliliter for milliliter with blood.

  3. Class III or IV

      a. A Class III or IV hemorrhage requires blood as well as NS.

      b. Whole blood is preferred if available.

      c. Blood is transfused in aliquots of 10 to 15 mL/kg with the goal of restoring hemodynamic stability and raising hemoglobin to >7 g/dL.

C. Blood replacement therapy

The replacement of blood for the child in hemorrhagic shock begins as soon as possible.

  1. Fresh whole blood:

      a. Fresh (<48 hours old) whole blood contains red blood cells, platelets, and clotting factors.

      b. When available and crossmatched, it is the ideal replacement product.

      c. Unfortunately, it is rarely available, and stored (*banked*) blood components usually are used instead.

      d. A full crossmatch takes about 1 hour to accomplish.

  2. Packed red blood cells (PRBCs)

      a. PRBCs are red cell concentrates (250 to 300 mL) with a Hct between 50% and 70%.

      b. They contain no platelets and very little factors V and VIII.

      c. To maintain shelf life, packed cells are stored in solutions that bind calcium.

      d. Potassium levels may be high, particularly if blood has been stored for more than 20 days.

  3. Red cell replacement (**Table 6-6**)

      a. Estimated blood volume (EBV) is given by the following equation:

$$EBV = weight\ in\ kg \times blood\ volume\ (in\ mL/kg\ from\ Table\ 6\text{-}6)$$

      b. Volume of PRBCs required to achieve a desired Hct is given by the equation:

$$Volume\ of\ cells\ (mL) = \frac{(EBV) \times (Hct\ desired - Hct\ present)}{Hct\ of\ PRBCs}$$

TABLE 6-6

ESTIMATED BLOOD VOLUME PER KILOGRAM OF BODY WEIGHT

Age	Blood Volume (mL/kg)
Premature	100
Term infant	90
Child	80
Adult	60-70

    c. Type-specific blood
      (1) In life-threatening shock situations, type-specific blood can be given without a full crossmatch.
      (2) The incidence of major transfusion reactions with crossmatched blood is 1:10:000; with the type-specific, uncrossmatched blood, it is 1:1000.
    d. Universal donor: Type O blood
      (1) If type-specific blood is unavailable, type O blood is given. Type O-negative blood should be reserved for females to avoid Rh sensitization.
      (2) Type O-positive blood can be used in males until type-specific blood becomes available.

D. Massive transfusion
  1. Definition: A blood transfusion requirement of 1 blood volume (~80 to 100 mL/kg) in 24 hours or ~50% of blood volume (40 to 50 mL/kg) in 3 hours
  2. Potential adverse events (see Section VI.E. for management strategies)
    a. Hypothermia
    b. Dilutional thrombocytopenia
    c. Dilution of plasma coagulation factors: Coagulation factor deficits are reflected in prolonged prothrombin time, activated partial thromboplastin time, and decreased fibrinogen.
    d. Hypocalcemia
    e. Hyperkalemia

E. Adjuncts to red cell replacement
  1. Blood filters: Routinely administer all blood products through blood filters (170 micron) to remove platelet and fibrin aggregates, which may reduce the risk of pulmonary microembolization.
  2. Warming blood
    a. Blood from the blood bank is refrigerated and should be warmed, prior to or during transfusion, particularly if large transfusions are anticipated.
    b. Cold blood is associated with a higher incidence of arrhythmias and contributes to coagulopathy.
  3. Platelets
    a. PRBCs do not contain factors V and VIII, or platelets.
    b. Empiric platelet transfusions (10 mL/kg) are often necessary because they contain the depleted clotting factors as well as platelets.
  4. Fresh-frozen plasma (FFP): If the platelet count has been normalized, but massive hemorrhage persists and coagulation studies suggest multiple coagulation factor deficiencies (i.e.,

disseminated intravascular coagulopathy [DIC]), then FFP,
10-15 mL/kg, may be given).
5. Cryoprecipitate: Continued bleeding secondary to
hypofibrinogenemia and DIC are treated with cryoprecipitate
after platelets and FFP have been given.
6. Recombinant activated factor VII (VIIa, NovoSeven)
    a. Factor VIIa has been given for life-threatening post-
       traumatic, postoperative, pulmonary, and intracerebral
       hemorrhage.
    b. Outcomes data suggest prompt hemostasis and decreased
       transfusion requirements. However, survival has not
       improved.
7. Calcium
    a. PRBCs and platelets contain calcium-binding (chelating)
       agents.
    b. With massive transfusion, hypocalcemia may produce
       hypotension.
    c. Calcium chloride (10 mg/kg) or calcium gluconate
       (100 mg/kg) is used in symptomatic patients, those with
       unexplained BP instability, or following transfusion of
       >100 mL/kg of blood.
    d. Preferentially, calcium chloride should be given through a
       central venous catheter.
8. Vitamin K (phytonadione)
    a. Hepatic dysfunction in shock and sepsis may
       acutely affect vitamin K dependent coagulation
       processes.
    b. Vitamin K dose: Neonates and infants 0.5 mg
       subcutaneous (SC)/IV; children, adolescents, adults 2 mg
       SC/IV
    c. Evaluate if continued therapy is needed. IV vitamin K has
       been associated with anaphylaxis.
9. Hyperkalemia
    a. Because of cell lysis, potassium rises in direct proportion
       to storage time of stored blood.
    b. If multiple transfusions are expected and/or patient is
       sensitive to K^+ (e.g., neonates, patients receiving digoxin),
       use the freshest blood available.
    c. Monitor plasma K^+ levels and be prepared to treat
       arrhythmia with medications that counteract hyperkalemia
       (calcium chloride, sodium bicarbonate, insulin, glucose).
10. Graft-versus-host disease (GVHD)
    a. PRBCs contain white cells, which can result in GVHD in
       immunocompromised or potentially compromised hosts
       (e.g., newborns).
    b. Routine irradiation of blood products prevents GVHD.

6

VII. Distributive shock
   A. Definition
      1. Distributive shock is characterized by hypotension caused by diminished or absent sympathetic activity and loss of vascular tone.
      2. It is typically seen following transection of the spinal cord in the cervicothoracic region. However, anaphylaxis and some forms of septic shock follow a distributive shock pattern.
   B. Pathophysiology
      1. Reduced peripheral vascular tone leads to pooling of blood in the extremities and inadequate venous return.
      2. Initially, the patient has warm extremities, low diastolic pressure, and a very wide pulse pressure.
      3. Ultimately, perfusion pressure falls and acidosis develops.
   C. Management of neurogenic shock
      The goal of management is to restore blood flow to vital organs.
      1. ABCs
         a. Upper airway control
            (1) The patient with spinal cord injury may also have bulbar injury.
            (2) Therefore, assess patient's level of consciousness and ability to handle secretions.
         b. Cough and gag reflex
            (1) Assessment of the cough and gag reflex in the child with a full stomach requires clinical judgment and extreme care.
            (2) When in doubt, it is safer to intubate the trachea rather than elicit a gag reflex in a patient with a full stomach and an unprotected airway.
         c. Development of pulmonary edema
            (1) If there is concomitant head trauma, anaphylaxis, or septic shock, the patient may develop pulmonary edema or respiratory insufficiency.
            (2) Supplemental O_2 should always be provided.
         d. Tracheal intubation if patient is comatose, has poor secretion control, or has marginal O_2 saturation (Sao_2)
      2. Trendelenburg position (head down, legs elevated) and compressive leg wraps
      3. NS in 20-mL/kg aliquots
      4. Vasopressor drugs to treat low SVR
         a. Phenylephrine (Neo-Synephrine)
            (1) Action: Direct α_1-adrenergic agonist (vasoconstriction)
            (2) Single dose: 10 mcg/kg
            (3) Duration: 5 to 10 minutes
            (4) Continuous infusion: 0.5-10 mcg/kg/min

       b. Norepinephrine (levophed)

         (1) Action: Indirect α_1 much greater than β-adrenergic agonist

         (2) Dose: Continuous infusion 0.05-1 mcg/kg/min

D. Management of anaphylactic shock

  1. Remove or stop the triggering agent.

  2. Epinephrine (1:1000 solution) intramuscular (IM) or SC

    a. Recommended dose is 0.01 mg/kg (0.1 mL/kg of 1:1000 solution)

    b. General dosing guideline: 0.1 mL in <1 year old; 0.2 mL 1-10 years old; 0.3 mL >10 years old

    c. Effect may last only 20 min; may need repeat dosing.

    d. IM injection of epinephrine in the anterolateral thigh achieves more rapid absorption than SC injection.

  3. Place patient in the Trendelenburg position.

  4. Respiratory management

    a. Apply 100% O_2 by face mask.

    b. Intubate the trachea immediately if patient has stridor, facial edema, or respiratory distress.

    c. Racemic epinephrine (nebulized)—via face mask or endotracheal tube if the patient exhibits stridor

  5. Obtain IV access and bolus NS in 20-mL/kg aliquots until BP improves.

  6. If no improvement, start epinephrine infusion, 0.05 to 1 mcg/kg/min.

  7. If patient remains hypotensive and flushed in appearance, start norepinephrine, 0.05 to 1 mcg/kg/min.

  8. Adjunctive therapies

    a. H1 antihistamine—(e.g., diphenhydramine [Benadryl]) 1 mg/kg (max 50 mg) IV, relieves itching but does *not* treat shock.

    b. Methylprednisolone, 2 mg/kg/day IV—divided every 6 hours. Discontinue after 4 to 5 days without a taper.

    c. H2 antihistamine—(e.g., ranitindine [Zantac]) 2-4 mg/kg (max 50 mg) IV.

  9. Monitoring: Patients should be monitored carefully for at least 24 hours after anaphylactic shock because recurrent symptoms are possible within the first 24 hours (rarely, up to 72 hours).

VIII. Septic shock

  A. Definition

    Septic shock results from overwhelming infection (i.e., bacterial, viral, fungal, peritonitis, pneumonia), resulting in vascular and/or myocardial dysfunction.

B. Pathophysiology
1. Initially, the clinical picture is similar to neurogenic shock, except there is evidence of sepsis.
2. The peripheral tissues may be initially well perfused (warm shock), with an elevated pulse pressure (bounding pulses) and low diastolic pressure.
3. Unlike neurogenic shock, there is an accumulation of interstitial fluid and edema, especially in dependent tissues, and pulmonary and/or cerebral edema as a result of endothelial disruption.
4. Ultimately, perfusion fails, leading to lactic acidosis, hypotension with cold extremities (cold shock), and multi-organ system failure.

C. Signs and symptoms
1. Clinical suspicion or evidence for infection
2. Temperature instability (hyperthermia or hypothermia)
3. Tachycardia, bradycardia; tachypnea, apnea
4. Coagulopathy (DIC)
5. Impaired organ system function
   a. Peripheral hypoperfusion: Low BP, signs of poor cardiac output
   b. Decreased level of consciousness
   c. Oliguria
   d. Hypoxemia
   e. Acidosis
   f. Pulmonary edema

D. Management
1. Oxygenation
   a. Apply high-flow O_2 by face mask.
   b. If SaO_2 >90% cannot be maintained, apply noninvasive (continuous positive airway pressure or bi-level positive airway pressure) or invasive ventilation (via endotracheal intubation).
2. Obtain IV access (two large bore) or IO access.
3. Initial resuscitation
   a. Push normal saline in 20-mL/kg aliquots until BP and peripheral perfusion improve.
   b. This may require massive fluid administration (50 to 100 mL/kg).
   c. Discontinue fluid boluses if hepatomegaly or rales develop.
   d. Fluid resuscitation should be completed within the first 15 minutes.
4. Antibiotic therapy is dependent on the age of the patient (see Chapter 19). The neonate in shock requires acyclovir to treat for the potential of herpes simplex sepsis.

   5. Correct hypoglycemia and hypocalcemia.
   6. Use ketamine (with atropine) to sedate the patient during intubation (or during central venous cannulation). Etomidate use may increase mortality in septic shock and is not recommended.
   7. Fluid-refractory shock: Goal is to restore peripheral perfusion and BP with inotropes
      a. Dopamine, 5 to 20 mcg/kg/min; titrate to reverse cold shock.
      b. Epinephrine, 0.05 to 1.0 mcg/kg/min; titrate if resistant to dopamine.
      c. Norepinephrine, 0.05 to 1.0 mcg/kg/min for warm shock
      d. Catecholamines may be given via peripheral IV or IO routes until central venous access is established.
   8. Catecholamine-resistant shock
      a. Begin hydrocortisone, 2 mg/kg/day for stress coverage, up to 100 mg/day titrated to reversal of shock, if at risk for absolute adrenal insufficiency.
      b. Consider obtaining endogenous cortisol levels with and/or without ACTH (cosyntropin) stimulation to evaluate for absolute or relative adrenal insufficiency.
      c. Adrenal insufficiency is a risk factor for patients with purpura fulminans, congenital adrenal hyperplasia, prior recent steroid exposure, and hypothalamic-pituitary abnormality.
   9. Escalate to invasive monitoring using central venous and arterial lines with the goal of normalizing BP, central venous pressure, and central venous SaO_2 >70%.
   10. Monitor for the development of coagulopathy (DIC) and end-organ failure.
   11. Advanced monitoring and therapies (**Fig. 6-1**, pages 124-125)
IX. Endocrinologic shock
   The management of endocrinologic emergencies, such as hypoadrenalism, hypothyroidism or hyperthyroidism, and hypovolemia from acute diabetes mellitus is discussed in Chapter 10.
 X. Cardiogenic shock
   See Chapter 7.
XI. Obstructive shock
   See Chapter 7.

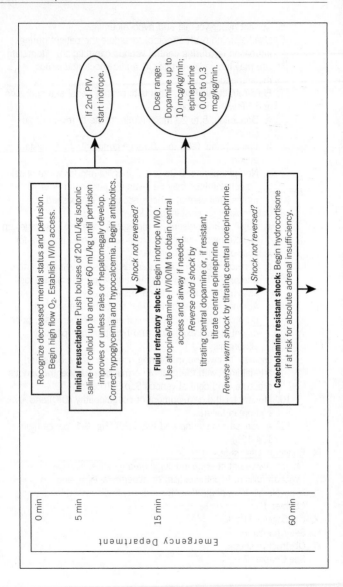

0 min Recognize decreased mental status and perfusion. Begin high flow O₂. Establish IV/IO access.

5 min **Initial resuscitation:** Push boluses of 20 mL/kg isotonic saline or colloid up to and over 60 mL/kg until perfusion improves or unless rales or hepatomegaly develop. Correct hypoglycemia and hypocalcemia. Begin antibiotics.

If 2nd PIV, start inotrope.

Shock not reversed?

15 min **Fluid refractory shock:** Begin inotrope IV/IO. Use atropine/ketamine IV/IO/IM to obtain central access and airway if needed.
Reverse cold shock by titrating central dopamine or, if resistant, titrate central epinephrine
Reverse warm shock by titrating central norepinephrine.

Dose range:
- Dopamine up to 10 mcg/kg/min; epinephrine 0.05 to 0.3 mcg/kg/min.

Shock not reversed?

60 min **Catecholamine resistant shock:** Begin hydrocortisone if at risk for absolute adrenal insufficiency.

Emergency Department

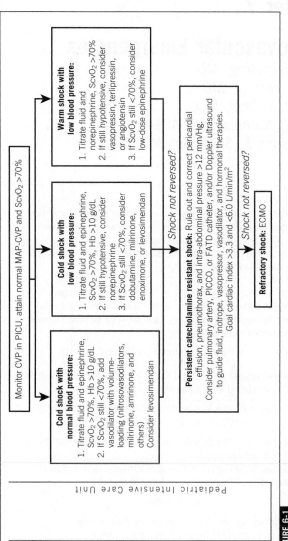

Pediatric Intensive Care Unit

Monitor CVP in PICU, attain normal MAP-CVP and ScvO₂ >70%

Cold shock with normal blood pressure:
1. Titrate fluid and epinephrine, ScvO₂ >70%, Hb >10 g/dL
2. If ScvO₂ still <70%, add vasodilator with volume-loading (nitrosovasodilators, milrinone, amrinone, and others)
Consider levosimendan

Cold shock with low blood pressure:
1. Titrate fluid and epinephrine, ScvO₂ >70%, Hb >10 g/dL
2. If still hypotensive, consider norepinephrine
3. If ScvO₂ still <70%, consider dobutamine, milrinone, enoximone, or levosimendan

Warm shock with low blood pressure:
1. Titrate fluid and norepinephrine, ScvO₂ >70%
2. If still hypotensive, consider vasopressin, terlipressin, or angiotensin
3. If ScvO₂ still <70%, consider low-dose epinephrine

Shock not reversed?

Persistent catecholamine resistant shock: Rule out and correct pericardial effusion, pneumothorax, and intra-abdominal pressure >12 mm/Hg. Consider pulmonary artery, PICCO, or FATD catheter, and/or Doppler ultrasound to guide fluid, inotrope, vasopressor, vasodilator, and hormonal therapies.
Goal cardiac index >3.3 and <6.0 L/min/m²

Shock not reversed?

Refractory shock: ECMO

FIGURE 6-1

Algorithm for time-sensitive, goal-directed, stepwise management of septic shock in infants and children. *(Modified from Brierley J, Carcillo JA, Choong K, et al. Clinical practice parameters for hemodynamic support of pediatric and neonatal septic shock: 2007 update from the American College of Critical Care Medicine. Crit Care Med 2009;37:666–688.)* *CVP,* Central venous pressure; *ECMO,* extracorporeal membrane oxygenation; *FATD,* femoral artery thermodilution; *Hb,* hemoglobin; *IM,* intramuscular; *IO,* intraosseous; *IV,* intravenous; *MAP,* mean arterial pressure; *PICCO,* peripherally inserted central catheter occlusion; *PICU,* pediatric intensive care unit; *PIV,* peripheral IV; *ScvO₂,* central venous oxygen saturation.

Chapter 7

Cardiovascular Emergencies

Arthur Smerling, MD,
Allan J. Hordof, MD,
Janet N. Scheel, MD,
David G. Nichols, MD, MBA,
and Charles L. Schleien, MD, MBA

I. Overview
   A. Definition
      1. These are acute, life-threatening conditions characterized by inadequate delivery of oxygen (O_2) to tissues and/or severe elevations of venous or arterial pressure.
      2. Cardiac arrest and shock are discussed separately in Chapters 5 and 6, respectively.
   B. Physiology
      1. The function of the heart is to deliver O_2 to the tissues.
      2. **Oxygen delivery** is the product of cardiac output (CO) and arterial oxygen content (CaO_2) and must be sufficient to meet the body's metabolic needs:

      $$O_2 \text{ delivery} = CO \times CaO_2$$

      3. Arterial oxygen content (mL O_2/dL blood) is the concentration of O_2 in the blood and is determined by this formula:

      $$CaO_2 = (1.34 \times SaO_2 \times \text{hemoglobin concentration [g/dL]}) + (0.003 \times PaO_2 \text{ [mm Hg]})$$

      where SaO_2 is the O_2 saturation and PaO_2 is the partial pressure of O_2 in arterial blood.
      4. Cardiac output or blood flow is determined by the product of heart rate (HR) and stroke volume (SV):

      $$CO = HR \times SV$$

      a. Stroke volume may be altered by the following:
         (1) Preload (or impaired ventricular filling)
         (2) Afterload (or resistance to forward flow)
         (3) Contractility (or myocardial dysfunction)
      b. HR abnormalities or arrhythmias that alter CO include the following:
         (1) Tachyarrhythmias (with inadequate diastolic filling time)
         (2) Bradyarrhythmias (with inadequate SV frequency)

        (3) Abnormalities of atrioventricular synchrony (with loss of atrial contribution to ventricular loading)

    5. The mean arterial pressure (MAP) is determined by cardiac output and systemic vascular resistance (SVR):

$$MAP = CO \times SVR$$

    A low blood pressure (**hypotension**) occurs in the presence of low CO, low SVR, or both.

II. Signs and symptoms of heart disease

   These are based on physiologic derangement.

   A. Decreased O_2 delivery
     1. Cyanosis
     2. Exercise intolerance, fatigue
     3. Failure to thrive
     4. Agitation or lethargy
     5. Oliguria

   B. Heart failure

     Heart failure is defined here as inadequate ventricular contractility and/or valvar competence associated with pulmonary or systemic venous congestion.
     1. Respiratory signs and symptoms
       a. Exercise intolerance
       b. Dyspnea (especially on exertion or during feeding in infants)
       c. Wheezing
       d. Tachypnea
       e. Rales
     2. Cardiovascular signs and symptoms
       a. Tachycardia
       b. Delayed capillary refill time (>3 to 4 sec)
       c. Cool, clammy extremities
       d. Sweating
       e. Peripheral edema
       f. Cardiomegaly
       g. Gallop rhythm
       h. Jugular venous distension
     3. Other
       a. Hepatomegaly
       b. Failure to thrive

   C. Radiographic signs of heart disease (**Table 7-1**)

III. Arrhythmias

   A. Overview
     1. Arrhythmias may cause a variety of cardiovascular emergencies, ranging from palpitations and syncope to shock and cardiac arrest caused by poor CO.
     2. The acute management of arrhythmias requires continuous electrocardiographic and SaO_2 monitoring.

TABLE 7-1	
CHEST RADIOGRAPHIC FINDINGS SUGGESTIVE OF HEART DISEASE	
Sign	Differential Diagnosis
Cardiomegaly (>50% thoracic diameter)	• Decreased ventricular function • Pericardial effusion • Valvar insufficiency • Large left-to-right shunt
Increased pulmonary vascular markings	• Pulmonary overcirculation (left-to-right shunt)
Diffuse alveolar infiltrates	• Left ventricular failure • Massive pulmonary overcirculation (large left-to-right shunt) • Mitral valve insufficiency or stenosis • Pulmonary vein stenosis or anomalous pulmonary venous connection
Lobar infiltrate	• Pneumonia (may be associated with left-to right shunt)
Pleural effusion	• Decreased ventricular function • Systemic venous hypertension after Fontan procedure • Chylothorax

3. Management of unstable arrhythmias begins with the ABCs of resuscitation—that is, ensuring a patent airway and breathing 100% O_2.
4. If pulses are not palpable, begin cardiopulmonary resuscitation pending application of specific antiarrhythmic therapy.

B. Factors predisposing to arrhythmias
   1. Congenital heart disease
   2. Isolated conduction system disorders—Wolff-Parkinson-White (WPW) syndrome, Brugada syndrome, prolonged QT syndromes
   3. Associated systemic illness: Myocarditis, Kawasaki disease, dilated cardiomyopathy, muscular dystrophies, collagen vascular diseases, endocrine diseases
   4. Drug toxicities: Adriamycin, tricyclic antidepressants, cocaine, amphetamines, digoxin, beta blockers, asthma medications (see Chapter 17)
   5. Other: Blunt trauma to chest or head, increased intracranial pressure (ICP)

C. Bradyarrhythmias
   1. Sinus bradycardia
      a. Rate: Slow (**Table 7-2**)
      b. Rhythm: Regular
      c. P wave: Sinus (upright in leads I, II, aVF)
      d. Causes: Hypoxia, hypoglycemia, increased ICP, hyperkalemia, acidosis, vagal maneuvers, hypothermia

TABLE 7-2	
ABNORMALLY SLOW HEART RATES IN CHILDREN	
Age (yr)	Heart Rate (beats/min)
<2	<90
2-6	<80
6-11	<70
>11	<60

    e. Drug intoxication: Digoxin, beta blockers, amiodarone, calcium channel blockers

    f. Management: Treat underlying cause.

       (1) Atropine; 0.02 mg/kg intravenous (IV), intraosseous (IO), intramuscular (IM) (maximum, 1 mg)

       (2) Epinephrine, 1 mcg/kg IV/IO (maximum 1 mg)

2. Sinus arrest

    a. Rate: Slow (see Table 7-2)

    b. Rhythm:

       (1) Irregular (pause in rhythm; multiple of sinus cycle length)

       (2) Pause often followed by nodal or ventricular escape beat

    c. P wave

       (1) Sinus (upright in leads I, II, aVF)

       (2) Unexpectedly prolonged P-P interval

    d. Cause: Sick sinus syndrome

    e. Management: Treat underlying cause.

       (1) Atropine 0.02 mg/kg, IV, IO, IM (maximum, 1 mg),

       (2) Epinephrine 1 to 10 mcg/kg, IV, IO

       (3) Consider pacing if pause >3 seconds.

3. First-degree atrioventricular block

    a. Rate: Slow or normal (see Table 7-2)

    b. Rhythm: Regular

    c. P wave: Prolonged P-R interval

    d. Causes: Benign variant if electrocardiogram (ECG) is otherwise normal

    e. Management: Observe.

4. Mobitz type I second-degree atrioventricular (AV) block (Wenckebach)

    a. Rate: Slow or normal (see Table 7-2)

    b. Rhythm: Irregular

    c. P wave: Gradual prolongation of P-R interval prior to nonconducted P wave (dropped QRS)

    d. Causes: May be benign (during sleep) or may be a prelude to higher degrees of AV block if observed when awake

    e. Management: Observe closely if it occurs when awake.

5. Mobitz type II second-degree AV block
    a. Rate: Slow or normal (see Table 7-2)
    b. Rhythm: Irregular
    c. P wave: Constant PR interval prior to nonconducted P wave
    d. Causes
        (1) Myocardial disease
        (2) Drug intoxication
        (3) Lyme disease
    e. Management
        (1) Atropine, 0.02 mg/kg, IV, IO, or isoproterenol, 0.05 to 1 mcg/kg/min infusion acutely, if ventricular escape rate is slow
        (2) Permanent pacemaker if rhythm persists >1 week and ventricular escape rate is slow
6. 2:1 (or higher) AV block: Similar to Mobitz type II AV block, except that the P:QRS ratio is constant (e.g., 2:1, 3:1)
7. Complete (third-degree) heart block
    a. Rate: Slow
    b. Rhythm: Regular or irregular
    c. P wave: No relationship to QRS (P waves "march through" the QRS; AV dissociation)
    d. Causes
        (1) Congenital heart disease
        (2) Cardiac surgery
        (3) Maternal lupus
        (4) Lyme disease
    e. Management: Atropine, 0.02 mg/kg IV, or isoproterenol, 0.05 mcg/kg/min infusion acutely
    f. Transcutaneous pacing (**Fig. 7-1**) or temporary transvenous pacing if unstable
    g. Permanent pacemaker if rhythm persists for >1 week
D. Narrow complex tachyarrhythmias
    1. Sinus tachycardia
        a. Rate: Fast (100 to 230 beats/min, age-dependent)
        b. Rhythm: Regular
        c. P wave: Sinus (upright in leads I, II, aVF)
        d. Causes
            (1) Hypovolemia
            (2) Fever
            (3) Anemia
            (4) Hypercarbia
            (5) Pain
            (6) Heart failure
            (7) Hyperthyroidism
        e. Management: Treat underlying cause.

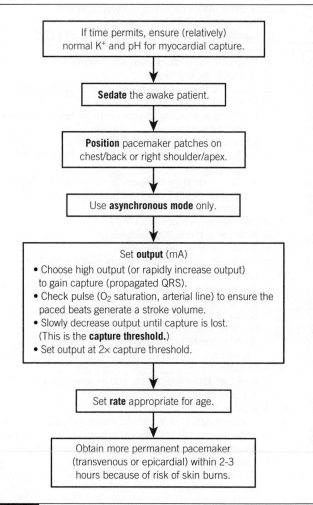

If time permits, ensure (relatively) normal K⁺ and pH for myocardial capture.

Sedate the awake patient.

Position pacemaker patches on chest/back or right shoulder/apex.

Use **asynchronous mode** only.

Set **output** (mA)
- Choose high output (or rapidly increase output) to gain capture (propagated QRS).
- Check pulse (O₂ saturation, arterial line) to ensure the paced beats generate a stroke volume.
- Slowly decrease output until capture is lost. (This is the **capture threshold.**)
- Set output at 2× capture threshold.

Set **rate** appropriate for age.

Obtain more permanent pacemaker (transvenous or epicardial) within 2-3 hours because of risk of skin burns.

FIGURE 7-1

Algorithm for use of a transcutaneous pacemaker.

2. Orthodromic AV reciprocating tachycardia (AVRT)
   a. Rate: Fast (~250 to 300 beats/min)
   b. Common form of supraventricular tachycardia (SVT) in infants
   c. P wave: Variable; often retrograde P waves (on ST segment) in leads II, III, aVF, and V_1
   d. Causes: Accessory pathway (including WPW syndrome)
   e. Management
      (1) Consider vagal maneuvers: Ice to the face or unilateral carotid massage
      (2) Adenosine, 100-400 mcg/kg, rapid IV push
      (3) Synchronized cardioversion (0.5 to 1 J/kg) if blood pressure (BP) unstable
      (4) Contraindication: Verapamil is contraindicated in the treatment of SVT in infants because of the risk of sudden death.
3. AV node reentry tachycardia (AVNRT)
   a. Rate: fast (~160 to 300 beats/min)
   b. Common form of SVT in children
   c. P wave: Retrograde P wave usually buried in QRS or terminal S wave (best detected in lead V_1)
   d. Cause: Dual AV nodal pathway
   e. Management:
      (1) Vagal maneuvers: Ice cold towel on forehead
      (2) Adenosine, 100-400 mcg/kg IV, rapid push
      (3) Synchronized cardioversion (0.5 to 1 J/kg) if BP unstable
4. Atrial flutter
   a. Rate: Fast (atrial rate, 200 to 500 beats/min, with 1 : 1, 2 : 1, or higher block)
   b. Rhythm: Regular
   c. P wave: Indistinct or isoelectric. Always consider atrial flutter in the presence of unexplained narrow complex tachycardia with indistinct P waves.
   d. Causes
      (1) Congenital heart disease
      (2) Cardiac surgery
      (3) Myocarditis
   e. Management
      (1) Synchronized cardioversion (0.5 to 1 J/kg)
      (2) If flutter recurs after cardioversion and patient is stable:
         (a) Diltiazem, 0.25 to 0.5 mg/kg IV (over 2 min), *or*
         (b) Procainamide, 15 mg/kg IV load over 30 minutes (1 gm maximum) followed by 20 to 80 mcg/kg/min IV infusion *plus* diltiazem 0.5 mg/kg IV (over 2 min) *or*

(c) Esmolol (to control ventricular rate), 500 mcg/kg IV load over 1 to 3 minutes, followed by 25 to 200 mcg/kg/min infusion

5. Atrial fibrillation
   a. Rate: Atrial rate, 350 to 600 beats/min; ventricular rate variable and slower
   b. Rare in infants and children
   c. Rhythm: Irregularly irregular
   d. P wave: Indistinct
   e. Causes
      (1) Repaired congenital heart disease (e.g., Fontan) in teenager
      (2) WPW syndrome
   f. Management
      (1) Echocardiography to rule out atrial thrombus
      (2) If no atrial thrombus, administer synchronized cardioversion
         or
      (3) Procainamide, 15 mg/kg IV load over 30 minutes (1 gm maximum), followed by 20 to 80 mcg/kg/min IV infusion
      (4) If atrial thrombus is present, start heparinization **without** cardioversion

6. Junctional ectopic tachycardia
   a. Rate: 110 to 250 beats/min (usually >150 beats/min in infants)
   b. Rhythm: Regular or irregular
   c. P wave: AV dissociation
   d. Cause: Congenital heart surgery (postoperative)
   e. Management
      (1) Discontinue catecholamine infusions.
      (2) Amiodarone, 5 mg/kg IV load over 20 minutes, max 300 mg dose; then infusion, 5 to 15 mcg/kg/min
      (3) Mild to moderate hypothermia (34° to 35° C)
      (4) Overdrive atrial or AV sequential pacing

7. Atrial (ectopic) tachycardia
   a. Rate: 150-250 beats/min
   b. Rhythm: regular
   c. P wave: Different from sinus morphology
   d. Causes: Automaticity at site within the atria different from sinus node
   e. Management
      (1) Amiodarone, 5 mg/kg IV load over 20 minutes (maximum 300 mg/dose) then infusion 5 to 15 mcg/kg/min
      (2) Radiofrequency or surgical ablation
      (3) Cardioversion or overdrive pacing not effective

E. Wide complex tachycardias
   1. Ventricular tachycardia (V Tach)
      a. Rate: More than three premature ventricular contractions at rate >10% faster than sinus rate
      b. Rhythm: Regular
      c. QRS
         (1) Usually widened (especially beyond infancy)
         (2) Uniform (monomorphic) or variable (polymorphic) morphology
         (3) May be narrow complex in infants
         (4) AV dissociation or fusion beat distinguishes V Tach from SVT with aberrancy
      d. Causes
         (1) Prolonged QT interval
         (2) Hyperkalemia
         (3) Myocarditis
         (4) Cardiomyopathy
         (5) Drug intoxication
      e. Management
         (1) Wide complex tachycardia is V Tach until proven otherwise
         (2) If unstable, immediate synchronized cardioversion, 0.5 to 1 J/kg
         (3) Amiodarone, 5 mg/kg IV load over 20 minutes, followed by 5 to 15 mcg/kg/min infusion
         (4) Treat underlying cause.
         (5) For torsades de pointes (polymorphic V Tach with twisting polarity around isoelectric baseline) start cardioversion and give magnesium sulfate, 25 to 50 mg/kg IV over 5 minutes.
   2. SVT with aberrant ventricular conduction (bundle branch block): See earlier, AVRT or AVNRT.
   3. Ventricular fibrillation (V Fib)
      a. Rate, rhythm: Extremely rapid, chaotic rhythm
      b. QRS: Very low amplitude
      c. Causes
         (1) Degenerating V Tach or SVT
         (2) Cardiac arrest
         (3) Prolonged QT syndrome
         (4) WPW
      d. Management
         (1) Defibrillation, 2 to 4 J/kg (for monophasic or biphasic defibrillators)
         (2) If V Fib persists, restart CPR immediately while preparing to repeat dose.

TABLE 7-3

BLOOD PRESSURE BY AGE (99TH PERCENTILE)

Age	Blood Pressure (mm Hg)	
	Systolic	Diastolic
<7 days	106	
7-30 days	110	
1 mo-2 yr	118	82
3-5 yr	124	84
6-9 yr	130	86
10-12 yr	134	90

(3) Automatic external defibrillator (AED)
  (a) In children older than 8 years: Use standard preset energy dose.
  (b) In children 1 to 8 years: Use attenuated pediatric dose if available; otherwise, use standard dose.
(4) Treat underlying cause.

IV. Hypertensive emergency
  A. Definition
    1. A hypertensive emergency is characterized by severe hypertension (BP >99% for age, height, and weight; **Table 7-3**) and possible evidence of end-organ damage (e.g., stroke, encephalopathy, pulmonary edema, retinopathy).
    2. Some use the term *malignant hypertension* to denote a severe hypertensive emergency associated with retinal hemorrhages.
  B. Causes and manifestations (**Table 7-4**)
    1. Activation of the renin-angiotensin system associated with renovascular disease
      a. Most common cause of a hypertensive emergency in children
      b. Specific lesions
        (1) All types of glomerulonephritis
        (2) Reflux nephropathy
        (3) Renal artery stenosis
        (4) Hemolytic uremic syndrome
    2. Drug intoxication
      a. Immunosuppressive drugs (e.g., corticosteroids, tacrolimus, cyclosporine)
      b. Sympathomimetic drugs (e.g., cocaine, amphetamines, phenylephrine)
    3. Increased ICP—Cushing response: Hypertension, bradycardia, and irregular respirations
    The most important management decision is whether the presenting encephalopathy is the primary cause of the

TABLE 7-4

CAUSES AND MANIFESTATIONS OF HYPERTENSIVE CRISES IN CHILDREN

Causes	Manifestations
Renovascular disease	Obtundation, coma, blurry vision
	Edema (peripheral and/or pulmonary)
	Urinary discoloration (tea-colored, bloody), oliguria
Increased intracranial pressure	Headache, nausea, and vomiting
	Heart rate changes (usually bradycardia but sometimes tachycardia)
	Irregular respirations (may be subtle hypoventilation)
	Neurogenic pulmonary edema
Sympathomimetic drug intoxication	Palpitations
	Seizures, coma
Immunosuppressive drug intoxication	Obtundation, coma (posterior reversible encephalopathy syndrome)
Pregnancy (eclampsia)	Obtundation, coma
Coarctation of aorta	Differential upper, lower extremity blood pressure
Thyrotoxicosis	Palpitations
	Sweating
Pheochromocytoma	Obtundation, coma
	Palpitations
	Sweating

hypertension (Cushing response) or a secondary manifestation of the hypertension, which is usually renovascular in origin. If brain injury is the cause of systemic hypertension, then vasodilating antihypertensive drugs are contraindicated.

4. Coarctation of the aorta
5. Endocrine disease, including thyrotoxicosis and pheochromocytoma, are rarer causes. The causes and manifestations of hypertensive emergencies are summarized in Table 7-4.

C. Management
1. Goal: Reduce BP by 25% within 1 hour with antihypertensive medications.
2. Antihypertensive medications (**Table 7-5**)
   a. Mechanism of action is either vasodilation or beta blockade
   b. Contraindicated for increased ICP
3. Management of increased ICP (see Chapter 15)

V. Congestive heart failure
A. Causes
1. Congenital heart disease
   a. Volume overload (e.g., ventricular septal defect, mitral regurgitation)
   b. Pressure overload (e.g., coarctation of the aorta, aortic stenosis, tetralogy of Fallot)

TABLE 7-5

ANTIHYPERTENSIVE MEDICATIONS

Drug	Dose	Route	Comments
Nifedipine	0.25-0.5 mg/kg	PO, sublingual, IV	Predictable, can be drawn up as liquid from capsule for IV administration
Nicardipine	0.5-4 mcg/kg/min	IV	Easily filtrated; short half-life
Labetalol	0.1-0.25 mg/kg *or* 0.4-1 mg/kg/hr	IV	Titrate infusion for persistent hypertension; contraindicated in asthma patients
Esmolol	500 mcg/kg/min × 2 min, then 25-200 mcg/kg/min	IV	Contraindicated in patients with asthma or who have received calcium channel blockers
Nitroprusside	0.5-8 mcg/kg/min	IV	Intra-arterial monitoring required
Hydralazine	0.1-0.5 mg/kg	IV	
Diazoxide	0.1-0.5 mg/kg	IV	Repeat at 10- to 15-min intervals; causes hyperglycemia

IV, Intravenous; *PO,* orally.

2. Infections
   a. Myocarditis (adenovirus, coxsackie, enterovirus, *Mycoplasma*)
   b. Endocarditis (*Staphylococcus*, *Streptococcus*)
3. Ischemia
   a. Anomalous left coronary artery syndrome
   b. Kawasaki syndrome
   c. Reperfusion injury following cardiopulmonary bypass or cardiac arrest
4. Dilated cardiomyopathies (e.g., Duchenne muscular dystrophy)
5. Uncontrolled tachyarrhythmia
6. Myocardial contusion
7. Drug toxicity
   a. Tricyclic antidepressants
   b. Mushrooms and other anticholinergics
   c. Anthracyclines
   d. Digoxin
   e. Beta blockers
   f. Organophosphates
   g. Carbon monoxide
   h. Cyanide
   i. Cocaine and other sympathomimetics
B. Evaluation
   1. Vital signs and ABCs
   2. Physical examination
      a. Assess for hypoxemia by color and pulse oximetry.

      b. Assess for increased work of breathing and rales (left ventricular failure).

      c. Assess for hepatomegaly (right ventricular failure)

      d. Assess for poor perfusion

         (1) Lethargy

         (2) Oliguria

         (3) Delayed capillary refill time (>3 seconds)

   3. Laboratory studies

      a. Serum chemistries and complete blood count

      b. ECG: Rhythm, axis, ST segments, intervals (including QTc)

      c. Chest radiograph

         (1) Heart size and shape

         (2) Pulmonary vascular markings

         (3) Position of bronchi

         (4) Lung fields

      d. Echocardiograph

         (1) Structural heart disease

         (2) Ventricular function

         (3) Pericardial effusion

C. Management of decompensating congestive heart failure (CHF)

   1. 100% O_2 by face mask or nasal cannulae

   2. Full noninvasive monitoring

      a. Continuous electrocardiography

      b. Pulse oximetry

      c. Automatic BP measurement every 2 to 5 minutes

   3. Contact a pediatric referral center as soon as decompensating CHF (e.g., lethargy, increased work of breathing, decreased SaO_2) is identified, because these patients may be refractory to pharmacologic management.

   4. Continuous positive airway pressure or bilevel positive airway pressure

      a. These forms of noninvasive ventilation decrease afterload to the left ventricle by increasing intrathoracic pressure.

      b. This is accomplished without the need for sedation and endotracheal intubation.

   5. Optimize preload.

      a. Judicious IV fluid: Give normal saline (NS), 5 mL/kg bolus, if the history and/or physical examination suggest dehydration.

      b. Monitor before and after fluid bolus for signs of fluid overload, including hepatomegaly and rales.

      c. Stop fluid administration if increased signs of CHF or no improvement in perfusion.

   6. Start inodilators if BP is in normal range.

      a. Milrinone: Loading dose, 25-50 mcg/kg over 30-60 minutes followed by infusion, 0.25 to 0.75 mcg/kg/min, *or*

      b. Dobutamine: 5 to 20 mcg/kg/min

TABLE 7-6

SEDATIVE DRUG OPTIONS IN CHILD WITH DECOMPENSATING HEART FAILURE

Drug	IV Dose	Risks
Fentanyl	1-2 mcg/kg	Hypotension if the patient combines heart failure and hypovolemia
Etomidate	0.3 mg/kg	Provides cardiovascular stability during intubation, but possible adrenal suppression and increased 28-day mortality in those with adrenal suppression
Ketamine	1 mg/kg	• Tachyarrhythmia • Increased intracranial pressure • Hypotension in patients with chronic heart failure and catecholamine depletion • Contraindicated in patients with PVCs (may precipitate V Tach)
Propofol	1-2.5 mg/kg	Hypotension (usually mild)
Midazolam	0.1 mg/kg	Hypotension • Usually mild if given as sole agent • Severe if given in combination with other sedatives to a patient with decompensating CHF
Thiopental		Contraindicated because of extreme hypotension risk

CHF, Congestive heart failure; *PVC,* premature ventricular contractions; *V Tach,* ventricular tachycardia.

7. Consider tracheal intubation and mechanical ventilation if the patient has not responded to these measures.
   a. Sedation and intubation are hazardous in this setting and consultation with pediatric intensive care physicians is recommended if time permits. Transport to a pediatric intensive care facility should be expedited.
   b. Resuscitation drugs should be immediately available.
   c. All sedative drugs have risks in the patient with decompensating heart failure (**Table 7-6**).
   d. Fentanyl, 1 to 2 mcg/kg IV, is recommended because it has the overall best risk-benefit profile in this setting.
8. Enhance monitoring
   a. Place central venous line for central venous pressure monitoring.
   b. Repeat echocardiography: Assess ventricular function, cardiac filling after therapies listed.
9. Inotropy, vasopressors
   a. The goal is to provide increased inotropy without excessively increasing myocardial O_2 consumption.
   b. The risks of a tachyarrhythmia or myocardial ischemia are high.
   c. Catecholamine infusions should only be attempted if other measures have failed to improve the condition.

      d. Catecholamine infusion options include the following:
         (1) Dopamine: 5 to 10 mcg/kg/min
         (2) Epinephrine: 0.05 to 0.5 mcg/kg/min
  10. Furosemide, 0.25 to 1 mg/kg IV: Used to treat pulmonary edema once adequate perfusion has been restored
  11. Extracorporeal membrane oxygenation (ECMO): Children with CHF who continue to decompensate after intubation may require mechanical circulatory assistance, including ECMO or a ventricular assist device (univentricular or biventricular).

VI. Management of obstruction to CO
  A. Left heart obstruction in the newborn
    1. Causes
      a. Hypoplastic left heart syndrome (HLHS)
      b. Critical coarctation of the aorta (CoA)
      c. Interrupted aortic arch (IAA)
    2. Presentation
      a. Associated with closure of the ductus arteriosus
      b. Signs of shock and CHF
         (1) Poor feeding, tachypnea (evolving over a few hours)
         (2) Pulmonary congestion in most cases
         (3) Cyanosis
         (4) Hepatomegaly
         (5) Diminished pulses in all extremities in HLHS
         (6) Usually diminished femoral pulses in critical CoA and IAA
    3. Diagnosis by echocardiography
    4. Management
      a. Prostaglandin E_1 (PGE$_1$), 0.025 to 0.1 mcg/kg/min IV to maintain ductal patency
      b. **Any newborn presenting in shock should be considered to have left heart obstruction until proven otherwise and should receive PGE$_1$ until an echocardiogram can rule out left heart obstruction.**
      c. Apnea occurs in 12% of infants receiving PGE$_1$.
         (1) Therefore, intubation and ventilator support equipment must be available immediately.
         (2) If prolonged transport or air transport is planned, the infant should be intubated prophylactically.
      d. Cautious fluid administration: 5 mL/kg NS
      e. Sodium bicarbonate for severe metabolic acidosis
      f. Close monitoring; treatment for glucose, potassium, calcium, and magnesium abnormalities
      g. Rule out sepsis.
         (1) Draw blood and urine cultures.
         (2) Administer antibiotics pending negative culture results.

       h. Ultimate goal: Present a stable patient for cardiac surgical repair.
- B. Left heart obstruction in the child and teenager
  - 1. Causes
    - a. Hypertrophic cardiomyopathy (HCM)
    - b. Aortic stenosis
  - 2. Presentation
    - a. Dyspnea on exertion
    - b. Angina
    - c. Syncope
    - d. Sudden death (especially during exercise)
  - 3. Management
    - a. For patients presenting with angina, history of syncope, or dyspnea on exertion:
      - (1) In general, prevent or treat tachycardia, which increases myocardial O_2 consumption
      - (2) NS, 10 mL/kg IV
      - (3) Topical cooling or antipyretics for hyperthermia or fever
      - (4) Rest
      - (5) Hospitalization for full cardiac workup, possible surgical repair, and/or implantation of an automatic defibrillator
    - b. For patients presenting with sudden death, presume a ventricular arrhythmia (see earlier and Chapter 5)
      - (1) ABCs and CPR
      - (2) Apply AED on the presumption of an arrhythmia
      - (3) NS, 20 mL/kg IV
      - (4) Phenylephrine 10 mcg/kg IV for hypotension
      - (5) Epinephrine may increase functional left heart obstruction and should be used only if all other therapies have failed.
      - (6) Hospitalization for full cardiac work-up, possible surgical repair, and/or implantation of an automatic defibrillator
      - (7) Chronic left heart obstruction from HCM may be treated with calcium channel blockers or beta blockers (but not both simultaneously).
- C. Right heart obstruction in the newborn
  - 1. Causes
    - a. Pulmonary atresia with intact ventricular septum
    - b. Tetralogy of Fallot with pulmonary atresia
    - c. Tricuspid atresia
  - 2. Presentation
    - a. Cyanosis and hypoxemia unresponsive to supplemental O_2 administration
    - b. Metabolic acidosis

3. Management
   a. PGE_1 infusion (see earlier)
   b. Ultimate goal: Cardiac surgical repair
D. Hypercyanotic spells (tet spells)
   1. Definition: Cyanotic spells occurring in patients with tetralogy of Fallot
   2. Pathophysiology: Increased right-to-left shunting caused by increased right ventricular (RV) outflow tract obstruction
   3. Management
      a. 100% O_2
      b. Knee-chest position increases SVR, resulting in decreased right-to-left shunting.
      c. IV fluid to increase preload
      d. Sedation: Morphine, 0.1 mg/kg IV, ketamine, or other calming maneuvers
      e. Phenylephrine, 1 to 10 mcg/kg IV, to raise SVR
      f. Esmolol, 500 mcg/kg, followed by 50 mcg/kg/min to decrease dynamic contribution of RV outflow tract
      g. Mechanical ventilation with heavier sedation, general anesthesia to break cycle of RV outflow tract obstruction
      h. Surgery: Complete repair or palliation with central aortic or subclavian to pulmonary artery (Blalock-Tausig) shunt.

Chapter 8

Electrolyte and Metabolic Disorders

Michael Wilhelm, MD,
and Charles L. Schleien, MD, MBA

I. Normal salt and water balance

The maintenance of normal circulating blood volume depends on normal salt and water balance. The extracellular fluid (ECF) volume is approximately 20% of body weight (40% in the newborn) and is divided 3:1 between the interstitial (15%) and intravascular (5%) spaces. Intracellular fluid (ICF) volume increases from approximately 35% of body weight in infants to 40% in adults. Individual ions are primarily located in one of these spaces (i.e., Na^+ in the ECF and K^+ in the ICF), which has important implications for management of these electrolyte disorders.

A. Maintenance fluid and electrolyte requirements

1. Maintenance fluid requirements (based on normal caloric expenditures):

   a. 4 mL/kg/hr for the first 10 kg of body weight
      PLUS

   b. 2 mL/kg/hr for the second 10 kg of body weight
      PLUS

   c. 1 mL/kg/hr for each additional kg (up to 100 mL/hr, maximum)

2. Maintenance electrolyte requirements

   a. Na^+: 3 to 4 mEq/100 mL

   b. K^+: 2 to 3 mEq/100 mL

3. **Never** use pure dextrose in water as the sole intravenous (IV) fluid therapy in children, because of the risk of symptomatic hyponatremia. The routine maintenance IV fluid in children consists of 5% dextrose (D5) 0.45% saline to which K^+ may be added if the patient has normal urine output.

II. Sodium disorders

Sodium is primarily distributed in the ECF where the normal Na^+ concentration ranges from 135 to 145 mEq/L. Alterations in total body sodium or total body water may result in an abnormal sodium concentration. Careful evaluation of the patient's volume status plays a critical role in establishing the appropriate diagnosis, as well as instituting effective therapy. Specific disorders, such as the syndrome of inappropriate antidiuretic hormone (SIADH), diabetes insipidus (DI), and adrenal insufficiency are covered separately in this chapter.

A. Hyponatremia

  1. Causes: True hyponatremia results from losses of salt in excess of water losses, retention of water in excess of salt retention, or deficiency of salt intake. Therefore, evaluation of the patient's volume status (especially weight loss or gain) is critical in arriving at the correct diagnosis.

    a. Sodium loss from renal or nonrenal sources

      (1) Renal sodium losses

        (a) Acute tubular necrosis

        (b) Cerebral salt wasting

        (c) Diuretic use or abuse

        (d) Mineralocorticoid deficiency (see Section II.C)

        (e) Prematurity

      (2) Extrarenal sodium losses

        (a) Vomiting, diarrhea

        (b) Burns

        (c) Cystic fibrosis

        (d) Nasogastric or cerebrospinal fluid (CSF) drainage

    b. Water retention

      (1) Primary

        (a) Water intoxication

        (b) Psychogenic polydipsia

        (c) SIADH

      (2) Iatrogenic

        (a) Desmopressin (DDAVP) therapy

        (b) Excessive replacement of isotonic fluid losses with hypotonic solutions

      (3) Compensatory

        (a) Hypoproteinemia (nephrotic syndrome, liver disease)

        (b) Congestive heart failure (CHF)

        (c) Capillary leak syndrome

    c. Dietary deficiency: Reconstitution errors for parenteral or enteral nutrition

    d. Factitious hyponatremia

      (1) Extreme hyperlipidemia, hyperglycemia, or hyperproteinemia may be associated with factitious hyponatremia (pseudohyponatremia).

      (2) This rarely occurs now because most laboratories use direct ion-selective electrode assays rather than flame photometry and indirect methods.

  2. Clinical manifestations

    a. Primarily result from effects of hyponatremia on excitable tissues (neurons)

  b. Lethargy or irritability may progress to seizures and coma.

  c. Gradual, chronic changes in sodium cause milder symptoms than rapid, acute changes.

  d. Symptoms may also result from associated alterations in volume status (i.e., dehydration, shock, CHF).

 3. Treatment

  a. Initial treatment should correct hypovolemic shock with normal saline (NS) using aliquots of 20 mL/kg.

  b. In symptomatic hyponatremic patients, sodium should be acutely raised to 120 to 125 mEq/L. The serum Na^+ level should *not* be increased by >12 mEq/24 hr or >18 mEq/48 hr.

  c. The rate of increase of the serum Na^+ level after treatment with hypertonic saline is often unpredictable. Therefore, the serum Na^+ level should be measured hourly during treatment of severe hyponatremia.

  d. Hypertonic saline is available in a variety of concentrations, all of which may promote phlebitis.

   (1) Either 2% or 3% hypertonic saline is used most commonly in children.

   (2) Therefore, the largest IV line available should be used for 2% hypertonic saline.

   (3) A central venous line should always be used for 3% hypertonic saline infusions.

  e. 3% Hypertonic saline dose

   (1) Give 1.2 mL/kg of 3% hypertonic saline/mEq/L desired increase in serum Na^+ level. The dose should be infused over 2 hours.

   (2) For example, a 10-kg infant with a serum Na^+ level of 115 mEq/L should receive 60 mL (1.2 [mL $\times$ kg^{-1}/mEq $\times$ L^{-1}] $\times$ 10 [kg] $\times$ 5 [mEq/L] = 60 mL) of 3% hypertonic saline to raise the serum Na^+ level to 120 mEq/L.

  f. Monitoring: Monitor vital signs, intake/output, serum Na^+, and serum glucose hourly for severe hyponatremia, with or without hypovolemia.

  g. In patients with free water excess (e.g., SIADH, water intoxication), therapy consists of fluid restriction and therapy of the underlying cause if possible.

  h. Therapy for salt wasting involves treatment of the underlying cause as well as adequate sodium and water replacement of the preexisting deficit and the ongoing losses.

B. Hyponatremic dehydration

 1. Causes: Typical vomiting and diarrhea from gastroenteritis

2. IV therapy
   a. Evaluate for shock (i.e., thready pulse, capillary refill time >3 seconds, lethargy) and give aliquots of NS, 20 mL/kg IV, until adequate perfusion restored.
   b. Treat symptomatic hyponatremia with hypertonic saline (see Section II.A.3).
   c. Estimate the extent of dehydration
      (1) <5% fluid volume (weight) loss: Mild dehydration
      (2) 5% to 9% fluid volume (weight) loss: Moderate dehydration
      (3) ≥10% fluid volume (weight) loss: Severe dehydration
   d. Replace preexisting volume deficit.
      (1) Based on known or estimated weight loss (e.g., from vomiting and diarrhea)
      (2) For example, a 10-kg infant with estimated 10% dehydration will receive 1 L of fluid to replace the preexisting volume deficit.
   e. Composition of IV fluid
      (1) NS
      (2) Add K^+ (20 mEq/L) after urine output established.
   f. Duration of fluid deficit replacement therapy: 24 hours (unless there are ongoing fluid losses)
3. Oral rehydration therapy
   a. Several oral rehydration solutions (ORSs) are available commercially. The World Health Organization formula (osmolarity, 245 mOsm/kg; glucose, 13.5 g/L, $[Na^+]$ = 75 mEq/L) remains the standard.
   b. Preferred over IV therapy for mild or moderate dehydration from gastroenteritis
   c. For mild dehydration, give ORS, 50 mL/kg over 4 hours. Then replace ongoing losses with ORS.
   d. For moderate dehydration, give ORS, 100 mL/kg over 4 hours. Then replace ongoing losses with ORS.
   e. Return to normal alimentation at maintenance rate as soon as possible.
   f. Contraindications: Coma, ileus, shock.

C. SIADH
Antidiuretic hormone (ADH) release from the posterior pituitary persists despite water retention and dilutional hyponatremia. The ADH release is therefore inappropriate. The resulting mild volume expansion also leads to Na^+ loss from the kidney.
1. Features
   a. Hyponatremia (serum Na^+ <130 mEq/L)
   b. Hypo-osmolality (serum osmolality <280 mOsm/kg)
   c. Urine osmolality >100 mOsm/kg (usually ~300 mOsm/kg)

The urine osmolality is inappropriately elevated (relative to low serum osmolality) reflecting the inability to dilute the urine maximally.

 d. Urine Na^+ >20 to 40 mEq/L

 e. Low blood urea nitrogen (BUN) level

2. Clinical presentation

 a. Asymptomatic

 b. Nausea, vomiting

 c. Mild hypervolemia (or euvolemia)

 d. Seizures (cerebral edema)

3. Conditions associated with SIADH

 a. Central nervous system disease or injury (infections, basilar skull fracture, ischemic insults, pituitary surgery)

 b. Burns

 c. Respiratory illness

4. Medications associated with SIADH

 a. Anticonvulsants (carbamazepine)

 b. Chemotherapeutics (cyclophosphamide, vincristine, cisplatinum)

 c. Antidepressants (serotonin reuptake inhibitors, haloperidol, amitryptyline)

 d. Antiarrhythmics (amiodarone)

 e. Certain hallucinogens (e.g., Ecstasy [3,4-methylene-dioxymethamphetamine])

5. Therapy: The choice of therapy depends on the severity of the hyponatremia and the presence of seizures.

 a. Fluid administration rate

  (1) Fluid (water) restriction should be used for all patients with SIADH. A two thirds maintenance fluid administration rate is adequate for the asymptomatic patient with mild hyponatremia ([Na^+] = 125 to 130 mEq/L).

  (2) Symptomatic patients with severe hyponatremia receive only half or even one third maintenance fluid administration.

  (3) A fluid administration rate of one third maintenance (400 mL/m^2/day) replaces only the insensible fluid losses.

  (4) Hyponatremia should be corrected slowly (48 to 72 hours).

 b. IV fluid composition

  (1) NS at the reduced (half to two thirds) maintenance rate is adequate for most patients.

  (2) Symptomatic patients with seizures or coma should receive hypertonic saline until serum Na^+ level increases to 120 to 125 mEq/L (see Section II.A.3).

    c. Diuretics
      (1) Consider furosemide for severe SIADH because it promotes excretion of hypotonic urine.
      (2) Then restrict isotonic fluids.
D. Adrenal crisis (acute adrenal insufficiency) presents with hyponatremia in addition to other clinical findings. It may present at any age and may be caused by primary problems of the adrenal gland or secondary to hypothalamic or pituitary dysfunction. Varying degrees of mineralocorticoid and glucocorticoid deficiency result.
  1. Causes (more common entities in bold)
    a. Infancy
      (1) **Adrenal hemorrhage**
      (2) Congenital adrenal hyperplasia (from 21-hydroxylase deficiency)
      (3) Adrenal hypoplasia (rare)
    b. Childhood
      (1) Abrupt withdrawal of exogenous corticosteroids
      (2) Adrenal hemorrhage from sepsis, particularly meningococcemia (Waterhouse-Friderichsen syndrome)
      (3) Autoimmune disease
      (4) Chronic infections (acquired immunodeficiency syndrome, tuberculosis)
      (5) Drugs that inhibit adrenal steroidogenesis (trimethoprim-sulfamethoxazole, etomidate, ketoconazole)
      (6) Adrenoleukodystrophy
  2. Clinical presentation
    a. Cardiovascular: **Shock** (may be refractory to fluid administration and catecholamines), dehydration, acidosis, hyponatremia, hyperkalemia, and hypercalcemia
    b. Gastrointestinal: **Vomiting,** anorexia, nausea, abdominal pain, weight loss
    c. Central nervous system: **Lethargy,** confusion
    d. Electrolytes: **Hyponatremia, hyperkalemia,** acidosis
    e. Endocrine: **Hypoglycemia**
    f. Hematologic: Eosinophilia, lymphocytosis
  3. Other signs: In cases of primary failure of glucocorticoid production, compensatory increases in adrenocorticotropic hormone (ACTH) and androgens may result in hyperpigmentation and virilization (in the male) or ambiguous genitalia (in the female).
  4. Differential diagnosis
    a. Pyloric stenosis: Presentation—vomiting, severe dehydration, and hypochloremic, hypokalemic, metabolic **alkalosis**

    b. Sepsis (especially urosepsis in the infant): Presentation—
       shock, vomiting, lethargy, hyponatremia, hyperkalemia,
       acidosis, hypoglycemia
  5. Evaluation
    a. Electrolytes, glucose, Ca^{2+}, arterial blood gas, complete blood
       count (CBC)
    b. Serum cortisol level
    c. ACTH stimulation test
    d. Electrocardiogram (ECG)
    e. Blood and urine cultures
    f. Urinalysis
  6. Treatment
    a. Treat shock with NS in 20-mL/kg aliquots. Patients may
       require large volumes of fluid and may be poorly responsive
       to vasoactive medications.
    b. Treat hypoglycemia: 25% dextrose (D25), 2 mL/kg IV. Then
       give D5 NS at maintenance rates.
    c. Treat hyperkalemia. See Section III.B.3 and **Tables 8-1** and
       8-2.
    d. Corticosteroid replacement (stress doses)
      (1) Hydrocortisone is the preferred corticosteroid to treat
          adrenal crisis because of mineralocorticoid activity in
          addition to glucocorticoid activity.
      (2) Doses: Hydrocortisone, 50 to 100 mg/m^2 IV bolus,
          followed by hydrocortisone 50 to 100 mg/m^2 per day
          divided in 4 doses; use intramuscular (IM) injection if IV
          route unavailable.
      (3) Typical steroid stress doses
        (a) Infant: Hydrocortisone 25 mg IV/IM; then 1 mg/hr
            continuous infusion

TABLE 8-1

CLASSIFICATION AND THERAPY OF HYPERKALEMIA

Degree of Hyperkalemia	Mechanism of Therapy	Therapy
Mild (5.0-6.0 mEq/L)	Decrease K^+ load	Remove K^+ from IVF. Discontinue spironolactone.
Moderate (6.0-7.0 mEq/L)	Enhance K^+ excretion	Kayexalate, 1 g/kg q6h PO or rectally Furosemide, 0.5-1 mg/kg IV q6h
Severe (>7.0 mEq/L, or symptomatic)	Redistribution of K^+ to intracellular space	β-agonists $NaHCO_3$, 1-2 mEq/kg IV Hyperventilate Insulin 0.1 units/kg and glucose 0.5 g/kg IV
	Inhibit effects of hyperkalemia on excitable membranes	Calcium IV (see Table 8-2 and text)

IV, Intravenous; *IVF*, intravenous fluid; *PO*, orally.

TABLE 8-2

EMERGENT THERAPY OF HYPERKALEMIA

Drug or Intervention	Dose (per kg)	Administration	Effect	Comment
Calcium	10-20 mg (chloride) or 100 mg (gluconate)	Slow IV push (central line for CaCl$_2$)	Stabilizes excitable membranes	Monitor ECG (see Section V.A.3)
Insulin + glucose	0.1 units and 0.5 g	Over 30 min IV	ECF → ICF	Monitor dextrose stick
Hyperventilation	N/A (Paco$_2$ < 30 mm Hg)	Rapid	ECF → ICF	Transient benefit
NaHCO$_3$	1-2 mEq	Slow IV push	ECF → ICF	See text
Albuterol	Unit dose	Nebulization	ECF → ICF	May repeat frequently

ECF, Extracellular fluid; *ECG*, electrocardiogram; *ICF*, intracellular fluid; *IV*, intravenous; *Paco$_2$*, partial pressure of carbon dioxide.

      (b) Child: Hydrocortisone 50 mg IV/IM; then 2 mg/hr continuous infusion
      (c) Adolescent: Hydrocortisone, 100 mg IV/IM; then 4 mg/hr continuous infusion
  E. Hypernatremia overview
    1. Causes: Hypernatremia results from water losses in excess of salt loss, excessive salt intake, or (rarely) salt retention; evaluation of the patient's volume status (especially weight loss or gain) is critical for determining the correct diagnosis.
      a. Free water loss occurs from renal or nonrenal sources.
        (1) Renal water losses result in a relatively dilute urine; causes include acute tubular necrosis-polyuric phase, diuretics (particularly osmotically active agents), and diabetes insipidus.
        (2) Nonrenal water losses result in compensatory concentration of the urine and include evaporative skin losses (especially in premature infants or after burns) and gastrointestinal losses.
      b. Sodium overload
        (1) Salt intoxication from exogenous sodium (enteral or parenteral), such as the following:
          (a) Hypertonic saline administration
          (b) Sodium bicarbonate treatment of metabolic acidosis
          (c) Hypertonic saline irrigation
          (d) Nutritional formula reconstitution errors
        (2) Mineralocorticoid excess rarely results in hypernatremia; typically, patients present with volume overload, hypertension, and normal serum sodium level.

  2. Hypernatremic dehydration therapy
     a. Treat shock with isotonic fluids, 15 to 20 mL/kg. Shock is
        very rare because hypernatremia expands the ECF
        volume.
     b. Correct hypernatremia **SLOWLY:**
        (1) Allow Na^+ level to decrease <0.5 mEq/L/hr to reduce the
            risk of seizures or cerebral edema.
        (2) For patients with serum Na^+ level = 150 to 165 mEq/L,
            this can usually be accomplished by replacing their fluid
            deficit over 48 to 72 hours with 0.45% saline.
        (3) With progressive hyperosmolarity, isotonic fluids may
            need to be given over a longer period of time.
  3. Salt intoxication therapy.
     a. Stop the source of excess Na^+ intake.
     b. For patients with normal renal function, natriuresis usually
        occurs spontaneously and will restore the normal serum Na^+
        level. If necessary, a small dose of furosemide will aid
        natriuresis.
     c. For patients with renal failure, consider dialysis.
  F. Diabetes insipidus
     1. Definition
        a. DI results from an inability to concentrate the urine in
           response to normal stimuli.
        b. The hallmark of DI is a serum Na^+ level >150 mEq/L, serum
           osmolarity >300 mOsm, simultaneous urine osmolarity
           <300 mOsm, and urine specific gravity <1.006. Patients
           present with polyuria.
        c. The infant or neurologically impaired patient cannot
           achieve a compensatory polydipsia and therefore
           appears severely dehydrated after sustained renal water
           losses.
     2. Causes: DI results from inadequate production of ADH (central
        DI) or an inability of the kidneys to respond to ADH
        (nephrogenic DI).
        a. Central DI: Absence of the pituitary, head trauma, global
           cerebral ischemia, intracranial infections (meningitis), brain
           tumors, neurosurgery involving the pituitary
        b. Nephrogenic DI: Congenital (X-linked dominant), renal
           tubular acidosis, sickle cell disease, obstructive uropathy,
           drugs (e.g., lithium, chemotherapeutic agents),
           hypercalcemia
     3. Treatment
        a. Treat hypovolemia with NS aliquots of 20 mL/kg until
           adequate perfusion is restored.
        b. Replace **preexisting water deficit** with 0.45% saline such
           that serum Na^+ level normalizes over 72 hours.

    c. Replace **ongoing excess urinary losses** milliliter for milliliter if urine output >4 mL/kg/hr. The Na^+ concentration in the urinary replacement fluid is adjusted based on urinary Na^+ losses to allow correction of hypernatremia over 72 hours.

    d. Replace insensible losses with D5/0.45% saline at one-third maintenance rates.

    e. Give vasopressin, 0.5 milliunits/kg/hr IV. Double the dose q30min until polyuria is controlled. Monitor serum Na^+ level and fluid balance meticulously and titrate therapy to maintain desired correction of hypernatremia and control of polyuria.

    f. Nephrogenic DI does not respond to exogenous ADH. Treatment consists of adequate fluid replacement and thiazide diuretics.

    g. Following pituitary surgery or acute brain injury, there may be alternating periods of DI, cerebral salt wasting, and SIADH, necessitating rapid changes in fluid management.

    h. Subacute or chronic central DI treatment
       (1) Use oral or intranasal desmopressin (DDAVP).
       (2) Exercise great care when prescribing, because the oral preparation has only 10% of the activity of the intranasal preparation.

III. Potassium disorders

Potassium is present predominantly in the ICF. Extracellular (including serum) potassium is tightly regulated. Minor changes in serum K^+ levels can produce life-threatening cardiac arrhythmias as well as affect neuromuscular function.

  A. Hypokalemia

    1. Causes
      a. Diuretics (particularly loop diuretics)
      b. Enema, laxative abuse (anorexia nervosa)
      c. Renal tubular dysfunction
      d. Renovascular disease (hyperreninemic states)
      e. Mineralocorticoid excess
      f. Alkalemia (causes an intracellular shift of K^+)
      g. Gastric fluid losses (pyloric stenosis, nasogastric tube suctioning)

    2. Manifestations
      a. Characteristic changes in the ECG, including atrial and ventricular ectopy (particularly in patients with congenital heart disease or after heart surgery) and U waves
      b. Enhanced digitalis toxicity
      c. Muscle weakness, cramping, paresthesias
      d. Paralytic ileus
      e. Metabolic alkalosis and paradoxical aciduria (caused by K^+-H^+ exchange in the renal collecting duct)

3. Therapy
   a. Symptomatic hypokalemia, particularly with electrocardiographic changes, requires urgent IV replacement. Replacement should not exceed 0.5 mEq/kg/hr in most cases because of the following:
      (1) Risk of hyperkalemia, particularly with acidosis or renal disease
      (2) KCl is irritating and can cause phlebitis.
         (a) Extravasation can result in significant skin injury.
         (b) Use a large, well-functioning IV, such as a central line or well-flowing antecubital vein.
   b. Because of the above cautions, enteral K^+ replacement is preferred in nonemergent situations.

B. Hyperkalemia
   1. Causes
      a. Renal failure
      b. Adrenal insufficiency (see Section II.D.)
      c. Hemolysis
      d. Tumor lysis syndrome
      e. Rhabdomyolysis (crush injury or electrical burns)
      f. Potassium-sparing diuretics
      g. Metabolic acidosis (for every 0.1-unit reduction in arterial pH, K^+ level increases 0.2 to 0.4 mEq/L)
      h. Factitious (hemolysis with sampling)
   2. Manifestations
      a. Slowly developing hyperkalemia may be asymptomatic and produce little ECG change.
      b. Rapidly rising serum K^+ level will produce alterations in cardiac conduction and repolarization (**Fig. 8-1**).
   3. Treatment (**Fig. 8-2**)
      Therapy of hyperkalemia involves antagonism of the effect of K^+ on excitable membranes, rapid redistribution of K^+ to intracellular stores, and elimination of K^+ from the body. The choice of therapy generally depends on the level of hyperkalemia, but symptomatic patients (i.e., electrocardiographic changes) must be treated as an emergency (Tables 8-1 and 8-2).
      a. Calcium
         (1) Restores a normal gradient between resting membrane potential and threshold membrane potential and thereby decreases myocardial excitability
         (2) Administer $CaCl_2$, 10 mg/kg, or calcium gluconate, 100 mg/kg **slow** IV push. $CaCl_2$ can cause significant tissue necrosis and **MUST** be given via a central line. (See Section IV.A.3.)

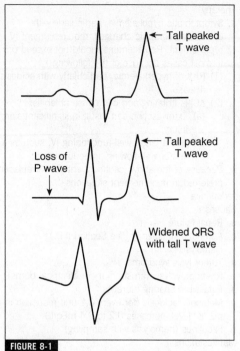

FIGURE 8-1

Electrocardiographic findings in hyperkalemia. There is progressive peaking of T waves, decreasing size of P waves, and prolongation of the QRS interval. *(From Slovis C, Jenkins R. ABC of clinical electrocardiography: conditions not primarily affecting the heart. BMJ 2002;324:1264-1267.)*

  b. Redistribution of K^+
    (1) Insulin, 0.1 unit/kg, and dextrose, 0.5 g/kg (2 mL/kg of D25W), over 20 minutes will redistribute K^+ to the intracellular space.
    (2) Alkalinization therapy with hyperventilation or $NaHCO_3$ (1 to 2 mEq/kg IV) should be used, even in the absence of acidosis.
    (3) Giving Ca^{2+} prior to alkalinization will help prevent ionized hypocalcemia. β-Agonists, including nebulized albuterol, cause K^+ to shift rapidly into the intracellular space and are useful if IV access is delayed.

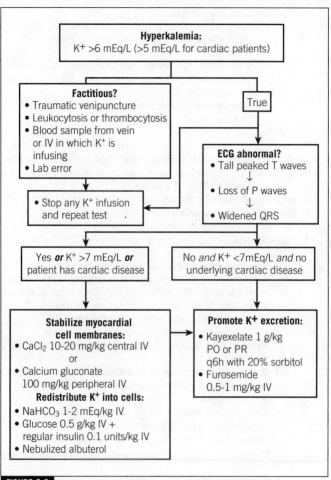

Hyperkalemia:
K^+ >6 mEq/L (>5 mEq/L for cardiac patients)

Factitious?
- Traumatic venipuncture
- Leukocytosis or thrombocytosis
- Blood sample from vein or IV in which K^+ is infusing
- Lab error

True

ECG abnormal?
- Tall peaked T waves
  ↓
- Loss of P waves
  ↓
- Widened QRS

- Stop any K^+ infusion and repeat test .

Yes *or* K^+ >7 mEq/L *or* patient has cardiac disease

No *and* K^+ <7mEq/L *and* no underlying cardiac disease

Stabilize myocardial cell membranes:
- $CaCl_2$ 10-20 mg/kg central IV
  or
- Calcium gluconate 100 mg/kg peripheral IV

Redistribute K^+ into cells:
- $NaHCO_3$ 1-2 mEq/kg IV
- Glucose 0.5 g/kg IV + regular insulin 0.1 units/kg IV
- Nebulized albuterol

Promote K^+ excretion:
- Kayexelate 1 g/kg PO or PR q6h with 20% sorbitol
- Furosemide 0.5-1 mg/kg IV

FIGURE 8-2

Hyperkalemia treatment algorithm. *ECG,* Electrocardiogram; *IV,* intravenous; *PO,* orally; *PR,* by rectum.

c. Enhance K+ excretion.
  (1) Polystyrene sulfonate (Kayexalate) 1 g/kg q6h, orally or rectally with 20% sorbitol, will enhance intestinal K+ elimination.
  (2) If the patient has residual renal function, loop diuretics (furosemide, 0.5 to 1 mg/kg IV) can be given to enhance K+ elimination.
  (3) Renal failure patients may require renal replacement therapy (dialysis, hemofiltration).

IV. Calcium disorders

Calcium exists in ionized (free) and protein-bound (total) forms. The ionized form exerts calcium's biologic effects and therefore should be measured when possible. Free serum calcium is tightly regulated by the counterbalancing effects of parathyroid hormone (PTH) secreted by the parathyroid glands and calcitonin secreted by the C cells in the thyroid. Additionally, normal vitamin D metabolism is required for efficient calcium absorption from the gastrointestinal (GI) tract.

A. Hypocalcemia

1. Causes
  a. PTH deficiency: Primary (DiGeorge syndrome, X-linked PTH deficiency, and CHARGE syndromes [coloboma of the eye, heart anomalies, choanal atresia, retardation, genital and ear anomalies]) or acquired (thyroid surgery, sepsis, burns, hypomagnesemia, and autoimmune disease)
  b. PTH resistance: Hypomagnesemia, receptor defect
  c. Renal wasting: Tubular dysfunction, aminoglycosides, loop diuretics
  d. Calcitriol (activated vitamin D) deficiency: Dietary deficiency, lack of sunlight, malabsorption, liver failure, renal failure, anticonvulsants
  e. Chelation, precipitation: Citrate (blood products), tumor lysis, pancreatitis, hyperphosphatemia, alkalosis (ionized hypocalcemia caused by increased Ca^{2+} binding to serum proteins)

2. Manifestations
  a. Neuromuscular: Tetany (Trousseau sign), hyperreflexia (Chvostek sign), paresthesias, weakness, irritability, seizures, muscle spasm
  b. Cardiovascular: Depressed myocardial contractility, hypotension, bradycardia, prolonged QTc, asystole, decreased response to catecholamines
  c. Respiratory: Laryngospasm, bronchospasm, weakness

3. Treatment
  a. Emergent IV therapy with a Ca^{2+} salt (calcium chloride or calcium gluconate) is required if the patient manifests the following:

       (1) Neuronal irritability (central or peripheral)

       (2) Electrocardiographic changes or arrhythmias

       (3) Hemodynamic collapse

   b. There is no clear therapeutic benefit of one Ca^{2+} salt over another.

   c. $CaCl_2$ causes significant sclerosis and tissue injury following extravasation. It should only be given via a central line (or large-bore, well-established IV in extreme emergencies).

   d. Administer calcium slowly and only in patients with electrocardiographic monitoring; calcium may cause arrhythmias, including bradycardia and asystole, particularly in digitalized patients.

   e. Dosage

       (1) Calcium chloride: 10 to 20 mg/kg IV slowly

       or

       (2) Calcium gluconate: 100 mg/kg IV slowly

   f. Refractory hypocalcemia may respond to magnesium supplementation.

   g. Correct significant hyperphosphatemia to prevent metastatic calcification.

B. Hypercalcemia

  1. Causes

   a. Hyperparathyroidism

   b. Malignancy

   c. Hypervitaminosis D

   d. Immobilization

   e. Thiazide diuretics

   f. Excessive parenteral calcium intake

   g. Williams' syndrome

   h. Milk-alkali syndrome

  2. Manifestations

   a. GI: Anorexia, nausea, abdominal pain

   b. Polyuria

   c. Lassitude

   d. Hypertension

   e. Renal calculi

   f. Pancreatitis

  3. Treatment

   a. Treat the underlying cause.

   b. Volume expansion with NS (10 to 20 mL/kg)

   c. Loop diuretic to enhance calciuresis

   d. Consider bisphosphonate therapy for protracted or severe cases.

8

TABLE 8-3

CHARACTERISTIC FINDINGS IN SOME INBORN ERRORS OF METABOLISM

Disorder	Manifestations
Organic acidemia	Anion gap acidosis, hyperammonemia, cytopenias
Urea cycle defect	Hyperammonemia, respiratory alkalosis, obtundation
Fatty acid oxidation defect	Nonketotic hypoglycemia
Carbohydrate disorder	Organomegaly, hypoglycemia, urinary-reducing substances, lactic acidosis

V. Inborn errors of metabolism

This section provides a brief general overview of the recognition, diagnosis, and initial management of inborn errors of metabolism (IEM). Although individually rare, the large number of different inborn errors makes their cumulative incidence an important consideration. Inborn errors may present at any age with a variety of signs and symptoms.

A. Presentation

1. The infantile presentations of IEMs include vomiting, lethargy, seizures, coma, shock, or cardiorespiratory arrest. The onset often occurs after dietary changes (e.g., the introduction of protein into the diet or fasting leading to hypoglycemia).

2. Older children often present with more insidious signs, such as loss of developmental milestones, failure to thrive, vomiting, lethargy, apnea or hyperventilation, seizures (may be intractable), hypotonia.

3. Clues to the diagnosis of an IEM (**Table 8-3**)

   a. Jaundice and/or hepatosplenomegaly
   b. Dysmorphic features
   c. Macrocephaly
   d. Cardiomyopathy
   e. Cataracts
   f. Characteristic color or odor of the urine

B. Initial laboratory evaluation

Laboratory studies are more likely to reveal a diagnosis if performed at the peak of illness (maximal metabolic derangement). Early consultation with a metabolic specialist will ensure proper handling of samples.

1. General laboratory tests: Electrolytes (and calculated anion gap), BUN, creatinine, glucose, liver function tests, CBC, arterial blood gases, ammonia, lactate, pyruvate, creatinine phosphokinase and aldolase, urinalysis; CSF, if obtained, should be frozen for metabolic analysis.

2. Specific metabolic tests: Freeze samples of urine and blood (in a green-topped tube) for organic and amino acids.

3. Fibroblast assays should be performed in case of death of an infant suspected of having an IEM. Ultimately this may provide more information than a complete autopsy. To obtain a viable skin biopsy sample, do the following:
   a. Obtain parental consent.
   b. Prepare the skin in a sterile fashion.
   c. Remove an ellipse of skin 0.5 × 1.0 cm.
   d. Place the skin in preservative-free saline.
   e. Store at room temperature.
C. Treatment
   IEMs cause symptoms because of hypoglycemia or the production of toxic metabolic byproducts. The goal of treatment is to prevent toxic metabolic byproduct accumulation and provide adequate glucose to prevent catabolism.
   1. Perform the ABCs of resuscitation (see Chapter 5).
   2. Stop enteral feeds.
   3. Give 10% dextrose, 0.45% saline, IV at maintenance rates. Use isotonic fluids if there is concern for cerebral edema (i.e., hyperammonemia).
   4. Treatment of hyperammonemia may require emergent dialysis or continuous venovenous hemodialysis.
   5. Consult a metabolic disease expert.

Chapter 9

Acute Renal Failure

*Charles L. Schleien, MD, MBA,
and David G. Nichols, MD, MBA*

I. Overview

Recent classification schemes refer to acute kidney injury to emphasize a spectrum of severity of which acute renal failure represents the most severe manifestation. The term *azotemia* implies an elevated level of urea and other nitrogenous compounds in the blood, which is the result of acute renal failure.

II. Definition

A. Rapid decline (hours, days, weeks) in glomerular and tubular functions
   1. With loss of ability to maintain fluid and electrolyte homeostasis
   2. With loss of ability to excrete organic solutes, including nitrogen waste products, drugs, and metabolites.
B. Manifestations
   1. Rising blood urea nitrogen (BUN) and serum creatinine levels
   2. Alteration in electrolyte concentrations, primarily of Na^+, K^+, Ca^{2+}, PO_4, bicarbonate
   3. Accumulation of extracellular fluid leading to interstitial edema and intravascular volume excess
   4. Oliguria may or may not be present.

III. Types of renal failure

Acute renal failure is caused by many diverse clinical conditions and is commonly categorized into three broad types: Prerenal, intrarenal, and postrenal (obstructive) renal failure.

A. Prerenal failure
   1. Characterized by decreased renal perfusion
   2. Glomerular and tubular function are normal
   3. Prerenal failure is the most common presenting form of acute renal failure in children. Causes include the following:
      a. Hypovolemia (e.g., from blood loss, diarrhea, burns, diabetes insipidus)
      b. Decreased renal perfusion secondary to abnormal systemic hemodynamics (e.g., septic shock, low cardiac output syndrome, hepatorenal syndrome)

    c. Drugs causing renal vasoconstriction (e.g., amphotericin B, catecholamine infusions, cyclosporine and tacrolimus)

    d. Drugs causing impaired renal autoregulation (e.g., angiotensin converting enzyme inhibitors, angiotensin II receptor blockers, nonsteroidal anti-inflammatory drugs [NSAIDs])

B. Intrarenal failure is characterized by disease or injury to the kidney itself—generally involving the vascular supply, glomerulus, interstitium, or tubule. Causes include the following:

    1. Renal ischemia (the most common precipitating event)

    2. Vascular obstruction (renal artery or vein obstruction)

    3. Glomerular disease

       a. The classification of glomerular disease begins with the clinical examination and urinalysis to divide glomerular disease into nephritic and nephrotic patterns.

       b. The nephritic pattern includes an active (inflammatory) urinary sediment with red cells, white cells, and casts, but only mild to moderate proteinuria.

       c. The nephrotic pattern of glomerular disease shows a relatively inactive urinary sediment without cells or casts but with very severe proteinuria, leading to hypoproteinemia and peripheral edema.

    4. Vasculitis

       a. Henoch-Schönlein purpura is the most common vasculitis with renal involvement in children.

       b. Other diseases include systemic lupus erythematosus, polyarteritis nodosa, and Wegener granulomatosis.

    5. Microangiopathy: Hemolytic-uremic syndrome and disseminated intravascular coagulation are common microangiopathic syndromes that may involve kidney injury.

    6. Acute tubular necrosis (ATN)

       a. Renal ischemia: ATN can follow prerenal azotemia after a series of additional insults occur, such as sepsis or persistent hypotension.

       b. Exposure to nephrotoxins (e.g., radiocontrast material, aminoglycosides, NSAIDs, uric acid, myoglobin)

    7. Interstitial nephritis

       a. Drug-induced (e.g., NSAIDs, aminoglycosides, amphotericin B, radiocontrast material)

       b. Nephrotoxic pigments (e.g., myoglobin, hemoglobin)

       c. Bilateral pyelonephritis

    8. Tubular obstruction

       a. Uric acid (tumor lysis syndrome)

       b. Drug-induced (e.g., acyclovir, ganciclovir, methotrexate)

C. Postrenal (obstructive) failure requires bilateral urinary tract obstruction or obstruction of the bladder or urethra.

1. In addition to congenital renal anomalies, such as posterior urethral valves, and ureteroceles, acquired obstructions such as stones or clot must be considered.
2. Unilateral ureteral obstruction may lead to renal failure if it occurs in the presence of significant underlying kidney disease or a single kidney.
3. Postrenal failure is often reversible.
4. Failure to diagnose obstructive renal failure is likely to lead to increased intraluminal pressure in collecting systems, hydroureter, renal ischemia, and intrinsic renal failure.
5. Major causes of obstruction at various sites in the urinary tract include the following:
   a. Urethral (e.g., posterior urethral valves, stricture)
   b. Bladder (e.g., blood clots, neurogenic bladder)
   c. Ureteral (e.g., stones, clots, fibrosis, extrinsic compression)

IV. Classification based on urine output: Oliguric versus nonoliguric
   A. Definitions
      1. Anuria: Complete absence of urine flow
      2. Oliguria: Urine flow <0.5 to 1.0 mL/kg/hr
      3. Polyuria: Average urine flow > average fluid intake over 24 hours
   B. Nonoliguric renal failure
      1. Often explained by higher glomerular filtration rate (GFR) than in oliguric renal failure; therefore, often associated with better prognosis
      2. Lower peak serum creatinine level than in oliguric renal failure
      3. Patients less likely to be fluid overloaded than oliguric renal failure patients
      4. Often induced by nephrotoxins
      5. Preservation of sufficient urine flow simplifies management and dialysis therapies may be unnecessary.
   C. Oliguric renal failure
      1. Oliguria is common in ATN and is often ischemia-related.
      2. More severe decrease of GFR than in nonoliguric renal failure
      3. Neither diuretics (furosemide, mannitol) nor dopamine infusion have proven of therapeutic benefit in the treatment of oliguric renal failure.
      4. Use of high-dose furosemide in this setting may be associated with ototoxicity.

V. Clinical presentation
   The signs and symptoms of acute renal failure may be nonspecific and reflect the manifestations of the disease that triggers renal failure or the hormonal and autonomic responses to renal injury. Specific diseases characterized by renal failure may have characteristic symptoms (**Table 9-1**).

TABLE 9-1

SYMPTOMS AND SIGNS ASSOCIATED WITH SPECIFIC DISEASE ENTITIES THAT INCLUDE ACUTE RENAL FAILURE

Symptoms and Signs	Severe Dehydration	Hemolytic-Uremic Syndrome	Glomerulonephritis	Henoch-Schönlein Purpura	Hepatorenal Syndrome	Goodpasture's Syndrome*	Posterior Urethral Valves
Vomiting	+	+ Abdominal pain		+ Also abdominal pain, ileus, intussusception			
Diarrhea	+	+					
Fever, sepsis	+	+					
Hemorrhage	+ Hemorrhagic shock	+ Bloody diarrhea		+ Guaiac-positive stool	+ Upper gastrointestinal bleed	+ (Hemoptysis)	+
Hypertension		+	+				
Rales, hypoxia			+		+	+	+ Lung hypoplasia
Rash			+ (Impetigo)	+ Red macules, petechiae (often on buttocks)			
Edema			+	+ Localized (e.g., periorbital)	+		
Urinary abnormalities		Anuria in 40% of cases	Red or tea-colored urine			Proteinuria and casts	Anuria in newborn

+ Symptom or sign is present.

*Antiglomerular basement membrane disease with pulmonary hemorrhage.

9

  A. Genitourinary signs and symptoms
    1. Oliguria or polyuria
    2. Urine discoloration
      a. Red urine: Hemoglobinuria or myoglobinuria
      b. Tea-colored urine: Glomerulonephritis
      c. Colorless urine (with polyuria): Diabetes insipidus
  B. Cardiovascular signs and symptoms
    1. Hypotension: Multiple causes (see Chapters 5, 6, and 7) that lead to decreased renal perfusion, kidney injury, and ultimately renal failure
    2. Hypertension: Associated with fluid overload from decreased urinary output and excess fluid intake
    3. Signs of low cardiac output: Tachycardia, gallop rhythm, diminished peripheral pulses, capillary refill time >3 seconds
    4. Signs of severe dehydration: Low cardiac output signs plus oliguria, dry mucous membranes, sunken fontanelle, and loss of skin turgor
  C. Respiratory signs and symptoms
    1. The respiratory signs and symptoms in the acute renal failure patient are usually associated with fluid overload and pulmonary edema.
    2. They consist of tachypnea, rales, and chest wall retractions.
    3. The patient may also exhibit hyperpnea as a compensatory reaction to metabolic acidosis.
  D. Neurologic signs and symptoms
    1. Somnolence, altered mental status
    2. Seizures
    3. Fatigue
  E. Gastrointestinal (GI) signs and symptoms
    1. GI bleeding (from platelet dysfunction)
    2. Nausea and vomiting
    3. Bloody diarrhea (may suggest hemolytic uremic syndrome or intussusception)
VI. Diagnostic studies
  A. Abnormalities of urine volume and urinalysis
    See **Table 9-2.**
  B. Renal failure indices
    1. Fractional excretion of sodium (FENa)
      a. Estimates the relative clearance of sodium and creatinine. When renal function is normal in oliguric states, more than 99% of filtered sodium is reabsorbed.
      b. Urine and serum Na and creatinine (Cr) levels are measured on simultaneously obtained specimens.

TABLE 9-2

URINE VOLUME AND URINALYSIS ABNORMALITIES IN ACUTE RENAL FAILURE

Parameter	Type of Renal Failure		
	Prerenal	Intrinsic	Postrenal
Urine volume	Oliguria	• Oliguria (most common) • Anuria • Polyuria	• Oliguria, • Anuria (complete obstruction) • Variable (intermittent obstruction)
Casts (urine sediment)	• Acellular • Hyaline casts	• Acellular • Granular casts (ATN) • Epithelial casts (ATN) • Red blood cell casts (GMN, vasculitis, or ISN) • White cell casts (ISN or PN)	• Usually none
Protein	None to mild	• Mild to moderate (ATN) • Severe (GMN)	• Usually none
Heme	Usually negative	• Positive (GMN) • Positive (rhabdomyolysis, hemoglobinuria)	• Positive if obstruction from blood clots
Leukocyte esterase	• Positive (UTI, PN)	• Positive (ISN or PN)	• Positive if obstruction from nephrolithiasis

ATN, Acute tubular necrosis; *GMN,* glomerulonephritis; *ISN,* interstitial nephritis; *PN,* pyelonephritis; *UTI,* urinary tract infection.

$$\text{FENa (\%)} = ([\text{urine Na/urine Cr}]/[\text{plasma Na/plasma Cr}]) \times 100$$

Rearranging:

$$\text{FENa (\%)} = (\text{urine Na/plasma Na}) \times (\text{plasma Cr/urine Cr}) \times 100$$

  c. FENa <1 is suggestive of prerenal azotemia. It indicates reabsorption of filtered Na in response to decreased renal perfusion.
  d. FENa <1 is also seen in acute glomerulonephritis or vasculitis. In these cases, the low FENa indicates a low GFR but normal tubular function.
  e. FENa >2 is suggestive of ATN. Other causes of increased FENa include diuretic administration, acute interstitial nephritis, and postrenal obstructive disease.
  f. FENa is less accurate in nonoliguric states.
  g. Newborn FENa values are higher; prerenal azotemia is associated with FENa <2.5 and ATN is associated with FENa >3.
 2. Serum BUN/Cr ratio
  a. Older children and adults

(1) Normal BUN/Cr = 10 to 15
(2) BUN/Cr >20 indicates prerenal azotemia
(3) The elevated BUN/Cr ratio is a less accurate predictor of prerenal azotemia than FENa.

b. Infants and young children: Because the normal serum creatinine level in the infant is only 0.3 to 0.5 mg/dL, BUN/Cr ratios are not useful in this age group.

3. Urine osmolality and specific gravity
   a. Measures of urinary concentrating ability
   b. Urine osmolality >500 mOsm/kg and urine specific gravity >1.020 suggest prerenal disease in the presence of compatible history, BUN, and creatinine.
   c. Loss of urinary concentrating ability (urine osmolality <350 mOsm/kg; urine specific gravity ≅1.010) is the classic finding in ATN. In practice, urine osmolality and specific gravity are highly variable in ATN.

C. Imaging
   1. Ultrasound
      a. The first imaging test indicated in every patient with acute renal failure of unknown cause
      b. Excellent test to rule out obstructive uropathy and congenital anomalies of the urinary tract, which may be reversible causes of acute renal failure
      c. Indicated in suspected pyelonephritis to rule out perinephric abscess.
      d. ATN and other diffuse renal diseases appear as nonspecific increased echogenicity (medical renal disease).
   2. Doppler ultrasound
      a. Color Doppler flow studies can identify arterial and venous thrombosis but have a low sensitivity.
      b. Renal resistive index
         (1) Increased renal resistive index (>0.7) indicates renal vasoconstriction from any cause (prerenal, intrarenal, or postrenal causes).
         (2) Common indications for measurement of renal resistive index include suspected renal transplant rejection, urinary tract obstruction, and renal artery thrombosis.
   3. Radiocontrast administration
      a. Studies requiring radiocontrast administration (e.g., intravenous pyelography) are contraindicated in suspected acute renal failure.
      b. Ultrasound and helical computed tomography scan (for nephrolithiasis) provide equivalent or better data.

VII. Prevention
   A. Intravascular volume maintenance and repletion
      1. Because severe dehydration and hypovolemic shock are major causes of acute renal failure, rapid restoration of intravascular volume is a key preventive measure.
      2. Administer normal saline (NS), 20 mL/kg, intravenous (IV) or intraosseous (IO) rapidly to patients with severe dehydration or hypovolemia (see Chapter 6).
      3. The saline bolus administration may be repeated twice in the presence of severe hypovolemia.
      4. Restrict fluid administration if there are any signs of hypervolemia (e.g., rales, hypertension, peripheral edema, liver enlargement, gallop rhythm, or increased body weight compared with known baseline weight).
   B. Nephrotoxic drugs
      1. Nephrotoxic drugs (e.g., aminoglycosides, amphotericin B, cyclosporine, tacrolimus, radiocontrast agents) are major causes of acute renal failure.
      2. The prevention strategy includes using these drugs only if absolutely necessary and then monitoring serum levels, if possible.

VIII. Management
   Once intravascular volume has been restored, the immediate therapeutic objectives are to treat life-threatening metabolic abnormalities and decide on renal replacement therapy.
   A. Hyperkalemia
      See Chapter 8.
      1. Definition
         a. For patients **without** underlying cardiac disease: Serum K^+ >6 mEq/L
         b. For patients **with** underlying cardiac disease: Serum K^+ >5 mEq/L
         c. Any patient with electrocardiographic evidence of hyperkalemia (peaked T waves, prolonged PR interval, widened QRS)
      2. Highest risk scenarios
         a. Tumor lysis syndrome
         b. Rhabdomyolysis
      3. Immediate resuscitation
         a. Calcium gluconate, 100 mg/kg IV or IO **or** calcium chloride, 10 mg/kg via central line only. Administer by **slow** injection.
         b. 25% dextrose, 2 mL/kg, *plus* regular insulin, 0.1 unit/kg IV
         c. Sodium bicarbonate, 1 mEq/kg IV or IO
         d. Albuterol inhalation if no IV access available
         e. Verify that the patient is **not** receiving potassium supplementation.

    4. Increase K$^+$ excretion.
      a. Polystyrene sulfonate (Kayexalate), 1 g/kg q6h, orally or rectally with 20% sorbitol
      b. Furosemide, 1 mg/kg IV or IO (if patient is still producing urine)

B. Hyperphosphatemia
    1. High-risk scenarios: Tumor lysis syndrome, rhabdomyolysis, phosphate poisoning (e.g., laxatives, phosphate enemas).
    2. Risk of calcium-phosphate precipitation
      a. Determined by the calcium-phosphate product: Serum calcium concentration × serum phosphate concentration >60 mg^2/dL^2 results in increased risk of calcium-phosphate precipitation
      b. Calcium phosphate precipitation in the renal tubules may lead to renal failure
      c. Calcium phosphate precipitation in the heart may result in arrhythmias
    3. Treatment
      a. For nonoliguric patients, give NS at twice maintenance rates until serum phosphate normalizes (~12 hours).
      b. For anuric or oliguric patients with severe hyperphosphatemia, renal replacement therapy (hemodialysis or continuous venovenous hemofiltration with dialysis) will be necessary because saline administration is likely to worsen fluid overload and hypocalcemia (dilution).

C. Hypocalcemia
    1. Often associated with hyperphosphatemia, probably because of parathyroid hormone inhibition
    2. If calcium administration in the hypocalcemic patient does not increase the calcium phosphate product >60, then administer calcium as described earlier (see Section VIII.A.3).
    3. Asymptomatic hypocalcemia is not treated with calcium administration if there is a risk of calcium phosphate precipitation (see Section VIII.B.2).
    4. Symptomatic hypocalcemia (e.g., tetany or seizures), should be treated with supplemental calcium, even if there is a risk of calcium phosphate precipitation. Simultaneously, renal replacement therapy should be activated as fast as possible to normalize the serum phosphate concentration.

D. Acidosis
    1. Causes
      a. Inability to excrete acid
      b. Underlying disease may be associated with increased acid production (e.g., sepsis or shock)
    2. Treatment
      a. For patients with underlying cardiac disease, give sodium bicarbonate, 1 mEq/kg IV or IO.

      b. For patients without underlying cardiac disease, bicarbonate should **not** be given **unless** the acidosis is very severe (pH <7.0 to 7.2) or symptomatic. The risks of bicarbonate administration include hyperosmolality, hypernatremia, and hypercapnia.

E. Other electrolyte abnormalities

    See Chapter 8.

F. Urinary drainage

   1. Place a Foley catheter in the bladder to rule out urethral obstruction as the cause of oliguria or anuria.

   2. Measure hourly urine output.

G. Fluid management

   1. For hypovolemic patients: Restore normovolemia with NS boluses, 20 mL/kg IV or IO.

   2. For euvolemic patients

      a. Administer IV fluids equal to insensible fluid losses plus urine output.

      b. Insensible loss replacement fluid: 5% dextrose (D5) 0.45% saline, 40 mL/kg/day

      c. Insensible losses may vary greatly. Hence, the patient should be weighed q12-24h and examined frequently for signs of hypervolemia or hypovolemia.

      d. Measure serum and urinary sodium levels frequently (e.g., q4h until stable)

      e. Replace urine output milliliter for milliliter with 0.45% or 0.9% saline.

      f. If patient develops signs of hypervolemia, decrease urine replacement to 0.5 mL/mL urine output.

   3. For hypervolemic patients

      a. Attempt diuresis with furosemide, 1 mg/kg IV. Do not repeat if there is no response.

      b. Administer D5 0.45% saline IV at 40% of maintenance requirements (for insensible losses) plus 0.5 mL NS/mL urine output.

      c. Consider renal replacement therapy.

H. Indications for renal replacement therapy

   1. Electrolyte disorders refractory to medical management

   2. Uremic complications (e.g., encephalopathy, pericarditis)

   3. BUN >100 mg/dL

   4. Severe fluid overload (e.g., hypertension, congestive heart failure)

   5. Hyperammonemia (rapidly rising or refractory to lactulose administration)

Chapter 10

Endocrine Emergencies: Diabetic Ketoacidosis, Hypoglycemia, and Thyroid Storm

Lisa Grimaldi, MD,
George P. Chrousos, MD, MACE, MACP, FRCP,
and David G. Nichols, MD, MBA

I. Overview

Diabetic ketoacidosis (DKA) is one of the most frequently encountered metabolic diseases in the pediatric age group, occurring in 25% to 40% of children with newly diagnosed type I diabetes mellitus. It remains a significant source of morbidity and mortality in all age groups. This chapter provides the principles, pathophysiology, differential diagnosis, and most effective therapies for DKA, as well as the other most common endocrine emergencies in pediatric patients.

II. Diabetic ketoacidosis

A. Definition

DKA may be the initial presentation of a new onset diabetic or a complication in a known diabetic. It is defined by the following conditions and laboratory findings in a diabetic patient with a history compatible with diabetes mellitus:

1. Hyperglycemia (glucose >300 mg/dL)
2. Ketonemia (ketones present at >1:2 dilution)
3. Metabolic acidosis (pH <7.3 or HCO_3^- <15 mmol/L)
4. Ketonuria
5. Glucosuria

B. Signs and symptoms

1. Polyuria
2. Polydipsia
3. Dehydration with weight loss
4. Abdominal pain
5. Vomiting without diarrhea
6. Kussmaul respirations
7. Fruity breath
8. Altered mental status, ranging from clouded sensorium to coma (see Section II.G)

C. Pathophysiology
1. Diabetes mellitus is caused by inadequate amounts of insulin. The absence of insulin results in the following:
   a. Decreased
      (1) Glucose utilization
      (2) Ketone utilization
   b. Increased
      (1) Glycogenolysis
      (2) Gluconeogenesis
      (3) Proteolysis
      (4) Lipolysis
      (5) Ketogenesis
2. Osmotic diuresis and dehydration: The resultant hyperglycemia and ketonemia produce an osmotic diuresis (water, sodium, potassium, phosphate, and calcium loss), dehydration, and metabolic acidosis (ketoacidosis and lactic acidosis).
3. Shock (rare)
   a. Shock from dehydration alone is rare in DKA. Presence of shock should prompt emergent evaluation for other causes (e.g., cardiogenic, septic).
4. Altered mental status
   a. Hyperosmolality and acidosis lead to lethargy in most patients.
   b. Approximately 1% of patients may develop frank cerebral edema secondary to osmotic shifts of water into the brain, cerebral ischemia, and impaired cerebral autoregulation.
D. Fluid and electrolyte changes
1. Dehydration (usually 10% to 15% of body weight)
2. Elevated serum osmolality
   Serum osmolality (mOsm/L) =

$$(2 \times \text{sodium [mEq/L]}) + (\text{glucose [mg/dL]}/18) + (\text{BUN [mg/dL]}/2.8)$$

where BUN is blood urea nitrogen.
3. Sodium (Na^+)
   a. The admission serum Na value is the net result of two opposing forces.
      (1) Hyperglycemia and hyperosmolality lead to movement of water from the intracellular space to the extracellular space, thereby tending to lower the serum Na level.
      (2) Conversely, the osmotic diuresis (polyuria) results in more water than salt loss, thereby tending to raise the serum Na level.
   b. A low-normal serum Na level, or mild hyponatremia, characterizes most DKA patients at the time of admission, although some patients may present with hypernatremia.

c. The serum Na level usually rises during rehydration with normal saline (NS) and treatment with insulin.

d. Hyponatremia and failure of the serum Na to rise as expected during correction of hyperglycemia may be risk factors for cerebral edema.

e. Calculation of expected rise in serum Na level during correction of hyperglycemia:

(1) It is estimated that serum sodium is reduced by 1.6 to 2.4 mEq/L for each 100 mg/dL rise in glucose above 100 mg/dL (**Sample Calculation 1**).

(2) This relationship can be used to estimate the *expected* serum sodium level once the serum glucose has returned to normal.

f. Pseudohyponatremia: Severe hyperlipidemia may lead to a measurement artifact so that the measured serum Na^+ is lower than the true serum Na^+.

4. Potassium (K^+)

a. Total body potassium depletion characterizes all patients with DKA. This deficit must be repleted.

b. The serum K concentration is variable, depending on the K^+ losses from polyuria versus the extent of acidosis, which moves intracellular K^+ ions to the extracellular space, thereby raising serum K^+ concentration.

c. Serum K^+ concentration will fall with administration of insulin as K^+ moves back into cells.

5. Hypophosphatemia: This depresses red blood cell 2,3-diphosphoglycerate levels and may result in muscle weakness and easy fatigue.

E. Management

1. Fluids and electrolytes

a. Clinically assess the degree of dehydration (**Table 10-1**).

b. The typical signs of dehydration may be less obvious in DKA because the hyperosmolar state tends to support circulating blood volume.

Sample Calculation 1

If glucose is 600 mg/dL and sodium is 132 mEq/L:

Serum glucose difference (SGD) above normal (N) = 600 − 100 = 500 mg/L

Ratio of SGD to N = 500/100 = 5

Expected increase in serum Na = 5 × 1.6 = 8 mEq/L

Final expected serum Na after treatment = 132 + 8 = 140 mEq/L

TABLE 10-1

CLINICAL ASSESSMENT OF DEHYDRATION

	Fluid Deficit		
Severity	**Infants**	**Children**	**Clinical Examination**
Mild	5% (50 mL/kg)	3% (30 mL/kg)	Slightly dry mucous membranes, normal skin turgor, tears present, mild tachycardia
Moderate	10% (100 mL/kg)	6% (60 mL/kg)	Dry mucous membranes, tenting skin, reduced tear production, moderate tachycardia, irritability
Severe	15% (150 mL/kg)	9% (90 mL/kg)	Cracked lips, clammy skin, sunken fontanelles, no tears, severe tachycardia, hypotension, delayed capillary refill, lethargy

    c. Administer NS, 10 mL/kg over 1 hour for moderate dehydration (may administer 5 mL/kg if mild and 20 mL/kg if severe).

    d. For shock

       (1) Administer NS, 20 mL/kg over 1 hour and repeat as needed until perfusion returns to normal.

       (2) Start dopamine infusion if no improvement.

       (3) Obtain echocardiogram as well as blood and urine cultures to search for other causes of shock.

    e. Total fluid deficit and rate of rehydration

       (1) Calculate based on degree of dehydration (see Table 10-1) and maintenance fluid requirements based on weight.

       (2) Replace remaining deficit (after deducting initial bolus) over 48 hours in addition to providing maintenance fluid (**Sample Calculation 2**).

Sample Calculation 2

For 20-kg child who is clinically assessed to be 10% dehydrated:

$$\text{Initial bolus} = 10 \text{ mL/kg} = 10 \times 20 = 200 \text{ mL NS}$$

$$\text{Fluid deficit (replace over 48 hr)} = \text{total deficit} - \text{initial bolus}$$

$$= 100 \text{ mL/kg} = 100 \times 20 = 2000 \text{ mL} - 200 \text{ mL} = 1800 \text{ mL/48 hr}$$

$$= 38 \text{ mL/hr} \times 48 \text{ hr}$$

$$\text{Maintenance fluid} = 4 \text{ mL/hr for first 10 kg} = 40 \text{ mL/hr} +$$
$$2 \text{ mL/hr for second 10 kg} = 20 \text{ mL/hr} = 60 \text{ mL/hr}$$

$$\text{Total fluid (for first 48 hr)} = \text{deficit} + \text{maintenance} = 38 \text{ mL/hr} +$$
$$60 \text{ mL/hr} = 98 \text{ mL/hr (including insulin drip)}$$

    f. Intravenous (IV) fluid composition
      (1) Start with 0.9% saline.
      (2) Then change to 0.45% saline once serum sodium
          approaches normal range.
      (3) 40 mEq/L of potassium (divided equally between
          KCl and KPO_4) should be added once serum K^+
          <5.5 mEq/L.
    g. Contraindications to K^+ administration
      (1) K^+ >5.5 mEq/L
      (2) Oliguria or anuria
      (3) Do not continue KPO_4 if patient becomes hypocalcemic
         or hypomagnesemic.
    h. Rehydration rate for high-risk patients:
      (1) Replace the fluid deficit over 72 hours if there is
         increased risk for cerebral edema, including children
         younger than 3 years, prolonged prodrome and severe
         dehydration (BUN >40 mg/dL), severe acidosis
         (pH <7.0), severe hyperglycemia (serum glucose
         >1000 mg/dL), or severe hyperosmolality (serum
         osmolality >320 mOsm/kg).
      (2) Replacement of ongoing urinary losses:
         (a) Replacement of ongoing losses is controversial and
            requires meticulous monitoring and clinical
            judgment.
         (b) If polyuria is so severe that urinary output
            exceeds intake of maintenance and deficit
            replacement fluids, then urinary replacement is
            indicated.
         (c) An acceptable regimen is to replace all urine output
            >2 mL/kg/hr with 0.45% saline (i.e., 1 mL 0.45%
            saline for each mL of urine >2 mL/kg/hr).
         (d) The regimen is then adjusted based on meticulous
            monitoring of intake and output and serum and
            urinary electrolyte levels.
  2. Sodium bicarbonate
    a. In general, bicarbonate administration should be avoided
      during DKA treatment. Insulin and rehydration will correct
      acidosis for the vast majority of DKA patients.
    b. Possible indication for bicarbonate therapy: If the initial pH
      is <7.0 and the patient has cardiac instability, give sodium
      bicarbonate, 1 mEq/kg IV over 1 to 2 hours.
    c. **Never give bicarbonate as an IV bolus (IV push).**
  3. Insulin
    a. Continuous insulin infusion
      (1) Use a continuous IV infusion to administer insulin during
         DKA.

        (2) There is less risk of a precipitous fall in glucose level and serum osmolality, thereby potentially reducing the risk of cerebral edema.

    b. Bolus insulin

        (1) Bolus insulin before starting the infusion is controversial.

        (2) We no longer recommend bolus insulin during DKA because of data suggesting increased cerebral edema risk.

    c. Timing of insulin infusion: Start the insulin infusion after 1 to 2 hours of IV hydration have been completed (usually after 10 mL/kg of NS).

    d. Insulin infusion dose

        (1) Start insulin infusion at 0.1 units/kg/hr.

        (2) Rarely, titrate insulin to as high as 0.2 units/kg/hr if glucose falls at a rate of <50 mg/dL/hr.

        (3) If glucose falls to >100 mg/dL/hr or if the patient remains ketotic, continue insulin at 0.05 to 0.1 units/kg/hr but add glucose (D5) to the maintenance IV solution.

    e. Discontinuation of insulin infusion

        (1) Discontinue the insulin infusion only after ketonemia or ketonuria has resolved.

        (2) At this point, the serum glucose should be <200 mg/dL, the venous pH should be >7.3, and the patient should be able to eat and drink.

        (3) Subcutaneous insulin can now control blood sugar.

  4. Glucose

    a. Measure serum glucose hourly. The rate of glucose level decrease should not exceed 100 mg/dL/hr.

    b. As glucose approaches 300 mg/dL, add D5 to the IV solution.

  5. **Remember:** Ketosis often fails to resolve if the following occur:

    a. Infection is present.

    b. Fluids are inadequately replaced.

F. Monitoring

  1. Vital signs and glucose level hourly for all patients

  2. Check pH, Na^+, and K^+ every 1 to 2 hours until pH >7.3 and Na^+ and K^+ are stable and in the normal range. The frequency of monitoring depends on the severity of DKA and risk of cerebral edema.

  3. Calcium and phosphorus every 4 hours

  4. All urine for ketones

  5. Intake and output and hydration status every hour

  6. Electrocardiogram: Look for peaked T waves consistent with hyperkalemia or flattened T waves with U waves seen with hypokalemia.

  7. Neurologic examination hourly

G. Progressive cerebral edema
1. Incidence: 0.5% to 1% of DKA cases
2. Mortality rate: 20% to 25%
3. Risk factors for cerebral edema
   a. Younger age (<3 to 5 years)
   b. Severe dehydration (prolonged polyuria, elevated BUN level)
   c. Severe acidosis (pH <7.0): Hyperventilation and the use of bicarbonate may be markers for the severity of acidosis.
   d. Rapid correction of dehydration and hyperglycemia
   e. Failure of serum Na^+ level to rise during DKA therapy
4. Signs and symptoms
   a. Increasing lethargy
   b. Worsening headache or vomiting
   c. Irritability
   d. Decreasing Glasgow Coma Scale (GCS) score or GCS <8: See Chapter 16 and Table 16-1.
5. Management
   a. Timing
      (1) Begin management based on clinical findings.
      (2) Computed tomography scan evidence of cerebral edema may be a late finding.
   b. Airway and breathing
      (1) Secure airway to prevent aspiration if GCS <9.
      (2) Because DKA patients hyperventilate while breathing spontaneously, mechanical ventilatory settings should attempt to achieve approximately the same minute ventilation and partial pressure of carbon dioxide as during spontaneous breathing.
   c. Osmolar therapy with mannitol: Administer mannitol, 0.25 to 1 g/kg IV.
   d. Osmolar therapy with hypertonic saline: Administer 2% hypertonic saline, 8 to 10 mL/kg IV over 20 minutes to increase serum Na^+ level by 5 mEq/L.
6. Prevention of complications
   a. Lower blood glucose slowly, <80 to 100 mg/dL/hr.
   b. Do not perform lumbar puncture if any of the signs or symptoms of cerebral edema (see earlier) are present.
III. Hypoglycemia
   A. Neonates
   1. Definition
      a. Serum glucose level normally falls from maternal levels (>100 mg/dL) to 50 mg/dL at 2 hours of age.
      b. The exact level at which hypoglycemia may have clinical manifestations remains unclear and most likely varies with the child's age, size, and clinical situation.

    c. The threshold glucose level for treating hypoglycemia in the first 24 hours of life is defined as follows:

      (1) Premature, very low birth weight, sick: <50 mg/dL

      (2) Full-term, healthy: <40 mg/dL

    d. Beyond 24 hours of life, values <40 to 50 mg/dL should be treated.

    e. All high-risk infants (see later) should be screened for hypoglycemia.

    f. Any low value obtained by bedside testing should be confirmed by a definitive laboratory test, but therapy should not be withheld while awaiting results.

    g. All patients with persistent or recurrent low serum glucose values or hypoglycemia after 1 week of age should undergo diagnostic workup.

  2. Causes

    a. Transient

      (1) Small for gestational age

      (2) Infant of diabetic mother

      (3) Asphyxia

      (4) Infection, sepsis

      (5) Respiratory distress syndrome

      (6) Polycythemia

      (7) Hypothermia

    b. Persistent

      (1) Inborn errors of metabolism (e.g., carbohydrate, amino acid, lipid)

      (2) Endogenous insulin excess

        (a) Nesidioblastosis

        (b) Beckwith-Wiedemann syndrome

        (c) β cell or islet cell hyperplasia

      (3) Adrenal insufficiency (glucocorticoid deficiency)

      (4) Growth hormone deficiency

      (5) Panhypopituitarism

B. Infants and children

  1. Definition

    a. Blood glucose <45-60 mg/dL

    b. Persistent or recurrent low values should be confirmed and patient should undergo diagnostic workup.

  2. Causes (two thirds idiopathic, cause found in approximately one third of cases)

    a. Insulin excess (sudden cessation of total parenteral nutrition, Munchausen syndrome by proxy, side effect of insulin treatment in diabetes mellitus type 1)

    b. Inborn errors of metabolism

    c. Adrenal insufficiency (glucocorticoid deficiency)

    d. Growth hormone deficiency

10

      e. Panhypopituitarism

      f. Liver disease

      g. Toxins (e.g., ethanol, aspirin, oral hypoglycemic agents, sulfonamides)

      h. Starvation

C. Signs and symptoms

   1. Neonates

      a. Neurologic: Jitteriness, hypotonia, lethargy, seizure, abnormal cry

      b. Respiratory: Apnea, tachypnea

   2. Infants and older children

      a. Gastrointestinal: Nausea, abdominal pain

      b. Neurologic: Anxiety, headache, weakness, seizure

      c. Catecholamine excess: Diaphoresis, pallor, tachycardia

D. Therapy

   1. Dextrose, glucose

      a. Dosage: 0.5 g/kg as 25% solution (2 mL/kg D25) via IV push

      b. Followed by constant IV infusion of 10% dextrose at maintenance level

         (1) Neonate, infant: 4 to 8 mg/kg/min

         (2) Large adolescent: 2 to 3 mg/kg/min

      c. Titrate infusion rate to maintain glucose in the normal range.

      d. May require 8 to 15 mg/kg/min; central access may be necessary to deliver hypertonic 15% to 20% glucose solution.

   2. Glucagon

      a. Requires glycogen stores and the enzymes to break down glycogen; not useful in neonate, starvation, or glycogen storage diseases.

      b. Temporizing measure only; must follow with dextrose, as indicated earlier

      c. Dose: 0.1 to 0.3 mg/kg (maximum dose, 1 mg) IV, intramuscular

   3. Diazoxide

      a. Used for hyperinsulinemic states

      b. Side effects include fluid retention, hypertrichosis, coarse facial features, thrombocytopenia

      c. Dosage: 5 to 20 mg/kg/day orally (PO), divided into three doses

      d. Surgical removal of most of the pancreas may be indicated for hyperinsulinemia refractory to medical therapies (e.g., diazoxide, octreotide)

   4. Hydrocortisone

      a. Should be used in cases of cortisol insufficiency or hypoglycemia refractory to IV glucose

      b. Dosage: 5 mg/kg/day, divided into two doses (**Table 10-2**)

TABLE 10-2

PHARMACOLOGIC THERAPY FOR HYPOGLYCEMIA

Drug	Indications	Dosage
Dextrose	All causes of hypoglycemia	2 mL/kg 25% dextrose IVP, followed by infusion of 10% dextrose, 4-8 mg/kg/min
Glucagon	Temporizing measure until IV access obtained	0.1-0.3 mg/kg (maximum, 1 mg) IM or IV
Diazoxide	Hyperinsulinemic states	5-20 mg/kg/day PO divided q8h
Hydrocortisone	Adrenal crisis	Infant: 25 mg IV or IM stat, then 1 mg/hr IV infusion
		Child: 50 mg IV or IM stat, then 2 mg/hr IV infusion
		Adolescent: 100 mg IV or IM stat, then 4 mg/hr IV infusion

IM, Intramuscular; *IVP*, intravenous push; *PO*, orally.

IV. Thyroid storm
   A. Definition
      1. A life-threatening complication of hyperthyroidism that is **rare** in children and may progress to coma and death if not treated promptly.
      2. Most patients will have the general findings of hyperthyroidism, including goiter, exophthalmos, and hypertension.
      3. 50% of episodes are precipitated by a stressor (surgery, infection).
   B. Signs and symptoms
      Thyroid storm is characterized by acute onset of thyrotoxic symptoms, including the following:
      1. Autonomic: Fever
      2. Cardiovascular: Tachycardia, arrhythmias, high-output heart failure
      3. Gastrointestinal: Vomiting, diarrhea, abdominal pain
      4. Neurologic: Agitation, tremor, psychosis, seizure, coma
   C. Treatment
      Blood sample should be obtained for thyroid function tests (triiodothyronine [T_3], free thyroxin, thyroid-stimulating hormone, antithyroid antibodies) before treatment is initiated (**Table 10-3**).
      1. Propranolol
         a. Many of the hypermetabolic effects of hyperthyroidism are mediated by β-adrenergic receptors.
         b. Inhibits peripheral thyroid hormone effects
         c. Dosage: 10 mcg/kg IV over 10 minutes, followed by 0.5 to 2 mg/kg/day PO, divided q8h

TABLE 10-3		
PHARMACOLOGIC THERAPY FOR THYROID STORM		
Therapy	**Mechanism of Action**	**Dosage**
Propranolol	Beta blocker; inhibits peripheral thyroid hormone effects	10 mcg/kg IV over 10 min, followed by 0.5-2 mg/kg/day PO, divided q8h
Propylthiouracil	Prevents thyroid hormone synthesis and conversion to active form	5-7 mg/kg/day PO, divided q8h
Lugol's iodide	Rapidly terminates thyroid hormone release	5 drops PO, q8h
Acetaminophen	Decreases temperature and metabolic rate	15 mg/kg PO or PR, q8h

IV, Intravenous; *PO,* orally; *PR,* by rectum.

2. Propylthiouracil
   a. Prevents thyroid hormone synthesis and inhibits conversion of thyroxine to the more active form, T_3
   b. Should be given in addition to propranolol
   c. Dosage: 5 to 7 mg/kg/day PO, divided q8h
   d. May substitute with methimazole, 0.6 to 0.7 mg/kg/day PO, divided q8h
3. Iodide
   a. Rapidly terminates thyroid hormone release
   b. Dose: Lugol's iodide, 5 drops PO q8h
4. Measures to decrease temperature and metabolic rate
   a. Tepid sponging or cooling blanket
   b. Acetaminophen for fever reduction
V. Adrenal crisis
   See Chapter 8.

Chapter 11

Gastrointestinal Emergencies

Maria Oliva-Hemker, MD,
Paul M. Colombani, MD, MBA, FACS, FAAP,
and Myron Yaster, MD

I. Acute abdominal pain
   A. Overview
      1. Whether acute abdominal pain occurs in a healthy child or in a child with a chronic illness, the suddenness and severity of the pain often results in the parent seeking immediate evaluation by a pediatrician or emergency room physician.
      2. Although many cases of acute abdominal pain are benign, a major diagnostic challenge for the clinician is to identify diseases that require urgent treatment (see Chapters 22, 23, and 32).
   B. Differential diagnoses
      1. The most common operative cause of acute abdominal pain in children is appendicitis, and the most common medical cause is gastroenteritis.
      2. More than 25% of patients with acute abdominal pain have no clear cause.
      3. Referred pain from pneumonia mimics abdominal pain and can be ruled out with a chest radiograph.
      4. **Table 11-1** lists some common causes of abdominal pain by age and severity.
   C. Assessment
      In most cases, acute abdominal pain can be diagnosed through the history and physical examination. The initial goal should be to determine whether a condition exists that will require immediate surgical intervention (**Boxes 11-1** and **11-2**).
      1. History: Focus on frequency, sequence, and timing of symptom progression; related or aggravating factors; recent trauma; past operations; location; concurrent illnesses and, in girls, gynecologic and sexual history.
      2. Location
         a. Epigastric
            (1) Peptic ulcer
            (2) Esophagitis
            (3) Hiatal hernia
            (4) Pancreatitis

TABLE 11-1

ACUTE ABDOMINAL PAIN DIAGNOSES IN CHILDREN RANKED APPROXIMATELY BY AGE AND SEVERITY

Diagnosis	Age Group	Potentially Life-Threatening	Comments
Necrotizing enterocolitis	Infant	Yes	Premature infants with abdominal tenderness, vomiting, apnea, hypotension; older full-term infants with congenital heart disease
Midgut volvulus	Infant	Yes	Underlying malrotation of bowel; vomiting is presenting symptom; may have very large third space fluid losses
Intussusception	Infant (2 mo-2 yr)	Yes	Intermittent severe, crampy pain; vomiting; bloody ("currant jelly") stool; decreased level of consciousness may be presenting sign, so high index of suspicion needed
Incarcerated inguinal hernia	Infant	Yes	Hernias overall more common in boys; girls more likely to have incarcerated hernia involving ovary; firm, tender inguinal mass extending into scrotum or labia (more common on the right side)
Meckel diverticulum	Infant	Rare	Abdominal pain with rectal bleeding
Infantile colic	Infant	No	No other symptoms; normal examination findings
Hirschsprung disease associated enterocolitis	Infant, child	Yes	Abdominal pain, distention, bilious vomiting, diarrhea, fever; x-ray shows dilated colon with air-fluid levels, gasless rectum
Foreign body ingestion	Child	Yes	Abdominal pain after ingestion of sharp or large (>5 cm) object or button battery; indicates need for surgical evaluation
Henoch-Schönlein purpura	Child	No	Colicky abdominal pain with bloody stools, purpuric rash on buttocks and lower extremities
Ectopic pregnancy	Female teenager	Yes	Abdominal pain, amenorrhea, and vaginal bleeding, typically 6-8 wk after a missed menstrual period
Pelvic inflammatory disease	Female teenager	Rare	Bilateral lower abdominal pain, worse during menses or intercourse; life-threatening if sepsis, tubo-ovarian abscess, or other intra-abdominal infection

TABLE 11-1

ACUTE ABDOMINAL PAIN DIAGNOSES IN CHILDREN RANKED APPROXIMATELY BY AGE AND SEVERITY—cont'd

Diagnosis	Age Group	Potentially Life-Threatening	Comments
Inflammatory bowel disease	Child, teenager	Rare	Abdominal pain often with bloody diarrhea, weight loss, and nonintestinal manifestations (e.g., arthritis, rash)
Diabetic ketoacidosis	All	Yes	Abdominal pain with history of polydipsia and polyuria
Gastroenteritis	All	Yes (in poor environment)	Abdominal pain accompanied by diarrhea; massive watery diarrhea in infants leads to dehydration, shock; bloody diarrhea (Shigella, Salmonella, Escherichia coli) can lead to life-threatening complications (e.g., seizures, hemolytic-uremic syndrome)
Adhesions	All	Yes	Abdominal pain, distension, vomiting in patient with history of previous abdominal surgery
Peptic ulcer disease	All	Yes	Hemorrhage and perforation more likely in younger children; most common causes—corticosteroids, NSAIDs, critical illness (burns, head trauma, etc.); Helicobacter pylori less common than in adults
Appendicitis	All (especially teenagers)	Yes	Periumbilical pain migrates to right lower quadrant (RLQ); RLQ pain elicited on rectal examination
Pneumonia	All	Yes	Abdominal pain, often with fever and tachypnea
Pancreatitis	All	Yes	Epigastric pain often associated with fever and vomiting; history may include trauma, gallstones, medications, multiple organ dysfunction
Sickle cell disease—vaso-occlusive crisis	All	Rare	Highly variable pain patterns often triggered by dehydration, infection, stress; 50% of cases associated with other objective signs and symptoms (fever, tenderness, vomiting, tachycardia)
Urinary tract infection	All	No	Abdominal pain associated with fever, dysuria, frequency, vomiting (infants), and flank pain (children)
Constipation	All	No	Less than three stools/wk; fecal incontinence in severe cases; colicky pain
Pharyngitis	All	No	Abdominal pain combined with fever, sore throat

---

BOX 11-1

CONDITIONS TYPICALLY REQUIRING SURGICAL INTERVENTION

- Appendicitis
- Intestinal obstruction
- Perforated viscus
- Incarcerated hernia
- Volvulus
- Nonreduced intussusception
- Torsion of testicle or ovary
- Necrotic pancreatitis
- Toxic megacolon
- Acute cholecystitis

BOX 11-2

INDICATIONS FOR SURGICAL CONSULTATION WITH ACUTE ABDOMINAL PAIN

History of significant abdominal trauma
Bilious or feculent vomitus
Severe or worsening abdominal pain with clinical deterioration
Abdominal rigidity or guarding
Rebound abdominal tenderness
Marked abdominal distention
Acute fluid or blood loss into abdomen

---

    b. Periumbilical
      (1) Appendicitis
      (2) Cholangitis
      (3) Pancreatitis
      (4) Inflammatory bowel disease
    c. Left upper quadrant
      (1) Splenic abscess
      (2) Malignancy
    d. Right upper quadrant
      (1) Hepatitis
      (2) Cholecystitis
      (3) Cholangitis
      (4) Tumors
    e. Lower quadrant
      (1) Appendicitis
      (2) Inflammatory bowel disease
      (3) Tubo-ovarian abscess
      (4) Acute ovarian torsion
      (5) Pelvic inflammatory disease
      (6) Ectopic pregnancy
    f. Suprapubic
      (1) Urinary tract infection
      (2) Urolithiasis
      (3) Uteropelvic obstruction
      (4) Pregnancy
      (5) Pelvic inflammatory disease
      (6) Dysmenorrhea

3. Examination
    a. Examining the child with acute abdominal pain requires patience and gentleness to gain the child's trust.
    b. In addition to the abdomen, a full examination of the patient is essential, including the lungs, testes and scrotum, inguinal regions, rectum, and costovertebral areas.
4. General appearance and vital signs
    a. Pallor, diaphoresis, restlessness, or rigidity can all be clues to the severity or cause of the underlying disorder.
    b. The child with visceral pain may writhe when experiencing peristaltic waves, whereas the child with peritonitis may be quiet and resist movement.
    c. Fever may indicate underlying infection or inflammation.
    d. Tachycardia, hypotension, and delayed capillary refill may indicate hypovolemia.
5. Abdominal examination
    a. Evaluate for contour, scars, hernias, vascular pattern, presence or absence of bowel sounds, skin hyperesthesia, and areas of maximal tenderness or presence of rebound tenderness.
    b. Attempt deeper palpation to evaluate for masses or organomegaly.
    c. Rare signs may be noted, such as periumbilical discoloration (Cullen sign), suggesting intraperitoneal bleeding, or flank discoloration (Grey Turner sign), suggesting retroperitoneal bleeding.
6. Rectal and pelvic examinations
    a. These should be limited to one or at most two examiners and when significant information is expected to be obtained.
    b. A digital rectal examination may provide useful information about tenderness, sphincter tone, and presence of masses, stool, or blood in the stool.
    c. Examination of the external male genitalia may reveal penile and scrotal abnormalities.
    d. In girls, pelvic examination may reveal purulent vaginal or cervical discharge, cervical motion tenderness, and/or uterine or adnexal masses.
7. Associated extra-abdominal signs
    a. Iliopsoas and obturator tests suggest an inflamed or ruptured appendix, peritonitis, or an iliopsoas abscess.
        A positive iliopsoas test: In the left lateral decubitus position, flank pain is elicited during passive hyperextension of the right thigh while the examiner applies counter-pressure to the right hip.
        A positive obturator test: In the supine position with the right hip and knee flexed and counter-pressure applied to

the lateral aspect of the right knee, abdominal or pelvic pain is elicited during internal rotation of the right thigh combined with lateral movement of the lower leg.
   b. Murphy sign: A positive Murphy sign (pain with deep inspiration during palpation of the right subcostal area) suggests acute cholecystitis.
   c. Jaundice: Jaundice suggests hemolysis or liver disease.
   d. Purpura and arthritis: Purpura and arthritis suggest Henoch-Schönlein purpura.
8. Laboratory and radiographic studies
   a. Studies to be obtained depend on the diagnosis under consideration (**Tables 11-2** and **11-3**).
   b. Commonly obtained initial tests include a complete blood cell count and urinalysis.
   c. A negative pregnancy test should be documented in postmenarchal girls before ordering radiographs or computed tomography (CT) scans.

TABLE 11-2

RECOMMENDED SCREENING LABORATORY STUDIES FOR EVALUATION OF ACUTE ABDOMINAL PAIN

Test	Finding	Suggested Diagnosis
Complete blood count	Leukocytosis	Bacterial gastroenteritis, pyelonephritis, pancreatitis, appendicitis, peritonitis
	Anemia	Peptic ulcer disease, varices, Meckel diverticulum, sickle cell anemia, inflammatory bowel disease
Urinalysis	Positive leukocyte esterase, positive nitrites, positive Gram stain, or >10 WBCs/mm³	Urinary tract infection
	Positive glucose and ketones	Diabetic ketoacidosis
Chemistry panel	Hypokalemia and hypochloremia	Duodenal or gastric outlet obstruction leading to vomiting
	Hyponatremia or hypernatremia	Any cause of diarrhea
	Acidosis	Gastroenteritis → dehydration; diabetic ketoacidosis
	Elevated BUN level	Dehydration, intussusception, hemolytic-uremic syndrome
	Elevated serum aspartate, AST, and ALT levels	Acute hepatitis (viral or drug-induced)
	Elevated alkaline phosphatase and bilirubin levels	Gallbladder disease, bile duct obstruction, cholangitis
	Elevated amylase and lipase levels	Pancreatitis
Other	Positive pregnancy test (hCG)	Ectopic pregnancy
	Positive gram stain and culture of vaginal or urethral discharge	Sexually transmitted disease

ALT, Alanine aminotransferase; *AST*, aspartate aminotransferase; *BUN*, blood urea nitrogen; *hCG*, human chorionic gonadotrophin; *WBC*, white blood cells.

TABLE 11-3

RECOMMENDED RADIOGRAPHIC STUDIES FOR EVALUATION OF ACUTE ABDOMINAL PAIN

Test	Comments
Abdominal radiography	To evaluate for free air in peritoneal cavity (perforation), mass, air-fluid levels (Hirschsprung disease or toxic megacolon), gasless bowel, foreign bodies, appendicolith (appendicitis); obtain supine and upright views and lateral, if necessary
Chest radiography	Obtain two views for lower lobe pneumonia
Abdominal ultrasonography	To evaluate for mass, appendicitis, intussusception, ovarian pathology, bowel wall thickening, free fluid
CT or MRI of abdomen	Indications similar to ultrasonography; pancreatitis visualized much better with CT scanning than with ultrasound

CT, Computed tomography; *MRI,* magnetic resonance imaging.

    d. In additional to abdominal radiographs, other radiologic studies may be indicated after surgical consultation for patients with a surgical acute abdomen.

  D. Management

    1. Treatment of acute abdominal pain should be directed at the underlying cause.

    2. Traditionally, the use of analgesics has been discouraged in patients with abdominal pain because of the fear that it would interfere with accurate evaluation and diagnosis, but we disagree.

    3. Judicious use of analgesics may permit a more thorough examination of the patient and lead to a more timely and correct diagnosis.

II. Vomiting

  A. Differential diagnoses

    1. The causes of nausea and vomiting are vast and include infections (Chapter 19), intestinal obstructions (Chapters 23 and 32), metabolic disorders (Chapter 8), toxins (Chapters 15 and 16), neurologic problems (Chapter 17), endocrine disorders (Chapter 10), psychological disorders, pregnancy, and postoperative or postanesthesia problems.

    2. The initial primary goal is to diagnose and treat the particular disorder causing vomiting and treat or prevent dehydration. Treating the symptom is also important for common non–life-threatening causes of vomiting such as after general anesthesia, opioids, certain psychological disorders, or mild gastroenteritis.

  B. Symptomatic management

    1. A wide variety of drugs with different mechanisms of action have been used to treat or prevent opioid-induced nausea and vomiting.

TABLE 11-4

RECOMMENDED DOSING OF THE MOST COMMONLY USED ANTIEMETICS

Antiemetic	Dosing Frequency	Maximum Dose (mg)	Route of Administration		
			IV (mg/kg)	PO	Rectal
Ondansetron	q4-6h	8	0.15	8-15 kg: 2 mg 15-30 kg: 4 mg >31 kg: 8 mg	
Diphenhydramine	q4-6h	50	1	1 mg/kg	
Promethazine (contraindicated age <2 years)	q4-6h	25	0.25-1	0.25-1 mg/kg	0.25-1 mg/kg
Prochlorperazine (contraindicated age <2 years)	q8-12h	5 (PO, rectal)	0.15	2.5 mg	2.5 mg
Metoclopramide	q2-4h	50	1-2	1-2 mg/kg	
Dexamethasone	Single dose	25	0.25-1		

IV, Intravenous; *PO*, oral.

  a. The most commonly used antiemetics are listed in **Table 11-4.**
  b. These include antihistamines (diphenhydramine, hydroxyzine), phenothiazines (prochlorperazine, promethazine), butyrophenones (haloperidol, droperidol), benzamides (metoclopramide), 5-HT$_3$ receptor antagonists (ondansetron, dolasetron, granisetron), and corticosteroids (dexamethasone).
 2. Many of the agents listed work synergistically. Although it does not make sense to combine two drugs that act via the same mechanism (e.g., two antihistamines such as diphenhydramine and hydroxyzine), combinations of drugs that act via different mechanisms (e.g., ondansetron, a selective inhibitor of type 3 serotonin receptors, and the steroid dexamethasone) can be effective.
III. Upper gastrointestinal bleeding
  A. Overview
   1. Upper gastrointestinal (GI) bleeding is defined as bleeding that originates above the ligament of Treitz.
   2. Although hematemesis (vomiting of bright red blood or dark, coffee ground–appearing material) can cause anxiety and distress in a child and parent, significant upper GI bleeding does not occur frequently in pediatric patients.
   3. Those at highest risk are acutely or chronically ill hospitalized children, particularly patients being cared for in an intensive care unit setting.
   4. Fatalities are very rare in children given their robust physiology and relatively low incidence of comorbid conditions.

TABLE 11-5

CAUSES OF UPPER GASTROINTESTINAL BLEEDING IN CHILDREN

Newborn	Infancy to Adolescence
Swallowed maternal blood	Swallowed blood (epistaxis)
Hemorrhagic disease (vitamin K deficiency)	Varices
Gastritis	Gastritis
Esophagitis	Esophagitis
Ulcer (gastric or duodenal)	Ulcer (gastric or duodenal)
Vascular malformation	Vascular malformation
Coagulopathy associated with infection	Coagulopathy
Congenital anomaly (web, duplication)	Gastrointestinal duplication, inflammatory bowel disease (Crohn's disease), Mallory-Weiss tear, caustic ingestion

B. Causes

Apart from disorders unique to the newborn, the causes of upper GI bleeding are similar in children of all ages (**Table 11-5**).

C. Assessment

1. The history is directed at possible underlying medical disorders, including gastroesophageal reflux disease, esophagitis, peptic ulcer disease, bulimia, inflammatory bowel disease, chronic liver disease, immunodeficiency, coagulopathy, renal insufficiency, congenital heart disease, use of medications (e.g., nonsteroidal anti-inflammatory drugs, corticosteroids, alcohol), and foreign bodies.

2. Stress ulcers can be seen in shock, sepsis, trauma, and burns.

3. Laboratory and radiologic studies are carried out, depending on differential diagnoses and to assess the degree of bleeding and hydration status (**Table 11-6** and **11-7**)

D. Physical examination

1. Determine heart rate (HR), blood pressure (BP), and capillary refill to assess severity of blood loss; evaluate for orthostatic changes

2. Inspect the following:

   a. Nail beds for delay in capillary refill

   b. Nasal mucosa and oropharynx for ulceration or bleeding

   c. Abdomen for distention, ascites, hepatosplenomegaly, caput medusae

   d. Skin for pallor, jaundice, or cutaneous abnormalities (spider hemangiomata)

E. Management

See **Figure 11-1**.

1. Most children have excellent cardiac, pulmonary, and renal function and can adapt to substantial blood loss without major effects on cardiopulmonary function. Hematocrit may take

---

TABLE 11-6

RECOMMENDED LABORATORY STUDIES FOR UPPER GASTROINTESTINAL BLEEDING

Test	Comments
Hematocrit, hemoglobin	Marker of acute or chronic blood loss
Platelet count	Low count may be seen with disseminated intravascular coagulopathy, hypersplenism, portal hypertension, or with severe hemorrhage; can be elevated in acute inflammation
Red blood cell indices	Indicators of bleeding chronicity or iron deficiency
Prothrombin and partial thromboplastin times	Elevated values could suggest underlying liver disease, vitamin K deficiency, disseminated intravascular coagulation, or coagulation disorders such as hemophilia
Testing of emesis or gastric lavage for blood	To confirm presence of blood in emesis or gastric lavage if unclear
Bilirubin	Elevated in liver disease or hemolysis (indirect bilirubin)
Alanine transaminase	Elevated in liver disease (primarily hepatocellular)
Aspartate transaminase	Elevated in liver disease (primarily hepatocellular)
Alkaline phosphatase	Elevated in liver disease (primarily cholestatic)

TABLE 11-7

RECOMMENDED DIAGNOSTIC STUDIES FOR UPPER GASTROINTESTINAL BLEEDING

Test	Comments
Plain abdominal radiography	To look for foreign body, distended bowel loops, or free intra-abdominal air, indicating perforation
Upper gastrointestinal series	May detect deep ulcer or other mucosal lesions but considered too insensitive to detect superficial mucosal lesions
Ultrasonography	If liver disease or portal hypertension suspected
CT or MRI	To evaluate for mass lesions
Esophagogastroduodenoscopy (EGD)	Permits visualization and biopsy of specific lesions and opportunity for immediate therapeutic intervention
^{99m}Tc-labeled red blood cells	To localize bleeding site
Angiography	To localize bleeding site (bleeding rate >0.5-1 mL/min required for adequate visualization of bleeding site)

CT, Computed tomography; *MRI,* magnetic resonance imaging.

---

approximately 24 hours to equilibrate; thus, the initial hematocrit may not be as accurate as the child's overall appearance, vital signs, perfusion, and color.

2. Place a large-bore nasogastric tube to lavage the stomach and obtain aspirate to look for recent or active bleeding.
   a. Lavage should be done with a sufficient quantity of room temperature normal saline (NS) to sample patient's gastric volume adequately.
   b. If lavage is negative, it may still not exclude a bleeding duodenal ulcer.
   c. Iced saline lavage is not recommended in children because of risk of hypothermia.

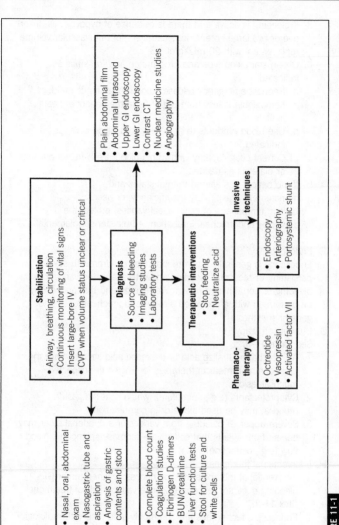

FIGURE 11-1

Management of gastrointestinal bleeding.

BUN, Blood urea nitrogen; *GI,* gastrointestinal; *CT,* computed tomography; *IV,* intravenous.

    3. If bleeding is active and there is evidence of hypovolemia, insert one or two large-bore venous catheters for intravascular volume replacement with 20 mL/kg of NS.

    4. Obtain stat blood type and crossmatch and transfuse as indicated.

       a. Request emergency release blood if bleeding is rapid, hemoglobin is less than 8 g/dL, and the patient appears acutely ill.

       b. Use blood products (e.g., packed red blood cells) as indicated.

       c. Correct coagulopathy with whole blood, fresh-frozen plasma, or platelets as needed.

    5. If the patient has altered mental status and hematemesis, respiratory insufficiency, or needs balloon tamponade of esophageal varices, protect the airway by endotracheal intubation. Administer supplemental oxygen.

F. Endoscopy

Endoscopy is generally recommended for children with severe, persistent, or recurrent bleeding and with suspected variceal bleeding or portal hypertension. We recommend that endoscopy be performed with a protected airway (endotracheal tube) under general anesthesia.

G. Pharmacotherapy

See **Table 11-8.**

    1. Agents that neutralize acid or decrease acid secretion are the most common medical therapies for known or suspected mucosal lesions.

    2. Cytoprotectants (e.g., sucralfate), which coat the gastric mucosa, may be used alone or in combination.

    3. Severe upper GI bleeding from varices or a duodenal ulcer may benefit from agents that selectively decrease splanchnic blood flow (e.g., octreotide).

H. Interventional therapies

    1. Interventional therapies may be necessary when upper GI bleeding does not respond to conservative medical treatment (**Box 11-3**).

    2. Endoscopic techniques are commonly tried first, with radiologic and surgical techniques reserved for situations in which endoscopy fails or is unavailable.

I. Liver disease

    1. In patients with liver disease, upper GI bleeding with or without hypotension can precipitate further hepatic dysfunction, ascites, and encephalopathy.

    2. See Chapter 12 for treatment details.

TABLE 11-8

PHARMACOTHERAPIES TO PREVENT UPPER GASTROINTESTINAL BLEEDING

Medication	Dose (Oral Unless Otherwise Indicated)
H$_2$ RECEPTOR ANTAGONISTS	
Ranitidine	4-10 mg/kg/day divided bid, tid; adult, 150-300 mg bid
	2-4 mg/kg/day IV divided bid, tid
Cimetidine	40 mg/kg/day divided tid, qid; adult, 400-800 mg bid
Famotidine	0.6-0.8 mg/kg/day divided bid, tid, to max 40 mg/day
	1 mg/kg/day IV divided bid
Nizatidine	10 mg/kg/day divided bid; adult, 150 mg bid or 300 mg at bedtime
PROTON PUMP INHIBITORS	
Omeprazole	0.7-3.3 mg/kg/day divided qd, bid; adult, 20-40 mg/day
Lansoprazole	15-30 mg/day divided qd, bid(for children and adults),
Pantoprazole	Limited data in children: 20 mg qd or 0.5-1 mg/kg qd (for children <20 kg); adult, 40 mg/day
CYTOPROTECTION	
Sucralfate	40-80 mg/kg/day divided bid, qid; adult, 1-4 g/day divided qid
Misoprostol (do not use in women or teenage girls because of reproductive risks)	Adult, 800 mcg/day divided bid, qid
VASOCONSTRICTION	
Octreotide	1 mcg/kg/dose IV (max, 100 mcg) bolus, followed by 1 mcg/kg/hr IV continuously
Vasopressin	2-10 milliunit/kg/min (0.002-0.010 unit/kg/min) IV continuously

BOX 11-3

INTERVENTIONAL THERAPIES FOR UPPER GASTROINTESTINAL HEMOSTASIS

ENDOSCOPIC TECHNIQUES

Electrocoagulation
Heater probe
Epinephrine injection
Sclerosant for varices
Elastic band ligator for varices

RADIOLOGIC TECHNIQUES

Angiographic embolization
Transjugular intrahepatic portosystemic shunt

SURGICAL TECHNIQUES

Oversewing ulcer bed
Portosystemic vascular shunts for intractable variceal bleeding

TABLE 11-9	
CAUSES OF LOWER GASTROINTESTINAL BLEEDING	
Newborn	**Infancy to Adolescence**
Gastrointestinal infection	Gastrointestinal infection
	Food protein allergy
Necrotizing enterocolitis	Meckel diverticulum
Allergic (e.g., cow milk/soy) proctocolitis	Intussusception
Hemorrhagic disease (vitamin K deficiency)	Polyps
Congenital anomalies (Hirschsprung disease)	Inflammatory bowel disease
Anal fissure	Anal fissure
Volvulus	Volvulus
	Hemolytic-uremic syndrome
	Angiodysplasia
	Bleeding diathesis
	Henoch Schönlein purpura

IV. Lower gastrointestinal bleeding
  A. Introduction
    1. Lower GI bleeding is defined as bleeding distal to the ligament of Treitz and is commonly encountered in clinical pediatric practice.
    2. Investigation of lower GI bleeding requires an understanding of the most likely causes based on the patient's age, amount and appearance of the blood loss, and associated clinical features (**Table 11-9**).
  B. Patterns of presentation of lower GI bleeding
    1. Maroon-colored stool suggests bleeding from the distal small intestine.
    2. Melanotic stool (black tarry stool, darker clots) suggests bleeding from the small intestine.
    3. Hematochezia (bright red blood per rectum) usually indicates bleeding from the colon rather than the small intestine or upper GI tract.
    4. Currant jelly stool (mixture of blood, mucus, and stool) suggests ischemic or inflammatory lesions, such as intussusception or acute colitis.
    5. Blood-streaked formed stool suggests a distal colonic lesion, such as an anal fissure, hemorrhoid, or juvenile polyp.
  C. Mimickers of gastrointestinal bleeding
    1. Red-appearing stools
      a. Exogenous blood
      b. Swallowed maternal blood (from cracked nipples in a breast-fed infant)
      c. Epistaxis
      d. Ingestion of red medications or foods (e.g., tomatoes, beets, punch, gelatin)

      e. *Serratia marcescens* in stool causing red pigmentation in soiled diapers

   2. Black-appearing stools

      a. Iron preparations

      b. Bismuth salicylate preparations

      c. Purple grape juice or grapes

      d. Spinach

      e. Chocolate

D. Assessment

   1. Obtain pertinent information regarding possible contributing factors, such as a history of constipation, crampy pain with diarrhea, passage of mucus with the stool; dietary factors such as iron supplements, other medications, or red foods that may alter stool appearance.

   2. If bleeding is melanotic or copious, also consider upper GI bleed as possible source.

   3. Laboratory and radiologic studies are carried out depending on the differential diagnoses and to assess degree of bleeding and hydration status.

E. Physical examination

   1. Determine HR and BP to assess severity of blood loss; evaluate for orthostatic changes.

   2. Inspect the following:

      a. Nail beds for delay in capillary refill

      b. Nasal mucosa and oropharynx for ulceration or bleeding

      c. Abdomen for mass distention, ascites, hepatosplenomegaly, caput medusae

      d. Perianal area for fissures

      e. Skin for jaundice

   3. Perform digital rectal examination and test for occult blood.

F. Diagnosis and management (**Table 11-10**)

See Figure 11-1.

   1. If lower GI bleeding is copious, consider the possibility of brisk upper GI bleed.

      a. Evaluate by placing a nasogastric tube to lavage the stomach and aspirate gastric secretions to look for recent or active bleeding.

      b. Lavage should be done with a sufficient quantity of room temperature NS to sample patient's gastric volume adequately.

   2. If lavage is negative, it may still not exclude a bleeding duodenal ulcer.

      a. The presence of blood-free bile in the aspirate more confidently excludes the possibility of ongoing bleeding proximal to the ligament of Treitz.

TABLE 11-10

DIAGNOSTIC STUDIES FOR LOWER GI BLEEDING

Test	Comments
Plain abdominal radiography	To look for foreign body or free intra-abdominal air indicating perforation
Barium enema	No role in initial evaluation unless intussusception is suspected
Ultrasonography	If liver disease or portal hypertension suspected
CT or MRI	To evaluate for mass lesions
Colonoscopy	Permits visualization and biopsy of specific lesions and opportunity for immediate therapeutic intervention
Enteroscopy	To evaluate small intestine
^{99m}Tc-pertechnetate (Meckel scan)	To detect ectopic gastric mucosa in Meckel diverticulum or intestinal duplications
^{99m}Tc-labeled red blood cells	To localize bleeding site
Angiography	To localize bleeding site—bleeding rate >0.5-1 mL/min required for adequate visualization of bleeding site
Intra-operative endoscopy	To localize bleeding site if other tests fail to identify source

CT, Computed tomography; *MRI,* magnetic resonance imaging.

b. Iced saline lavage is not recommended in the pediatric population because of risk of hypothermia.
3. If bleeding is active and there is evidence of hypovolemia, administer NS and blood products as described for upper GI bleeding (see earlier).
F. Therapy
1. Medical therapies depend on the diagnosis. Examples include use of antibiotics for infectious colitis, restriction of dietary protein for allergic colitis, and immunosuppressive and anti-inflammatory drugs for inflammatory bowel disease.
2. Endoscopic therapies in children are typically limited to polypectomy. However, other hemostatic techniques have been used in children for vascular colonic anomalies.
3. Surgical therapies are typically indicated to resect ischemic or necrotic bowel, Meckel diverticulum, or intestinal duplication or to treat a nonreducible intussusception (see Chapter 23). Patients with vascular anomalies may also require excision of focal lesions or resection of larger segments of involved intestine.
V. Acute pancreatitis
A. Definition
This is an inflammatory condition characterized by two or three of the following criteria:
1. Abdominal pain (usually radiating to the back)
2. Increased serum amylase level, more than three times normal
3. Abnormal pancreas on CT scan

B. Pathophysiology
  1. Acute pancreatitis is an autodigestive process that involves activation of trypsinogen to trypsin.
     a. This leads to release of all other enzyme precursors, which is an essential early step.
     b. This results in cell damage and necrosis, leading to pancreatic edema and inflammation.
  2. Oxidative stress, impaired microcirculation, and inflammatory cytokine release contribute to pancreatic injury and extrapancreatic complications.
C. Course
  1. The inflammatory process is self-limited (pancreatic and peripancreatic tissues) in 75% to 85% of cases, with resolution typically occurring in less than 1 week. In 15% to 25% of cases, multiple complications can occur.
  2. Mortality is very rare in children.
D. Causes
  1. The causes of acute pancreatitis in children include infections, anatomic abnormalities, medications (e.g., thiazides, corticosteroids, valproic acid, L-asparaginase) and biliary tract disease.
  2. Unlike adults, in which most cases of acute pancreatitis are caused by alcohol ingestion or gallstones, most episodes of severe pancreatitis in children are associated with multiple organ dysfunction (e.g., acute respiratory distress syndrome [ARDS], sepsis, hemolytic uremic syndrome, multiple trauma).
  3. Genetic diseases associated with pancreatitis include cystic fibrosis, diabetes mellitus, and certain hyperlipidemia syndromes.
E. Presentation of acute pancreatitis
  1. The most common presentation of acute pancreatitis is acute abdominal pain.
  2. Although most children will recover without sequelae, significant complications can occur (**Table 11-11**).
F. Laboratory abnormalities
  1. Leukocytosis
  2. Serum amylase level elevated to more than three times normal; may return to normal value by third day of illness
  3. Urine amylase level may remain elevated for longer period.
  4. Elevated serum lipase level; may remain elevated after serum amylase level normalizes
  5. Contrast-enhanced CT scan (especially, thin section multidetector row scans) show the pancreas with edema, heterogeneity of the parenchyma, or peripancreatic fluid collection.

TABLE 11-11

COMPLICATIONS OF ACUTE PANCREATITIS

Complication	Comments
Shock	Most lethal complications in first 24-48 hr after admission; results from transudation and exudation of fluid and myocardial depression caused by release of inflammatory mediators
Hypocalcemia	
Hypomagnesemia	
Jaundice	Seen in approximately 15%-20% of patients (total serum bilirubin usually <4 mg/dL unless coexisting liver disease or obstruction of biliary tree)
Hypoxemia	
Atelectasis	
Pleural effusions	
ARDS	
Acute renal failure	May require dialysis
Pancreatic necrosis	Has high infection rate; major risk factor for mortality in severe pancreatitis
Sepsis or abscess	
Pancreatic pseudocyst	May develop in approximately 15% of cases, especially traumatic pancreatitis

ARDS, Acute respiratory distress syndrome.

6. Ultrasound is generally an insensitive test for pancreatitis, but may detect an associated common bile duct stone.

VI. Foreign body ingestion
   A. Introduction
      1. Ingestion of a foreign body is a frequent occurrence in children but usually causes little morbidity.
      2. Most foreign body ingestions in children are not witnessed, so most may remain asymptomatic.
   B. General principles
      1. Coins are the foreign bodies most commonly swallowed by children.
      2. Most foreign body ingestions occur in children younger than 5 years.
      3. Most foreign bodies will be located in the stomach at initial evaluation.
      4. More than 80% of foreign bodies that come to medical attention will pass spontaneously. There is less chance of spontaneous passage from the GI tract in adults if the object is longer than 10 cm, in the older child if it is longer than 5 cm or wider than 2 cm, and in the infant if it is more than 2 cm in length or width.
      5. Perforation of the intestinal tract is rare, occurring in less than 1% of cases; sharp objects are associated with a higher perforation rate than nonsharp objects.
      6. Foreign bodies impacted in the oropharynx are usually sharp (e.g., bone), give rise to symptoms, and may cause significant

complications, such as perforation and retropharyngeal abscess.

C. Symptoms
   1. Symptoms of foreign body obstruction can be variable depending on the patient's age and location and size of the object.
   2. In young children, symptoms may be nonspecific, such as choking, drooling, and poor feeding.
   3. Respiratory distress may be the only symptom of a foreign body in the esophagus, particularly in the infant or toddler.

D. Common sites of foreign body obstruction in the GI tract in children
   1. Proximal esophagus at the level of the upper esophageal sphincter
   2. Proximal esophagus at the level of the thoracic inlet
   3. Distal esophagus at the level of the lower esophageal sphincter
   4. Pylorus
   5. Duodenal loop
   6. Ileocecal valve

E. Management
   1. As a general rule, objects that are sharp, large, located proximally to the duodenum, or producing pain should be considered for endoscopic removal.
   2. Biplane radiographs of the neck, chest, and upper abdomen are the initial laboratory investigations. Because of the risk of aspiration, endoscopy rather than contrast radiography should be used if there is a high suspicion of a radiolucent (approximately 35%) foreign body lodged in the esophagus.
   3. Emergent endoscopy is recommended for buttons, batteries, or sharp objects in the esophagus.
   4. Avoid using meat tenderizers to remove a food impaction because they can cause esophageal inflammation, ulceration, and perforation.
   5. Tissue injury can occur with battery ingestion because of pressure necrosis, low-voltage burns, or corrosive injury from leakage of the alkaline solution.
      a. Symptoms are uncommon following battery ingestion (<10% of cases).
      b. If a battery is ingested and remains in the stomach for 48 hours, consider endoscopic removal.
   6. Pushing a nonsharp object into the stomach with a bougie dilator or catheter may risk esophageal tear or perforation.
   7. If a blunt object remains in the stomach or intestines longer than 3 to 4 weeks or if the object remains in the same location on serial radiographs, consider endoscopic or surgical removal.

Chapter 12

Liver Failure

Michael A. Nares, MD,
and Steven J. Lobritto, MD

I. Definition
   A. Loss of primary liver functions
      This includes changes in protein synthesis, glucose homeostasis, bile excretion, lipid metabolism, drug detoxification, coagulation, urea clearance, and complement formation, culminating in the development of hepatic encephalopathy.
   B. Categorization
      These are classified as fulminant, subfulminant, or chronic, depending on the time in which hepatic encephalopathy develops in relation to the onset of clinical jaundice.
   C. Further subdivisions
      1. Hyperacute: Development of encephalopathy within 7 days of onset of biochemical abnormalities (potential for spontaneous recovery)
      2. Acute: Development of encephalopathy within 8 to 28 days of onset of biochemical abnormalities (potential for spontaneous recovery)
      3. Subacute: Development of encephalopathy within 5 to 12 weeks of onset of biochemical abnormalities (rarely recovers without transplantation)
      4. Late-onset liver failure: Development of encephalopathy within 2 to 6 months of onset of biochemical abnormalities
      5. Chronic liver failure: Development of encephalopathy more than 6 months after onset of biochemical abnormalities
II. Complications
   A. Hepatic encephalopathy
      1. Develops in children with liver failure at varying rates after insult and to varying degrees of severity
      2. Children with acute viral or toxic hepatic injury usually develop hepatic encephalopathy at a much faster rate than those with chronic liver injury.
      3. Five stages of hepatic encephalopathy in older children and adults:
         a. Stage I: Patient is alert and oriented but may have slow mentation; mild tremor may be identified.

      b. Stage II: Patient may be lethargic, confused, or agitated; intention tremor may be present; may be hyperventilating; asterixis can be easily elicited; pupillary response is normal.

      c. Stage III: Patient may be stuporous and may be aroused with verbal stimuli; muscle tone is increased and child is hyper-reflexic; there may be decreased spontaneous motor activity and a marked intention tremor may be identified; hyperventilation is present; asterixis is present if child is cooperative; pupillary response is normal.

      d. Stage IV: Child may be unarousable and spontaneous motor activity is absent; muscle tone is increased and child is hyper-reflexic; respirations are irregular; posturing (decorticate or decerebrate) may be observed; pupillary response is sluggish.

      e. Stage V: Child is unarousable and there is no spontaneous motor activity; apnea is present and the pupils are fixed.

   4. In the infant, these stages are more difficult to discern. Changes in motor tone, suck, reflexes, and arousability define the progression from one stage to the next.

   5. Mortality without liver transplantation:

      a. Stage II or III encephalopathy: 35%-65%

      b. Stage IV or V encephalopathy: >80%

B. Pathogenesis of hepatic encephalopathy

   1. Increase in serum ammonia level

   2. Accumulating neurotoxins that have not been cleared by the liver.

   3. Increased inhibitory neurotransmitters and decreased excitatory neurotransmitters.

   4. Inhibitory false neurotransmitter substances with γ-aminobutyric acid (GABA)—like activity (GABA is the most prominent inhibitory neurotransmitter in the central nervous system [CNS]).

C. Cerebral edema

   1. Present in 25% to 80% of children with fulminant hepatic failure

   2. No apparent correlation between cerebral edema and the time spent in grade IV encephalopathy, degree of hypoglycemia, hemorrhage, or hypotension

   3. Papilledema is an unreliable and late sign of cerebral edema.

   4. Computed tomography scan may be used to determine the presence of cerebral edema, but is not sufficiently sensitive to determine raised intracranial pressure.

   5. Pathology: Significant for swollen astrocytes

12

D. Coagulopathy
   1. Coagulopathy is common in liver failure; the liver is the main site of the production of coagulation factors and inhibitors of coagulation.
   2. Cholestasis predisposes to vitamin K deficiency, resulting in prolongation of both the prothrombin time (PT) and activated partial thromboplastin time (aPTT).
   3. The most common coagulation defects are decreased levels of the vitamin K—dependent cofactors (II, VII, IX, X) as well as factor V.
   4. Because there is hepatocyte damage, the coagulopathy is usually unresponsive to vitamin K replacement.
   5. Decreased levels of antithrombin III also contribute to activation of the coagulation cascade, exacerbating coagulopathy through consumption of factors.
   6. Disseminated intravascular coagulation (DIC) occurs as the liver is a site of inflammatory mediators; with the onset of DIC, platelets are consumed and thrombocytopenia may be present.
   7. Thrombocytopenia is common, caused by consumption (DIC), sequestration (hypersplenism), and infection (marrow suppression).
   8. Low fibrinogen levels result because of the combination of decreased production and increased consumption by the liver.
   9. The incidence of gastrointestinal (GI) bleeding increases when platelets drop below 50,000/mm^3.

E. Hepatorenal syndrome (HRS)
   1. Accounts for most cases of renal impairment associated with hepatic failure
   2. Defined as an unexplained progressive renal dysfunction in a patient with fulminant hepatic failure without evidence of parenchymal or obstructive kidney disease (by ultrasound)
   3. Characterized by sodium and water retention, low urinary sodium level (<10 mEq/L), benign urinary sediment without protein, cells, or casts; oliguria unresponsive to intravascular volume expansion.
   4. Pathogenesis is not known:
      a. May be related to a dysregulation of homeostasis between intrarenal vasodilators (prostaglandin I_2 and prostaglandin E_2) and vasoconstrictors (thromboxane A_2). However, levels of metabolites of these prostaglandins do not correlate with the presence of HRS.
      b. Another possible cause of HRS is altered renal perfusion secondary to a significant decrease in systemic vascular resistance. The proposed mechanism is a failure of the injured liver to metabolize and clear potent endogenous

vasodilating substances such as vasoactive intestinal peptide or substance P.

    5. HRS is reversible with the replacement of a functioning liver graft.

  F. Infection

    1. Low-complement state predisposes to infection.

    2. Venous access catheters provide portal of entry.

    3. Encourage a low threshold for empiric bacterial and fungal coverage.

III. Assessment and management of the child in acute liver failure

  A. Assessment and stabilization of the ABCs

  This is the first priority and focus of ongoing reassessment.

    1. Ensure patency of the airway (loss of airway reflexes), adequacy of breathing (apnea, adequate tidal volume, respiratory pattern), and circulation (signs of decreased cardiac output).

    2. Once the ABCs are adequate, intravenous access is obtained and blood sampling is done to determine the degree of liver impairment and metabolic disturbance.

  B. Monitoring

    1. If encephalopathy progresses to stage IV, placement of an intracranial pressure (ICP) monitor should be considered because of the risk of brain herniation.

    2. If an ICP monitor is to be placed, it should be done after correction of coagulopathy with activated factor VII, because of the risk of bleeding associated with placement of the device.

  C. Laboratory studies (**Table 12-1**)

    1. Serum chemistry (electrolyte and glucose levels, renal function)

    2. Complete blood count (evidence of infection, anemia, and thrombocytopenia)

    3. Serum albumin level (delayed reflection of hepatic synthetic dysfunction and poor nutritional state because half-life is 20 days).

TABLE 12-1

EARLY AND LATE LABORATORY ABNORMALITIES ASSOCIATED WITH LIVER FAILURE

Laboratory Study	Early Dysfunction	Later Dysfunction
AST	↑↑	Normal, or ↓
ALT	↑↑	Normal, or ↓
Bilirubin	Normal, ↑	↑↑
Glucose	Normal	↓, ↓↓
PT or INR	Normal, prolonged	Prolonged
aPTT	Normal, prolonged	Prolonged
Albumin	Normal	↓
Ammonia	Normal, ↑	↑↑
Lactate	Normal	↑

ALT, Alanine transaminase; *aPTT*, activated partial thromboplastin time; *AST*, aspartate transaminase; *INR*, international normalized ratio of the prothrombin time; *PT*, prothrombin time.

4. Liver enzyme levels (aspartate transaminase [AST], alanine transaminase [ALT], alkaline phosphatase, and γ-glutamyl transpeptidase [GTTP]; indicate degree of hepatocellular injury)

5. Coagulation times (PT, aPTT; best prognostic indicators of hepatic synthetic dysfunction)

6. Ammonia level (indicates hepatic metabolic or clearance function)

7. Bilirubin levels (total and direct)

8. Fibrinogen level (indicates hepatic synthetic function and consumption)

9. Prealbumin (more sensitive than albumin for hepatic synthetic function because half-life is only 2 days)

10. Serum osmolality (assists in fluid management and resuscitation)

IV. Treatment

A. Early management

1. Determine and stop ongoing exposure to hepatic toxins.

2. Monitor closely in a pediatric intensive care unit for neurologic, hemodynamic, and respiratory complications.

3. Perform rapid sequence intubation (see Chapter 2) once patient progresses to stage III or IV hepatic encephalopathy (stupor). Earlier intubation is advised if progression of encephalopathy is rapid.

4. Anticipate that the Pco_2 may rise after intubation if the patient was hyperventilating prior to intubation. Therefore, controlled hyperventilation may be necessary for a period of time after intubation if increased ICP is suspected and until other measures to control ICP can be instituted (see later, "Cerebral Edema").

5. Begin with two thirds maintenance intravenous (IV) fluids containing at least 5% dextrose.

a. IV fluids should be isotonic or hypertonic to minimize free water overload, which could exacerbate cerebral edema.

b. Determine serum glucose level every 1 to 2 hours.

(1) Dextrose concentration in the IV fluids should be adjusted to avoid hypoglycemia

(2) Dextrose concentration in peripheral IV fluids may be increased up to 12.5% to maintain normoglycemia.

(3) Higher dextrose concentration may be warranted, requiring a central venous line.

B. Ammonia-lowering therapies

1. Lactulose

a. Lactulose is a synthetic disaccharide that is neither absorbed nor metabolized in the upper GI tract.

    b. Intestinal bacteria degrade lactulose in the colon, causing acidification of the intestinal lumen.

    c. Acidification of the intestinal lumen enhances the conversion of ammonia (NH_3) to ammonium (NH_4^+), which is not reabsorbed, so excretion is enhanced.

    d. The goal should be two or three soft stools/day with a concomitant decrease in the serum ammonia level.

    e. The route of administration is oral or via a gastric tube if the patient is awake and cough and gag reflexes are intact.

2. Enteral antibiotics

    a. Enteral antibiotic-induced reduction in intestinal flora can lower bacterial protein metabolism and ammonia production.

    b. Although neomycin has been used for years, it is no longer recommended because there are no controlled trials showing it to be more effective than lactulose alone, and neomycin is also associated with nephrotoxicity and ototoxicity.

    c. Metronidazole is better tolerated than neomycin. If the serum ammonia concentration is not reduced with lactulose alone, start metronidazole.

3. Protein intake

    a. Because proteins rich in aromatic amino acids yield increased production of false neurotransmitters, limiting these elements in the diet may limit encephalopathy.

    b. Dairy and vegetable proteins are better tolerated than animal proteins.

    c. Adequate total protein intake must be maintained to prevent catabolism, protein breakdown, and subsequent ammonia production. Supplementation with formulas rich in branched-chain amino acids may have a role in the nutritional management of selected children.

4. Prevent GI bleeding.

    a. GI bleeding is a source of significant protein load and resulting increase in serum ammonia.

    b. The use of H_2 blockers or proton pump inhibitors to raise the gastric pH to >5 has been shown to decrease the incidence of GI bleeding and the need for subsequent red blood cell transfusions.

    c. If GI bleeding is suspected, an orogastric tube can be placed for removing blood and lowering the protein load, with careful attention to avoid undesirable elevations in ICP. (Extreme care is required if nasogastric tube insertion is attempted in a patient with coagulopathy.)

5. Correct hypokalemia and metabolic alkalosis.

    a. Hypokalemia increases renal ammonia production.

    b. Metabolic alkalosis facilitates ammonia entry into the brain.

   c. Therefore, administer supplemental KCl to correct
      hypokalemia in patients with adequate renal function.
C. Treatment of coagulopathy
   1. Vitamin K, 2.5 to 5 mg PO or 1 to 2 mg IV may be instituted.
      The response is usually poor with minimal correction of the PT
      and aPTT.
   2. Avoid routine prophylactic fresh-frozen plasma (FFP)
      administration because of the associated fluid load. FFP should
      be limited to treatment of clinical bleeding or as prophylaxis
      prior to an invasive procedure.
   3. Large-volume FFP replacement may be paired with
      plasmapheresis or CVVH (continuous venovenous
      hemofiltration) if the patient is fluid-overloaded.
   4. Transfuse platelets to maintain a platelet count >50,000 mm^3 if
      an invasive procedure is planned.
   5. Give recombinant factor VII (VIIa), 40 mcg/kg IV,
      if bleeding is severe or refractory to FFP or if the
      coagulopathy cannot otherwise be corrected prior to an invasive
      procedure.
D. Cerebral edema
   1. Deterioration of a child's neurologic status should prompt
      evaluation for cerebral edema and increased ICP.
   2. Frequent clinical examinations and close monitoring may be
      hindered by the need for tracheal intubation and mechanical
      ventilation.
   3. ICP monitoring may be indicated to guide therapy to prevent
      ongoing elevations in ICP. Conversely, there is a risk of bleeding
      with placement of an ICP monitor. Epidural catheters have the
      lowest risk of bleeding. Intraventricular and parenchymal
      catheters have the highest risks.
   4. Correction of coagulopathy with factor VIIa is critical prior to
      placement of an ICP monitoring device.
   5. If increased ICP is suspected (see Chapters 15 and 16):
      a. Ensure that airway is protected.
      b. Hyperventilate the patient if there is impending herniation.
         Otherwise, maintain normocapnia.
      c. Prevent hypotension.
      d. Avoid fluid overload.
      e. Increase serum osmolarity (to ~310-320 mOsm) with
         hypertonic saline or mannitol (if renal function is normal).
      f. Consider pentobarbital or thiopental infusion if other
         therapies have failed.
      g. Definitive treatment of increased ICP in the liver failure
         patient requires liver transplantation.
   6. The goal for ICP management should be to keep ICP
      <20 mm Hg and maintain a cerebral perfusion pressure

>50 mm Hg. Consider adding vasopressors to maintain mean arterial pressure and cerebral perfusion pressure.

E. HRS

1. Children with oliguria secondary to hypovolemia have similar findings to those with HRS, necessitating the careful monitoring (e.g., central venous pressure and partial normalization of the intravascular fluid status prior to making the diagnosis of HRS.

2. Once HRS is diagnosed, sodium and fluid restriction, as well as the use of CVVH, vasopressor medications (e.g., norepinephrine infusion), and replacement of albumin in hypoalbuminemic children may be indicated.

3. The goal is to maintain adequate intravascular volume and tissue perfusion without exacerbating cerebral edema and to correct acid-base and electrolyte abnormalities.

F. Hepatic encephalopathy

1. Avoid sedatives (benzodiazepines and barbiturates) if possible:
   a. These medications cause an alteration of consciousness that may cloud the assessment of the stage of hepatic encephalopathy.
   b. These medications specifically potentiate chloride channel opening caused by GABA binding, which worsens hepatic encephalopathy.
   c. Benzodiazepine and barbiturate metabolism and clearance are prolonged because of hepatic metabolic dysfunction.

2. Use of benzodiazepine antagonists
   a. Flumazenil is a benzodiazepine antagonist that has been reported to improve hepatic encephalopathy.
   b. This reversal is short-lived and does not reverse the underlying problem.

G. Transfer to regional transplantation center

1. After adequate initial stabilization, the child should be transferred to a regional transplantation center at the earliest possible opportunity for management as a potential transplant candidate.

2. Transfer should be considered early to avert transport during progression of the complications of liver failure (e.g., ICP elevation, coagulopathy, metabolic disturbances, encephalopathy).

Chapter 13

Hematologic Emergencies

Aaron L. Zuckerberg, MD,
Myron Yaster, MD,
and David G. Nichols, MD, MBA

I. Overview

The hematologic conditions in children that require rapid diagnosis, intervention, and management in the golden hour are limited and include sickle cell hemoglobinopathy presenting in crisis, immune (idiopathic) thrombocytopenia purpura (ITP), and nontraumatic bleeding.

II. Sickle cell disease

Sickle cell hemoglobinopathy is the most common single gene disorder in African Americans, affecting 1 in 500 individuals. Patients of Arabian, Mediterranean, and Indian descent may be affected as well. The most common variants of sickle cell disease, ranked in order of decreasing severity, are hemoglobin (Hb) SS [HbSS], HbS/β^0, HbSC, and HbS/β^+ thalassemia.

A. Pathophysiology: Red blood cells (RBCs) have

1. Decreased Hb affinity for oxygen (O_2)

2. Abnormal red cell shape and decreased flexibility

3. Hemolysis: Patients with sickle cell disease undergo continuous intravascular hemolysis, resulting in a chronic anemia. Hb concentration typically ranges between 6 and 9 g/dL.

4. Decreased endothelial and intravascular nitric oxide concentration → vasoconstriction, red cell sickling, and platelet and white blood cell adhesion

B. Clinical manifestations

1. Pathophysiology: Acute complications result from microvascular vaso-occlusion and hemolytic anemia.

2. Presenting symptoms: Common childhood complaints of fever, cough, abdominal pain, lethargy, and pallor.

3. Clinical course: Crises occur quickly and can progress rapidly to become life-threatening, so they should be evaluated and treated urgently.

4. Types of crises: Use the mnemonic **SHAPES.**
   Sepsis and other infectious complications
   Hemoglobin low—aplastic anemia
   Acute chest syndrome
   Painful crisis
   Engorgement: Splenic sequestration, priapism
   Stroke

TABLE 13-1

CLINICAL INFECTIONS AND RESPONSIBLE ORGANISMS

Infecting Organism	Type of Infection			
	Bacteremia	**Pneumonia**	**Osteomyelitis**	**Meningitis**
S. pneumoniae	Common	Less common		Common
Salmonella spp.			Common	
Mycoplasma pneumoniae		Common		
Chlamydia pneumoniae		Common		
Staphylococcus aureus	Less common		Less common	
H. influenzae	Less common			Less common
Escherichia coli	Less common			
Respiratory syncytial virus		Common		
Parvovirus		Less common		
Influenza A		Common		

C. Sepsis and other infectious complications
   1. Prevention: Immunization
      Children with sickle cell disease are functionally asplenic and are susceptible to overwhelming infection, particularly meningitis. They must routinely be immunized against pneumococcus, *Hemophilus influenzae*, hepatitis B, and Influenza virus (seasonal influenza A and H1N1).
   2. Prevention: Prophylactic antibiotics
      Ages 3 months-3 years: Penicillin VK, 125 mg orally (PO) bid
      Ages 3-5 years: Penicillin VK, 250 mg PO bid
      Age >5 years: Prophylactic antibiotics are at the discretion of the physician and parents.
   3. Clinical infections and the organisms responsible are shown in **Table 13-1.**
      a. Likely infecting organisms in patients with sickle cell disease are based on the site of infection.
      b. Empty cells in Table 13-1 indicate that the site is very rarely (or never) associated with the specific infecting organism.
D. Evaluation and treatment of infectious complications
   1. Fever (temperature >38.5° C) in a patient with sickle cell disease mandates an aggressive evaluation, including lumbar puncture, particularly in young children. The highest risk group has the following characteristics: HbSS or HbS/β^0 thalassemia genotype; fever >40° C; absence of chronic penicillin prophylaxis regimen.
   2. Laboratory tests in the febrile patients with sickle cell disease:
      a. Complete blood count (CBC)
      b. Blood and urine cultures

13

        c. Chest radiograph
        d. Lumbar puncture (if meningitis is suspected)
   3. Management
        a. Begin cefotaxime, 50 mg/kg intravenous (IV) q8h, stat.
        b. Add vancomycin if penicillin-resistant pneumococci are
           prevalent in the community.
        c. Some centers recommend ceftriaxone, 75-100 mg/kg
           intramuscular (IM), with observation in the emergency
           department for lower risk patients (HbSC, HbS/β^+
           thalassemia and fever <40° C). If stable for several
           hours, patients are discharged home to return in 24 hours
           for a second ceftriaxone dose. Given the very rare but
           potentially fatal risk of ceftriaxone-induced hemolytic
           anemia, we prefer to admit all sickle cell patients with
           possible bacteremia for IV antibiotics (cefotaxime ±
           vancomycin).
E. Aplastic anemia
   1. Pathophysiology
        a. Aplastic anemia: Results when the bone marrow's red cell
           production is temporarily decreased, usually as a
           consequence of infection with parvovirus B19.
        b. Presentation: As Hb drops precipitously, these children
           present in extremis—pale, lethargic, tachycardic, and in
           congestive heart failure.
        c. Duration: Marrow aplasia usually lasts only 7 to 10 days,
           during which these patients require intensive support until
           the bone marrow recovers.
   2. Evaluation
        a. CBC, with reticulocyte count
        b. Viral culture, nasopharyngeal, and rectal
        c. Electrocardiogram—rule out myocardial ischemia
   3. Management
        a. O_2
        b. RBC transfusion to Hb >6 g/dL
        c. Monitor for evidence of congestive heart failure during
           transfusions; may require partial exchange transfusions or
           judicious use of diuretics.
F. Acute chest syndrome (ACS)
   1. Presentation: Fever, new infiltrate on chest radiograph, increase
      in O_2 requirement, tachypnea, dyspnea, and chest pain
   2. Pathophysiology: Results from infection, infarction, or
      pulmonary fat embolism. Rib infarcts may be seen overlying the
      area of involvement. Some patients with sickle cell disease also
      have asthma as a comorbid disease and manifest airway
      hyperreactivity during ACS.

3. Clinical course: Sudden and potentially fatal deterioration is possible. Therefore, observation in an intensive care unit is indicated.
4. Evaluation
   a. Chest radiograph
   b. Blood culture
5. Management: aggressive, early treatment
   a. Supplemental O_2 to maintain Sao_2 >98%
      (1) Consider bilevel positive airway pressure if O_2 requirement >60%, or increasing work of breathing
   b. Exchange RBC transfusion:
      (1) Simple transfusion to increase hematocrit (Hct) to >30%
      (2) Partial exchange transfusion or erythrocytopheresis for patients with multilobar ACS or who are deteriorating rapidly. The goal is to reduce the HbS concentration to <30% of the total Hb. Consultation with a pediatric hematologist is required.
   c. Analgesia (see Chapter 20): IV opioids; patient-controlled analgesia (PCA); consider epidural analgesia.
   d. Antibiotics
      (1) Cefotaxime, 50 mg/kg IV q8h × 10 days
      (2) Vancomycin, 15 mg/kg IV q6-8h (until penicillin-resistant pneumococci are ruled out)
      (3) Azithromycin, 10-12 mg/kg PO on the first day and 5 mg/kg for the next 4 days
   e. Fluid management
      (1) Correct hypovolemia with normal saline (NS). Then give 0.45% saline, 20 mEq/L KCl, at maintenance rates.
      (2) Avoid excessive hydration
      (3) Treat pulmonary edema with furosemide
   f. Incentive spirometry
   g. Bronchodilators if wheezing is present
   h. Therapeutic bronchoscopy to remove inspissated secretions
G. Painful vaso-occlusive crises
   1. Definition: Microvascular occlusive and inflammatory events of bone and bone marrow, causing severe pain and usually localized to the lower back and extremities or manifested as abdominal pain
   2. Precipitated by dehydration, cold exposure, hypoxia, infection, inflammation, or overexertion
   3. Other clinical associations: Fever, leukocytosis, and lethargy. Hip or shoulder pain is suggestive of avascular necrosis, whereas right upper quadrant abdominal pain is suggestive of

13

cholelithiasis. Inadequately treated, these crises often progress to ACS and other systemic consequences, such as stroke.

4. Evaluation
   a. Site-specific imaging (abdominal ultrasound, magnetic resonance imaging [MRI], computed tomography [CT] scan)
   b. Sepsis, infection workup
   c. Close monitoring of O_2 requirements (for evolution to ACS) and mental status (for stroke) during treatment; liberal use of incentive spirometry

5. Management
   a. Judicious hydration: Avoid fluid overload with hypotonic solutions. Many patients have infarcted renal calyxes and therefore cannot concentrate urine, which leads to salt wasting.
   b. Analgesics: Nonsteroidal anti-inflammatory drugs (NSAIDs; see Chapter 20)
      (1) Ketorolac 0.5 mg/kg (maximum dose/30 mg)
      (2) Acetaminophen 15 mg/kg/dose (90 mg/kg/day)
      (3) Ibuprofen 6 to 10 mg/kg
   c. Analgesics: Opioids
      (1) Continuous IV infusions and ability to provide breakthrough supplemental dosing. Morphine and hydromorphone are most commonly used. Avoid meperidine.
      (2) IV PCA (see Chapter 20)
      (3) Transition to oral medications when pain is no longer severe and patient can tolerate oral feeding

6. Avascular necrosis management
   a. Avoidance of weight-bearing (e.g., bed rest, crutches)
   b. Physical therapy
   c. Pain control: NSAIDs
   d. Orthopedic consultation

H. Acute splenic sequestration
   1. Presentation
      a. Results from the rapid engorgement of the spleen by entrapped RBCs; usually follows an acute febrile illness
      b. Patients present with acute left upper quadrant pain, hypovolemia, dramatic splenomegaly, and profound anemia.
      c. Usually occurs before age 4 years in patients with HbSS disease; may occur later with other sickle variants
   2. Evaluation
      a. CBC with reticulocyte count
      b. Clinical evidence of hypovolemia and poor peripheral perfusion

3. Management
    a. NS, 20 to 30 mL/kg IV to rapidly restore effective circulating volume
    b. Emergency RBC transfusion, 10 to 20 mL/kg, to raise Hb levels to >6 g/dL

I. Priapism
    1. Definition: Priapism is a painful persistent erection that results from engorgement of the corpora cavernosa. *It is a medical emergency!* **Prompt simultaneous hematological treatment of the sickle cell crisis and urological treatment of the priapism is critical to achieve the best possible outcome for these patients.**
    2. Hematological management
        a. Aggressive IV fluid hydration
        b. Analgesics: IV PCA with continuous IV narcotic infusions
        c. Transfusions to minimize % HbS in circulation.
    3. Urology consultation
        a. Aspiration of blood from the corpora cavernosa followed by injection of an α-agonist (e.g., phenylephrine). Example:

        > Injection of phenylephrine (1 mL), diluted with NS to a concentration of 100 mcg/mL directly into corpora cavernosa every 5 minutes for 1 hour

        b. Emergency surgical intervention
        c. Outcome: Penile fibrosis and impotence risk are reduced if detumescence can be achieved within 4-12 hours.

J. Stroke
    1. Epidemiology: 10% of children with sickle cell disease have strokes, usually of the middle cerebral artery circulation.
    2. Presentation
        a. Usually after the age of 5 years, peaking between 6 and 9 years
        b. Acute presentation with severe headaches, seizures, visual disturbances, unresponsiveness, or extremity weakness.
        c. Subacute presentation with deterioration in school performance.
    3. Prevention
        a. Transcranial Doppler (TCD) can identify patients at risk.
        b. Regular elective exchange transfusions or chronic transfusion to maintain HbS <30% will decrease the risk of stroke.
    4. Evaluation
        a. CBC (severe anemia and ongoing hemolysis are risk factors for stroke in sickle cell disease).
        b. TCD ultrasound
           A focal increase in mean blood flow velocity suggests arterial stenosis and predicts an increased stroke risk.

13

      c. CT scan without contrast
         Excellent tool to localize intracranial hemorrhage, but
         may not localize infarction for >6 hours after onset of
         symptoms.
      d. MRI: Improved resolution and earlier identification of infarct
         compared with CT scan (within 2 to 4 hours of onset of
         symptoms).
      e. MR angiography: As good as angiography for identifying
         cerebrovascular disease
    5. Management
      a. Exchange transfusion often results in rapid neurologic
         improvement and prevention of a second stroke
      b. Supportive care including supplemental O_2 and
         anticonvulsant administration for seizures is important.
K. Transfusion therapy in sickle cell disease
    1. Simple transfusions: Simple red cell transfusions can be
      sufficient to stabilize or improve a child's clinical situation.
      An increase in O_2-carrying capacity helps abort the vaso-
      occlusive process and ACS and prevent end-organ
      complications. The target Hb level is 8 to 10 g/dL. Higher
      Hb levels can increase blood viscosity and exacerbate the
      vaso-occlusive process.
    2. Formula to calculate packed red cell volume for a simple
      transfusion:

$$\frac{(\text{Desired Hct} - \text{initial Hct}) \times \text{TBV}}{\text{Packed red cell Hct}}$$

    where the total blood volume (TBV) is given in **Table 13-2** and
    the packed red cell Hct is presumed to be 50% to 65%,
    depending on the preservative solution used.
    3. Double-volume exchange transfusion: The goal of a double-
      volume exchange transfusion is to decrease the HbS
      concentration to less than 30%, with a total Hb of 10 g/dL,
      thereby terminating the sickling crisis. This is also used to treat
      stroke, severe ACS, priapism, and aplastic crisis.

TABLE 13-2

TOTAL BLOOD VOLUME AS A FUNCTION OF AGE AND BODY WEIGHT

Age	Blood Volume (mL/kg) Body Weight
Premature neonate	100
Term neonate	85
Infant	75
3-6 yr	70
>6 yr	65

a. Manual method
   (1) Establish two large-bore IVs, using peripheral and/or central veins.
   (2) One catheter is placed to remove HbS blood and the other to replace an equal volume of HbA blood.
   (3) Alternatively, an intra-arterial catheter can be used for blood withdrawal.
b. Formula to calculate manual exchange blood volume:

$$\frac{(\text{Desired Hct} - \text{initial Hct}) \times \text{TBV}}{\text{Packed red cell Hct} - (0.5 \times [\text{initial Hct} + \text{desired Hct}])}$$

where packed red cell Hct is presumed to be the Hct of the unit of blood to be used in the exchange transfusion (usually 50% to 65%).
c. Automated pheresis machines
   (1) Erythrocytapheresis may be preferable to perform the exchange because it minimizes nursing workload, is more efficient in targeting a total Hb level, and is more efficient in lowering HbS level.
   (2) However, a large (>9 Fr) double-lumen central venous catheter is required for the procedure, which may prevent its use in small children.
d. Monitoring during exchange transfusion: Rapid changes in ionized calcium and blood glucose level can result in hemodynamic and neurologic changes during an exchange transfusion. Large volumes of old, packed RBCs may expose the patient to excessive potassium loads. Therefore, at regular intervals (four times during the exchange transfusion) measure the following:
   (1) Hct
   (2) Ionized calcium
   (3) Blood glucose level
   (4) Potassium level
   (5) Temperature

III. Immune (idiopathic) thrombocytopenic purpura
   A. Definition
      ITP is an acquired condition characterized by thrombocytopenia, leading to cutaneous or mucosal bleeding. Although it is usually benign and self-resolved, life-threatening intracranial hemorrhage occurs in ≈0.5% of patients.
   B. Epidemiology
      The most commonly acquired bleeding disorder in previously healthy children

13

C. Presentation

Usually follows a viral illness, with sudden onset of petechiae and bruising

D. Pathophysiology

Profound thrombocytopenia results when antibody-coated platelets are trapped and destroyed in the spleen.

E. Symptoms

1. Cutaneous bleeding (petechiae, purpura)
2. Mucosal bleeding (buccal, nasal)
3. Gastrointestinal (GI) and genitourinary sites are less common sites for mucosal bleeding.
4. No other constitutional symptoms or physical findings.
5. Although a life-threatening hemorrhage involving the central nervous system (CNS), airway, and GI tract is the major concern in these patients, it is uncommon. Brain hemorrhage occurs in less than 1% of episodes of thrombocytopenia.
6. Risk for severe hemorrhage if platelet count is <10,000 to 20,000/mm^3

F. Evaluation

1. CBC with differential, reticulocyte count, and peripheral smear
2. Hematology consult
3. Bone marrow aspirate to exclude infiltrative process of the bone marrow (leukemia, lymphoma). Some centers consider the bone marrow examination to be unnecessary if the clinical presentation, CBC, and smear are consistent with ITP.

G. Management

1. Option 1: Supportive care only
   a. Otherwise healthy children, with platelet count >10,000 to 20,000/mm^3 and with no evidence of life-threatening bleeding and no planned invasive procedures, may not require pharmacologic therapy.
   b. Bed rest is indicated for the first 48 hours and activity is restricted until the platelet count is >50,000/mm^3.
   c. Contact sports are strictly forbidden until full recovery.
   d. 80% of such patients will experience spontaneous recovery in a few months.
2. Option 2: Pharmacologic therapy
   a. Pharmacologic therapy may speed recovery and should be used in patients with severe bleeding or planned invasive procedures.
   b. Options include corticosteroids or IV immune globulin (IVIG) or anti-RhD immunoglobulin.
      (1) Corticosteroids
          (a) Prednisone 2 mg/kg/day PO, divided into three doses/day for 14 days. Prednisone is then tapered over 1 week

or

    (b) Methylprednisolone 30 mg/kg/day IV divided into 4 doses per day for 3 days

   (2) IVIG 1 g/kg/day (single daily dose) for 1 to 2 days

    (a) IVIG appears to be more effective than corticosteroids in preventing chronic ITP, but IVIG is also more expensive.

    (b) One approach is to use corticosteroids for cutaneous bleeding and reserve IVIG for severe mucosal bleeding.

   (3) Anti-RhD immunoglobulin, 75 mcg/kg IV for 1 day

    (a) Anti-RhD immunoglobulin may be associated with hemolysis, within 1 week of therapy.

    (b) Therefore, it should not be used in patients with Hb <10 g/dL or a positive Coombs test.

  3. Platelet transfusion

   Avoid platelet transfusion except for refractory ITP with life-threatening (usually intracranial) hemorrhage

IV. The bleeding child: Hemostasis, coagulation, and coagulopathy

  A. Overview

   The hemostatic system is designed to ensure the fluidity of blood until a vascular injury occurs; an explosive cascade of physiologic and biochemical reactions then limits the blood loss by sealing the defect in the vessel wall. Acquired nontraumatic causes of bleeding usually involve thrombocytopenia, qualitative platelet defects, or clotting factor deficiencies.

  B. Evaluation of the bleeding child

   1. Past medical history and family history: Past medical history clues to an underlying bleeding disorder include abnormal bleeding following brief trauma or surgery, recurrent epistaxis, easy bruising, or menorrhagia in the patient or family.

   2. Laboratory overview

    a. Traditionally, the coagulation cascade has been described by two pathways, the intrinsic and extrinsic pathways.

    (1) Clinically, the extrinsic pathway is the predominant clotting mechanism.

    (2) The activated partial thromboplastin time (aPTT) indicates the integrity of the intrinsic pathway, whereas the prothrombin time (PT) indicates the integrity of the extrinsic pathway.

    (3) The international normalized ratio (INR) allows standardization of the PT among different laboratories so that INR equals the PT ratio that would have been reported if a standard World Health Organization reference thromboplastin had been used in the PT determination.

13

TABLE 13-3				
DIFFERENTIAL DIAGNOSIS OF COAGULOPATHIES BASED ON LABORATORY RESULTS				
Disorder	**PT or INR**	**aPTT**	**Fibrinogen**	**Platelets**
DIC	↑	↑	↓	↓
Liver failure	↑	N or ↑	N or ↓	N or ↓
Vitamin K deficiency	↑	N	N	N
Heparin therapy	N (therapeutic) ↑ (supratherapeutic)	↑	N	N or ↓
Warfarin therapy	↑	N (therapeutic) ↑ (supratherapeutic)	N	N

↑, Increased; ↓, decreased; *aPTT*, activated partial thromboplastin time; *DIC*, disseminated intravascular coagulation; *INR*, international normalized ratio; *N*, normal; *PT*, prothrombin time.

    b. The net result of coagulation activation is the production of thrombin.
      (1) Thrombin then cleaves fibrinogen to form fibrin, and amplifies the cascade by activating earlier factors.
      (2) The tendency toward clotting is balanced by the action of the endogenous anticoagulants, antithrombin III, protein C, and protein S. Warfarin (Coumadin) and heparin are therapeutic anticoagulants that result in a predictable coagulation test profile (**Table 13-3**).
   3. Differential diagnosis of coagulopathies based on laboratory tests (see Table 13-3)
    a. Thrombocytopenia
      (1) Definition: Thrombocytopenia is a platelet count less than 150,000/mm^3.
      (2) Causes: Common causes of thrombocytopenia and bleeding include the following:
        (a) Massive blood transfusions
        (b) Sepsis
        (c) Disseminated intravascular coagulation (DIC)
        (d) Decreased bone marrow production
        (e) Increased platelet destruction from immune or mechanical causes (see earlier, section on ITP)
      (3) Treatment: Significant hemorrhage caused by thrombocytopenia is treated with platelet transfusion. The following considerations apply:
        (a) Hemorrhagic complications are rare when platelet counts are greater than 20,000/mm^3.
        (b) Patients undergoing invasive procedures should be transfused to >50,000/mm^3.
        (c) Patients undergoing intracranial procedures or with an ongoing CNS bleed should be transfused to >100,000/mm^3.

(d) Patients undergoing lumbar puncture should be transfused to >20,000/mm^3.

(e) One platelet unit/10 kg of body weight will raise the platelet count 30,000 to 40,000/mm^3 in the absence of platelet destruction or antiplatelet antibodies. A single apheresis unit contains the amount of platelets found in 6 to 10 routine platelet units in only 200 to 300 mL, thus minimizing the total volume to be given to the patient.

C. Qualitative platelet abnormalities

Despite adequate numbers of circulating platelets and clotting factors, patients with qualitative platelet defects have impaired platelet adhesion, aggregation, and clot retraction. The net result is the formation of a hemostatically inadequate platelet plug and purpuric bleeding. Acquired thrombocytopathies are the most common platelet abnormalities, although there are hereditary forms of qualitative platelet dysfunction.

1. Drug-induced platelet dysfunction

   a. Clinically relevant alterations of platelet responses are most commonly seen with use of aspirin and NSAIDs.

      (1) Aspirin causes irreversible inhibition of cyclooxygenase-1 (COX-1), which is required for platelet activation and aggregation. These effects persist for 1 week following the ingestion of a small dose of aspirin.

      (2) NSAIDs (e.g., ibuprofen, ketorolac) impair platelet function via reversible COX-1 inhibition. Effects are short-lived because of the reversible nature of this interaction. Platelet function is normal 6 hours after these drugs are discontinued.

   b. Treatment

      (1) Discontinue the offending drug.

      (2) If bleeding is present, desmopressin (DDAVP), 0.3 mcg/kg IV diluted in NS, may be infused. DDAVP should be given over 15 to 30 minutes.

2. Uremia

   a. Pathophysiology: Platelet dysfunction is the principle hemostatic defect in uremia, with profound impairment of platelet aggregation and activation.

   b. Presentation: Bleeding can be severe, presenting as purpura, epistaxis, or GI hemorrhage. On occasion, intracranial hemorrhage or hemorrhagic pericardial effusions can occur.

   c. Treatment

      (1) Platelet transfusion

      (2) DDAVP (0.3 mcg/kg IV over 30 minutes): DDAVP decreases the hemorrhagic diathesis of uremia for

13

up to 4 hours, permitting the placement of dialysis catheters.

    (3) Dialysis: Dialysis removes the uremic products that produce platelet dysfunction.

D. Disseminated intravascular coagulation

  1. Overview

    a. DIC is an acquired coagulopathy, which is triggered by an underlying condition that injures the vascular endothelium.

    b. As a result, the coagulation cascade is activated, which leads to intravascular thrombosis.

    c. Once clotting factors and platelets have been consumed, hemorrhage begins.

    d. Multiple organ failure results unless the underlying trigger is corrected.

  2. Conditions that may be associated with DIC:

    a. Sepsis

    b. Brain injury (PT > partial thromboplastin time [PTT])

    c. Malignancy

    d. Trauma

    e. Toxins

  3. Treatment: Treat the underlying disease.

    a. For DIC with significant bleeding: Fresh-frozen plasma (FFP), 10 mL/kg IV q12h

    b. For DIC with significant bleeding and severe hypofibrinogenemia: Cryoprecipitate, 10 mL/kg IV q6h

    c. For DIC with thrombosis, possible ischemic injury, and no bleeding: Heparin (unfractionated) 5 units/kg/hr IV. The use of heparin in DIC is extremely rare.

E. Vitamin K deficiency

  1. Normal physiology

    a. Vitamin K is obtained from vegetables and is produced by the intestinal flora.

    b. It is fat-soluble and requires bile salts for its absorption. Vitamin K is a coenzyme in the γ-glutamyl carboxylation of factors II, VII, IX, and X.

    c. Factor VII has the shortest half-life of 6 hours, which results in the excessive prolongation of PT compared with PTT.

  2. Causes

    a. Malnutrition

    b. Newborn (see Chapter 32)

    c. Biliary and liver disease

    d. Prolonged antibiotic therapy

  3. Management

    a. Vitamin K administration: IV vitamin K should be given slowly (over 15 minutes) to avoid anaphylactic reaction.

    (1) Infants, 1 mg IM or IV

    (2) Children, 2 to 5 mg IM or IV

    (3) Adolescents, 5-10 mg IM or IV

  b. FFP: If vitamin K deficiency is associated with significant bleeding, administer FFP 10 to 15 mL/kg initially, followed by FFP, 5 to 10 mL/kg IV q8h, as guided by clinical examination and coagulation studies.

F. Liver disease

 See Chapter 12.

 1. Pathophysiology: The coagulopathy associated with severe liver disease is a result of decreased factor synthesis, abnormal factor production, or primary fibrinolysis.

 2. Laboratory profile

  a. In some cases the routine coagulation profiles of liver disease and DIC may be identical (see Table 13-3).

  b. However, additional coagulation studies can distinguish liver disease from DIC.

  c. The levels of factors V and VIII are decreased in DIC but usually normal in liver disease. D-dimers (products of fibrinolysis) are usually markedly elevated in DIC, but normal or mildly elevated in liver disease.

 3. Management: See Chapter 12 for full details.

G. Massive blood transfusion

 1. Definition: Massive transfusion is defined as transfusion of >50% of the patient's blood volume (see Table 13-2) in 12 to 24 hours.

 2. Pathophysiology

  a. This coagulopathy is primarily caused by dilutional thrombocytopenia.

  b. Dilution of clotting factors also contributes to the coagulopathy because packed red cell units used for transfusion do not contain platelets or plasma.

  c. Acidosis and hypothermia, which are often associated with massive transfusion, inhibit the activity of clotting factors (acidosis and hypothermia) and platelets (hypothermia).

 3. Management

  a. Prevent coagulopathy by maintaining normothermia during massive transfusion.

  b. Anticipate coagulopathy once 50% of the blood volume has been transfused in 24 hours. Measure platelet count and coagulation profile.

  c. Transfuse nonconcentrated platelets 10 mL/kg IV if there is ongoing hemorrhage after loss of 50% of blood volume or if measured platelet count is <50,000 mm^3.

13

d. Transfuse FFP, 10 mL/kg IV, if hemorrhage continues despite correction of platelet count.

e. Administer cryoprecipitate, 5 to 10 mL/kg IV, if hemorrhage continues despite the measures cited and fibrinogen level is <100 mg/dL.

f. The following abnormalities should be looked for and treated as needed during massive transfusion: Hypothermia, metabolic acidosis, hypocalcemia, hyperkalemia, and hypoglycemia.

Chapter 14

Oncologic Emergencies

Katherine Biagas, MD, FCCM, FAAP,
Gustavo Del Toro, MD,
and Jeff C. Hoehner, MD, PhD

I. Common oncologic emergencies
   A. Conditions requiring immediate treatment
      1. Mediastinal mass and superior vena cava (SVC) syndrome
      2. Spinal cord compression
      3. Hyperleukocytosis
   B. Conditions with serious consequences
      1. Tumor lysis syndrome
      2. Fever and neutropenia
      3. Hypercalcemia
      4. Retinoic acid syndrome
      5. Typhlitis
      6. Hemorrhagic cystitis
      7. Complications of hematopoietic progenitor cell transplantation
II. Mediastinal masses
   See Chapter 23.
   A. Definition
      Mediastinal masses are space-occupying lesions located (or
      originating) within the mediastinal compartment.
   B. Cause and presentation
      1. Depends on the child's age
      2. Location of mass: Anterior, middle, or posterior mediastinum
      3. Benign lesions are more frequent in children <6 years old;
         malignant lesions are more frequent in children >6 years old.
      4. 50% of children presenting with a mediastinal mass are
         asymptomatic. Others may present with pain or respiratory
         symptoms.
   C. Differential diagnosis
      This is based on age and tumor location (see Chapter 23).
      1. Anterior and middle mediastinum: Germ cell tumors,
         lymphoma, thymic lesions, thyroid masses. Other
         nonmalignant lesions may include bronchogenic or enteric
         cysts.
      2. Posterior mediastinum: Usually a neurogenic tumor
         (e.g., neuroblastoma)

14

    D. Early clinical management: Safely establish the diagnosis
       1. Diagnostic procedures may include biopsy of extramediastinal nodes, aspiration of effusions for cytologic examination, and/or bone marrow aspiration.
       2. Needle biopsy alone is nondiagnostic in 50% of cases.
       3. If the diagnosis cannot be established by these means, open biopsy of the mediastinal mass may be indicated.
         a. The administration of general anesthesia may involve significant risk because of airway and/or vascular compression (pulmonary artery, superior and inferior vena cavae, and pulmonary veins). This risk is considered extreme if significant respiratory symptoms exist at rest (usually wheezing), or if >50% cross-sectional compression of the airway is evident by computed tomography (CT) scan.
         b. If general anesthesia is absolutely required, partial upright position with spontaneous respiration (withholding paralyzing agents) is necessary during induction. General anesthesia with cardiopulmonary bypass standby is also an option.
         c. If general anesthesia is contraindicated, corticosteroid administration and/or radiation therapy may rapidly reduce the size of the mass in many cases (i.e., lymphoma). Viable tissue may still remain to provide a precise diagnosis if biopsy is planned soon thereafter (i.e., within 48 hours).

III. SVC syndrome
    A. Pathophysiology
      Involves compression or obstruction of the SVC by a mass in the neck or anterior mediastinum
    B. Oncologic causes
       1. Non-Hodgkin lymphoma
       2. Hodgkin disease
       3. Acute lymphoblastic leukemia, particularly T-cell types
       4. Rare causes include malignant teratoma, thyroid cancer, thymoma (the remaining terrible Ts), a neuroblastoma, rhabdomyosarcoma, and Ewing's sarcoma.
       5. Occlusion of the SVC by a central venous catheter may be a secondary cause of SVC syndrome.
    C. Signs and symptoms
       1. Orthopnea, headache, facial swelling, dizziness, syncope, or sudden pallor
       2. Signs may be exacerbated with Valsalva maneuver.
         a. Pulsus paradoxus (drop in systolic blood pressure of >10 mm Hg) may be elicited with inspiration.
         b. In extreme cases, cardiorespiratory arrest may occur with change to supine posture.

D. Physical examination
  1. Facial edema and often plethora, jugular venous distention, or papilledema
  2. The most important aspect of evaluation is to determine the extent to which the mass involves mediastinal structures (see Section II and Chapter 23).

IV. Spinal cord compression
  A. Pathophysiology
  This is a tumor arising from or growing into the limited and rigid confines of the spinal canal, resulting in compression of the spinal cord.
  B. Tumor classification
    1. Intramedullary: Ependymoma or, less commonly, astrocytoma
    2. Extramedullary: More common than intramedullary but with a more diverse cause, including meningioma, nerve sheath tumors, primary bone tumors, or tumors of neural crest origin (e.g., neuroblastoma)
  C. Clinical presentation
  Pain is the most frequent symptom; weakness caused by spinal cord compression may be subtle.
  D. Diagnosis
  Magnetic resonance imaging is the diagnostic modality of choice.
  E. Treatment
    1. Immediate neurosurgical consultation if significant compression is noted.
    2. Subsequent urgent operative decompression is indicated. This includes laminectomy, clearing the spinal canal, and freeing the thecal sac and roots.

V. Hyperleukocytosis
  A. Pathophysiology
    1. Leukostasis: Large numbers of circulating leukocytes can cause significant morbidity, especially in the pulmonary and cerebral circulations and from tumor lysis syndrome.
    2. Hyperleukocytosis is considered clinically significant if leukocyte counts are as follows:
      a. >200,000/μL in acute myelogenous leukemia (AML)
      b. >300,000/μL in acute lymphoblastic leukemia (ALL)
      c. >300,000/μL in chronic myelogenous leukemia (CML)
      d. Threshold lower for patients with AML because of larger blast cells, creating vascular occlusion at lower white blood cell (WBC) counts than ALL or CML
    3. Most commonly seen in the following:
      a. Infant ALL
      b. AML
      c. T-cell ALL with a mediastinal mass
      d. Hypodiploid ALL

14

   B. Clinical syndromes
     1. Intracerebral hemorrhage: Blast proliferation within the cerebral vasculature and brain parenchyma leads to vessel damage and intraparenchymal hemorrhage.
     2. Intracerebral thrombosis: The increase in leukocyte volume increases blood viscosity, leading to blast aggregates and intravascular thrombus formation.
     3. Pulmonary leukostasis: Blast lysis in pulmonary vessels and parenchyma leads to release of intracellular contents, causing damage to alveoli.
     4. Tumor lysis syndrome (TLS): See Section VI.
     5. Coagulopathy
   C. Evaluation
     1. Physical examination
       a. Many patients are asymptomatic
       b. Mental status change
       c. Headache
       d. Blurred vision
       e. Seizure
       f. Coma
       g. Symptoms of stroke: Motor and sensory changes
       h. Ophthalmologic changes: Papilledema; retinal artery, vein distention
       i. Dyspnea
       j. Hypoxia
       k. Acidosis
       l. Cyanosis
       m. Priapism or clitoral engorgement
       n. Dactylitis
     2. Laboratory testing
       a. Electrolyte levels
       b. Calcium and phosphorus levels
       c. Blood urea nitrogen and creatinine levels
       d. Uric acid
       e. Coagulation profile
       f. Chest radiograph
   D. Treatment
     1. Begin management immediately for TLS (see Section VI).
     2. Intravenous (IV) fluids: 0.45% or 0.9% saline, with or without dextrose, at two to four times maintenance rate.
     3. Do not add potassium to IV fluids until WBC <75,000 cells/μL and K$^+$ <3.0 mEq/L.
     4. Do not add calcium to IV fluids until hyperphosphatemia has resolved (because of risk of calcium phosphate precipitation) unless frank tetany or hypocalcemic seizures are present.

5. Hypouricemic agents: Allopurinol or rasburicase (see Section VI.E for dosing).
6. Add sodium bicarbonate to IV fluids if acidosis is present or if using allopurinol.
7. Transfuse platelets to keep count >20,000/μL.
8. Transfuse packed red blood cells (PRBCs) to keep hemoglobin level >7 g/dL, but do not raise hemoglobin above 10 g/dL to avoid any significant increased viscosity.
9. Leukapheresis, exchange transfusion: Temporizing measure that can rapidly lower the WBC count
10. Begin appropriate antileukemic therapy as soon as the patient's clinical condition permits.

VI. Tumor Lysis Syndrome (TLS)
   A. Definition
      This is a metabolic emergency resulting from the death of tumor cells and release of their contents into circulation.
   B. Clinical findings
      1. Hyperuricemia
      2. Hyperphosphatemia
      3. Hyperkalemia
      4. Hypocalcemia
      5. Usually occurs 12 to 72 hours into initiation of chemotherapy in a patient with a large tumor burden; can occur before chemotherapy is started.
   C. Causes and pathophysiology
      This occurs in malignancies with a high tumor burden, rapid growth, and high sensitivity to chemotherapy.
      1. Usually presents with Burkitt lymphoma, lymphoblastic lymphoma, T-cell ALL
      2. Other malignancies that can present with TLS: Other types of ALL, neuroblastoma, medulloblastoma
      3. Hyperuricemia: Secondary to breakdown of released nucleic acids. Uric acid crystals may precipitate in the kidneys.
      4. Hyperphosphatemia: Occurs in part because of high content of phosphate in blast cells and by metabolic acidosis, which enhances release of intracellular phosphate into the extracellular space
      5. Hyperkalemia: Caused by potassium release from the high numbers of injured cells
      6. Hypocalcemia: Caused by formation of calcium phosphate secondary to hyperphosphatemia
      7. Acute renal failure: Caused by precipitation of uric acid crystals and calcium phosphate within the renal tubules and microvasculature

14

D. Evaluation and differential diagnosis
  1. Electrocardiogram (ECG): Essential if serum potassium is >5.5 mEq/L; may show QRS widening and peaked T waves
     a. Hypocalcemia can lead to a prolonged QTc interval on the ECG.
     b. Cardiac monitor for patients with electrocardiographic abnormalities
  2. Chest radiography to assess for mediastinal mass
  3. Abdominal ultrasound or CT scan
     If the patient has an abdominal or pelvic mass, assess for urinary tract obstruction, which can mimic TLS and will be exacerbated by aggressive IV hydration.
E. Therapy
  1. IV hydration: Two times maintenance rate, with a goal of >100 mL/m^2/hr of urine output
  2. Uric acid therapy
     a. Allopurinol: 300 mg/m^2/day orally (PO) or IV
        (1) Prevents formation of new uric acid
        (2) Has long been the standard drug used for hyperuricemia, but rasburicase now accepted as first-line treatment if TLS suspected
        (3) Alkalinization to solubilize the previously produced uric acid is now controversial because of the risk of calcium phosphate precipitation in any organ.
        (4) If metabolic acidosis is present, use 40 to 80 mEq/L of NaHCO$_3$ added to the IV fluids to keep the urine pH between 6.5 and 7.5.
        (5) Monitor urine pH carefully, because at a pH >7.5, xanthine, hypoxanthine, or calcium phosphate will deposit in the kidneys.
     b. Rasburicase: 0.15-0.2 mg/kg/day IV
        (1) Highly effective in reducing hyperuricemia
        (2) Does not require alkalinization because it works by converting uric acid to a soluble metabolite
        (3) Blood samples for uric acid level testing must be kept on ice because rasburicase will continue lowering the uric acid level on a room temperature sample, producing a falsely low value for the uric acid level.
  3. Weigh patient bid.
  4. Check electrolytes every 6 hours.
  5. Pharmacologic therapy
     a. Aluminum hydroxide, 15 mL PO every 8 hours, for severe hyperphosphatemia
     b. Sodium polystyrene sulfonate (kayexalate), 1 g/kg, for severe hyperkalemia

      c. Calcium gluconate, 100 to 200 mg/kg IV, for severe hyperkalemia

      d. Insulin, 0.1 unit/kg IV, followed by glucose (2 mL dextrose, 25%/kg IV) for severe hyperkalemia

      e. Calcium gluconate IV for severe symptomatic hypocalcemia only, because increased levels of calcium will induce the formation of further nephrotoxic calcium phosphate crystals

      f. Diuretics (furosemide 0.5 to 1.0 mg/kg IV or mannitol 0.25 g/kg IV) may be used in patients with third space accumulation of fluids and no evidence of intravascular fluid depletion.

    6. Dialysis

      a. Considered when fluid and electrolyte control is resistant to pharmacologic therapy

      b. Indications for dialysis in TLS

        (1) Volume overload with pleural/pericardial effusions

        (2) Acute renal failure

        (3) Intractable hyperkalemia

        (4) Hyperphosphatemia

        (5) Hyperuricemia

        (6) Severe symptomatic hypocalcemia

VII. Fever and neutropenia

  A. Definition

    1. Fever may be the only sign of infection in a neutropenic patient.

    2. General guidelines are a temperature >38° C with absolute neutrophil count ≤500 or >500/mm^3 but <1000/mm^3 and falling.

  B. Evaluation

    1. Detailed history and physical essential

    2. Areas requiring special attention on physical examination: Oropharynx, respiratory tract, perirectal area, central line sites, and sites of recent invasive procedures

    3. Blood culture from all lumens of central venous lines and peripheral venipuncture

    4. Urine culture

    5. Other cultures based on clinical exam

    6. Chest radiograph

  C. Treatment

    See Chapter 19.

    1. Begin broad-spectrum antibiotics promptly after evaluation (within 1 hour after arriving in clinic or emergency room).

2. Hospital admission for IV broad-spectrum antibiotics remains the standard of care but some centers manage their low-risk patients as outpatients, sometimes even with oral broad-spectrum antibiotics.

3. Infection is bacterial in origin in 85% to 90% of neutropenic patients with new-onset fever.

4. Choice of antibiotic or antibiotic combination ultimately depends on the following:
   a. Patient's prior infection history
   b. Predominant organisms at a given center or location
   c. Antibiotic sensitivity patterns at a given center

5. There is no clearly defined antibiotic or antibiotic combination as standard of care for fever and neutropenia.

6. Many centers use ceftazidime monotherapy as initial treatment.

7. Carbapenems (e.g., imipenem-cilastatin), other cephalosporins (e.g., cefepime), and extended-spectrum penicillins (e.g., piperacillin-tazobactam) are also popular monotherapies or used in combinations of empiric agents.
   a. Consider carbapenems as first choice in patients who present with source of potential anaerobic infections—perirectal abscess, gingivitis, cellulitis
   b. May add an aminoglycoside (e.g., gentamicin) initially for improved gram-negative coverage
   c. Use of vancomycin for initial management is controversial because of toxicity and risk of vancomycin-resistant organism production. Reasons for vancomycin use as part of initial empiric therapy include the following:
      (1) Institutions with high rates of gram-positive organisms leading to fulminant infections
      (2) Patients with signs of septic shock
      (3) Patients receiving high-dose ara-C or methotrexate; high risk of mucositis
      (4) Patients who recently underwent autologous or allogeneic hematopoietic progenitor cell transplantation (gram-positive bacteria most common cause of infection in these patients)
      (5) Patients with evidence of central line cellulitis
      (6) Patients with known colonization with vancomycin-only sensitive organisms

8. Fungal and viral causes of infection should be considered, particularly in those patients who are post-transplantation.

VIII. Hypercalcemia
   A. General considerations
      1. Hypercalcemia is a secondary phenomenon associated with less than 1% of pediatric tumors.
      2. Most often seen with ALL or alveolar rhabdomyosarcoma

B. Mechanisms
1. Increased bone resorption
2. Paraneoplastic syndromes with production of parathyroid-releasing hormone–related peptide, prostaglandin E2, or tumor necrosis factor, interleukin-1, osteoclastic-activating factor, or decreased renal excretion

C. Symptoms
1. Mild hypercalcemia (12 to 15 mg/dL total serum calcium): Weakness, nausea, vomiting, constipation, abdominal or back pain, polyuria
2. Severe (>15 mg/dL): Profound weakness, including weakness of respiratory muscles, severe nausea and vomiting, bradyarrythmias, coma, prolonged PR interval, and broad T waves

D. Treatment
1. General goals: Decrease the tumor burden, increase renal clearance, and decrease bone resorption.
2. For mild cases, the following are usually required:
   a. Replacement of volume deficit and maintenance of well-hydrated state
   b. Treatment of hypophosphatemia (oral phosphate, 10 mg/kg/dose, bid or tid)
3. For severe cases, the following are usually required:
   a. Hyperhydration (two to three times maintenance fluids) and furosemide (frequent doses of 1 to 2 mg/kg); increase renal clearance in severe cases.
   b. Glucocorticoids (prednisone, 2 mg/kg) may treat the primary tumor or interfere with osteoclastic-activating factor or prostaglandin.
   c. Calcitonin (4 international units/kg IM q12h) lowers serum calcium concentration by impeding osteoclast activity and increasing calcium excretion.
      (1) Rapid onset (4 to 6 hrs)
      (2) Minimal toxicity
      (3) Limited duration of action (48 hrs); longer-term therapy requires bisphosphonates.
   d. Bisphosphonates (pamidronate, 0.5 to 1.0 mg/kg, infused over 4 to 6 hours) impair attachment of osteoclastic precursors to mineralized bone.
      (1) Prolonged half-life in bone
      (2) Hypocalcemia may occur, especially after repeated doses.
      (3) Other important toxicities include fever, myalgias, lymphopenia, increased C-reactive protein levels, gastritis, and bone pain.

14

IX. Hemorrhagic cystitis
   A. Usual occurrence: As a sequela of chemotherapeutic treatment
      1. Usually associated with cyclophosphamide or ifosfamide; toxic metabolite precipitates in the bladder.
      2. Can occur hours to months after chemotherapy administration
      3. Can be caused by adenovirus, cytomegalovirus, JC virus, BK virus
   B. Evaluation
      1. Signs and symptoms are caused by bleeding and inflammation of the bladder, which can cause substantial blood loss and urinary obstruction.
         a. Dysuria
         b. Urgency
         c. Frequency
         d. Increased WBCs in urine
         e. Increased red blood cells in urine
         f. Clots in urine
         g. Bladder ultrasound: Edema, clots or hemorrhage, fibrosis
         h. Cystoscopy can locate large areas of hemorrhage.
   C. Treatment
      1. IV hydration
      2. Correction of thrombocytopenia—keep platelet count close to 100,000/μL
      3. Correction of coagulation abnormalities
      4. Transfusion of PRBCs.
      5. Hyperbaric oxygen treatment should be considered early in the treatment of hemorrhagic cystitis.
      6. Placement of double-lumen Foley catheter for bladder irrigation
      7. Initial bladder irrigation should be intermittent; may eventually require continuous bladder irrigation
      8. Control of bladder spasms with oxybutynin chloride, baclofen, belladonna, or opioids
      9. If no resolution after these measures, may need cystoscopy with electrocoagulation
      10. If electrocoagulation fails, may instill prostaglandin E2, 0.25% formalin, or alum.
X. Retinoic acid syndrome
   A. Cause
      1. This is seen in 25% of patients after treatment of promyelocytic leukemia with all-*trans* retinoic acid (ATRA).
   B. Clinical manifestations
      1. May develop days to weeks after ATRA
      2. Mortality: 5% to 13%

C. Signs and symptoms
1. Fever
2. Respiratory distress
3. Weight gain
4. Fluid retention
5. Pleural and pericardial effusions
6. Acute renal failure
7. Chest radiograph: Pulmonary edema/infiltrates and/or pleural effusions
D. Treatment
1. Dexamethasone, 0.5 to 1 mg/kg/dose q12h, with maximum of 10 mg/dose
2. Discontinue chemotherapy.

XI. Typhlitis
A. Definition
1. Typhlitis is an inflammatory condition of the intestine most commonly involving the right colon and less commonly involving other segments of the colon or small bowel.
2. It is also referred to as neutropenic colitis.
B. Findings
1. The neutropenic child most often presents with abdominal pain, nausea, anorexia, fever, abdominal tenderness and guarding, and dehydration.
C. Diagnosis
1. Abdominal plain films (flat and upright): To rule out free air (perforation) or pneumatosis coli
2. Abdominal CT scan: The diagnosis is most often and best confirmed by an abdominal CT scan, indicating edema and thickening of the bowel wall, with associated intraperitoneal fluid.
D. Treatment
1. Broad-spectrum antibiotics (including anaerobic coverage; see Chapter 19)
2. Bowel rest with IV hydration
3. Supplemental nutrition (total parenteral nutrition)
4. Operative intervention is reserved for patients with bowel perforation and/or continued clinical deterioration. Early surgical consultation is advisable.
E. Resolution
Clinical improvement typically parallels resolution of neutropenia.

XII. Sinusoidal obstructive syndrome (SOS)
A. Definition
1. Sometimes called veno-occlusive disease

  2. Most commonly seen after allogeneic hematopoietic progenitor cell transplantation, but can occur after chemotherapy in the autologous hematopoietic progenitor cell rescue and nontransplantation setting

  3. Usually occurs within 2 weeks of chemotherapy

 B. Signs and symptoms

  1. Right upper quadrant tenderness

  2. Hepatomegaly

  3. Fluid retention

  4. Jaundice

 C. Diagnosis

  1. Liver ultrasound with Doppler flow studies: Hepatomegaly, ascites, reversal of blood flow in the portal vein

  2. A normal liver ultrasound with Doppler does not rule out SOS; liver biopsy with measurement of the hepatic venous pressure gradient is the definitive diagnostic test.

 D. Treatment

  1. Preservation of intravascular volume in the presence of capillary leak, third spacing, and potential for hepatorenal syndrome

  2. Fluid restriction if intravascular volume is restored

  3. Aggressive diuresis

  4. All attempts should be made to provide treatment with defibrotide (not yet approved by the U.S. Food and Drug Administration) in confirmed severe cases.

 E. Outcome

 Severe SOS has an extremely high risk of mortality.

XIII. Acute graft-versus-host disease (AGVHD)

 A. Occurrence

 This develops within 100 days of allogeneic hematopoietic progenitor cell transplantation.

 B. Clinical findings: Include dermatitis, enteritis, hepatitis

  1. Dermatitis: Maculopapular rash with pink-red color

   a. Most common finding with AGVHD

   b. Can be painful

   c. Severe AGVHD skin rash: Bullae and extensive epidermal separation

   d. Definitive diagnosis of skin AGVHD made by skin biopsy

  2. Enteritis: Usually with diarrhea

   a. In severe cases, can be bloody and present with crampy abdominal pain

   b. Definitive diagnosis by intestinal biopsy

  3. Hepatitis

   a. Cholestatic picture with rise in bilirubin and alkaline phosphatase levels

   b. Definitive diagnosis by liver biopsy

   4. Gastrointestinal tract and/or liver AGVHD can occur in the absence of skin AGVHD.
C. Treatment
   1. Augmentation of post-transplantation immunosuppression
   2. Prednisone, 2 mg/kg/day, or equipotent steroid is first-line medication in patients who are not receiving steroids at the time of onset.
   3. If the presentation of new-onset AGVHD seems moderate to severe, treatment should be started emergently prior to confirmatory biopsy.
   4. Multiple alternatives (e.g., monoclonal antibodies, tacrolimus, and antithymocyte globulin) are available for steroid-refractory AGVHD, but the prognosis is poor overall.

14

Chapter 15

Head and Spinal Cord Trauma

Anne-Marie Guerguerian, MD, PhD,
Robert C. Tasker, MBBS, MD,
and Jayant K. Deshpande, MD, MPH

I. Overview
  A. Epidemiology
    1. The central nervous system is involved in 60% to 70% of all trauma-related injuries in children; traumatic brain injury (TBI) is the leading cause of death from injury.
    2. Almost 50% of these deaths occur within hours of injury.
    3. Acute and appropriate intervention may be lifesaving.
    4. Among children with trauma, the incidence of spinal cord injury (SCI) is approximately 1% to 2%.
  B. Causes
    1. Motor vehicle injury
    2. Falls
    3. Nonaccidental or inflicted injuries associated with child maltreatment or abuse, or firearm-related injuries.
  C. Outcomes
    1. The case fatality from TBI ranges from 6% to 35%. Factors associated with increased risk of mortality include:
      a. Severity: Initial worse severity of injury as measured by depth of coma classified according to Glasgow Coma Scale (GCS) score.
      b. Younger age
      c. Nonaccidental cause
    2. The attributable fatality from SCI is unclear, given that most SCI cases are associated with TBI; the average mortality associated with SCI is 20% but can be as high as 50% with atlanto-occipital dislocation.
II. Types of injuries
  A. Primary injury
    1. Involves immediate impact-related injury to brain tissue at the time of the insult
  B. Secondary injury
    1. Involves ongoing injury to brain tissue by hypoxia, hypotension, and cerebral edema after the primary injury has occurred.

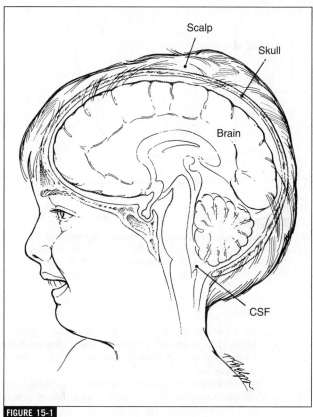

FIGURE 15-1

Sagittal view of the cranium. The child with head trauma is evaluated for injury
to all cranial components—scalp, skull, and brain.
CSF, Cerebrospinal fluid.

15

      2. The goal of therapy is to prevent or limit secondary injury. This
         is best accomplished by prompt and effective resuscitation
         followed by transfer to institutions providing comprehensive
         expertise in pediatric trauma, neurosurgery, and intensive
         care.
III. Pathophysiology
    A. Intracranial pressure (ICP)
      1. Intracranial compliance
        a. The cranium is a closed compartment filled with brain
          tissue, blood, and cerebrospinal fluid (CSF; **Fig. 15-1**).

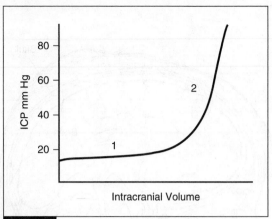

FIGURE 15-2

Intracranial compliance curve. Slope 1: Increases in intracranial volume only cause minor increases in ICP. Slope 2: Small increases in intracranial volume lead to marked increases in ICP. *ICP,* Intracranial pressure.

   b. The volume of one of these compartments can increase initially (e.g., brain edema) without causing changes in the ICP because of compensatory reductions in the volume of other components.
   c. Once these compensatory mechanisms are exhausted, the ICP will rise significantly with even small increases in blood, CSF, or brain volume (**Fig. 15-2**).
  2. Effects of increased ICP
   a. Rapid and/or sustained elevations in ICP compromise cerebral blood flow (CBF) leading to cerebral ischemia, further injury, cerebral edema, and further rises in ICP.
   b. Ultimately, herniation of the brain across the tentorium or through the foramen magnum occurs. Thus, control of ICP is one of the essential goals of TBI treatment.
   c. Elevated ICP may manifest itself as the Cushing reflex, a triad of the following:
     (1) Hypertension
     (2) Bradycardia
     (3) Abnormal breathing patterns
   d. The presence of this reflex indicates significant compromise of blood flow to the brain stem and impending herniation; it requires immediate therapeutic intervention.

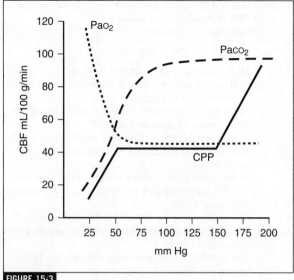

FIGURE 15-3

Relationships among CBF, CPP, PaO_2, and $PaCO_2$. **CBF and CPP,**
Autoregulation involves the ability of the cerebral circulation to maintain
adequate constant CBF in the face of changing CPP by altering
cerebrovascular resistance. In noninjured subjects, autoregulation is
maintained between 50 and 150 mm Hg. These thresholds may be different
in the injured brain, whether the changes are secondary to increases in ICP
or to decreases in MAP. **CBF and PaO_2,** CBF is unchanged until PaO_2
<60 mm Hg. **CBF and $PaCO_2$,** CBF increases almost linearly with $PaCO_2$ at
20 to 80 mm Hg, while hypocapnia induced with hyperventilation decreases
CBF.

CBF, Cerebral blood flow; *CPP,* cerebral perfusion pressure; *ICP,* intracranial
pressure; *$PaCO_2$,* partial pressure of arterial carbon dioxide; *PaO_2,* partial
pressure of arterial oxygen.

15

   e. Increased ICP should also be immediately suspected in the
    presence of the following:
     (1) Unilateral or bilateral dilated or fixed pupils
     (2) Posturing
     (3) Rapidly deteriorating level of consciousness or
       coma
  B. Cerebral blood flow
   CBF is determined by cerebral perfusion pressure (CPP; **Fig.
   15-3**), cerebral oxygen (O_2) demand, and arterial carbon dioxide
   (CO_2) and O_2 tension. Maintaining adequate blood flow and O_2
   delivery is a crucial determinant in maintaining the viability of

brain cells and preventing secondary injury. At the bedside, we target CBF by measuring the following:

1. Cerebral perfusion pressure

$$CPP = MAP - ICP$$

   a. MAP is measured mean arterial pressure.
   b. CPP may be reduced by an increase in ICP or a decrease in MAP (e.g., hypotension).
   c. Under normal conditions, ICP is low (<20 mm Hg) and CPP is primarily dependent on MAP.
   d. In the normal brain, CBF remains constant over a wide MAP range (50 to 150 mm Hg). This is called autoregulation.
   e. In TBI, autoregulation may be impaired and flow may become completely pressure-dependent; if ICP increases, it may impair CBF.
   f. Depending on age, a CPP >50 to 70 mm Hg suggests adequate CBF, whereas CPP <45 mm Hg suggests marked reduction in CBF.
   g. The lowest CPP threshold varies with age; it is likely patient-specific and dynamic over time.
   h. However, a CPP <40 mm Hg is associated with increased risk of mortality and should be avoided.
   i. Patients with GCS <9 require urgent neurosurgical consultation for direct measurement of ICP.

2. Cerebral O_2 consumption
   a. In the normal brain, CBF matches cerebral O_2 consumption—cerebral metabolic rate of oxygen ($CMRO_2$).
   b. Increase in $CMRO_2$ (e.g., seizures, pain, agitation) will lead to an increase in CBF, whereas a decrease in $CMRO_2$ (e.g., anesthesia, hypothermia) leads to a decrease in CBF. In TBI, this relationship may not be maintained.

3. Arterial CO_2 tension
   a. CBF is linearly related to the partial pressure of arterial carbon dioxide ($PaCO_2$) over the range of 20 to 80 mm Hg.
   b. Decreasing the $PaCO_2$ by 10 mm Hg decreases CBF by approximately 25% due to cerebral vasoconstriction.
   c. Cerebral vasodilation occurs within seconds of an increase in $PaCO_2$.
   d. Acutely, hypocapnia induced with hyperventilation (e.g., decreasing $PaCO_2$), will rapidly decrease CBF and cerebral blood volume, thereby decreasing ICP.
   e. However, excessive and sustained hyperventilation and hypocapnia may lead to brain ischemia.

4. Arterial O_2 tension
   a. CBF remains constant at partial pressure of arterial oxygen (PaO_2) >60 mm Hg.
   b. Hypoxemia, defined as PaO_2 <60 mm Hg or O_2 saturation (SaO_2) <90%, causes cerebral vasodilation and increases CBF, which can lead to increases in cerebral blood volume and ICP.
C. Therapeutic implications
   The goal of therapy in the head-injured child is to prevent or limit secondary brain injury by the following:
   1. Maximizing O_2 delivery and other substrates to the brain
   2. Maintaining CPP and CBF by supporting MAP and minimizing ICP. This may involve manipulation of $PaCO_2$, PaO_2, MAP, CSF, and level of consciousness.
   Principles applied to maximize O_2 delivery and perfusion pressure for TBI also apply to SCI.
IV. Evaluation: Primary survey—ABCs and disability
   A rapid, focused, and systematic physical examination (see Chapter 1) is the most important tool in assessment of the child with TBI and/or SCI. Airway, breathing, and circulation (ABCs) must be quickly assessed and treated simultaneously. Resuscitation and stabilization are performed while diagnosis, detail of the injury, and physical examination are concurrently assessed. In addition to the standard steps of the primary survey, assessment of GCS and spinal cord immobilization must be performed:
   A. GCS
      1. D for "disability" in the ABCs: The child's neurologic status can be rapidly classified according to the GCS score modified for infants and children (**Table 15-1**).
      2. Severe TBI is defined as a GCS <9; moderate, GCS = 9 to 12; mild, GCS = 13 to 15.
      3. Direct ICP measurement is recommended in children with severe TBI (GCS <9), GCS >8 but deteriorating level of consciousness, and GCS >8 and level of consciousness rendered invalid from anesthesia for surgical procedure.
   B. Spinal cord immobilization
      1. All children in whom the cause of trauma may be sufficient to lead to SCI, such as rapid acceleration-deceleration injuries related to motor vehicle accidents or sport-related injuries, multisystem trauma, falls or diving injuries, and potentially with shaking/impact-related injuries, should be considered to have SCI until proven otherwise.
      2. Additionally, children who have had GCS <15 at any time since the injury, who complain of neck pain, or who present with a focal neurologic deficit or paresthesias in the extremities should be suspected to have SCI. Spinal and cervical immobilization must be performed in all these children (see later).

15

TABLE 15-1

GLASGOW COMA SCALE SCORE

Response	Adolescents and Children	Infants	No. of Points
Eye opening	No response	No response	1
	To pain	To pain	2
	To voice	To voice	3
	Spontaneous	Spontaneous	4
Best verbal	No response	No response	1
	Incomprehensible	Moans to pain	2
	Inappropriate words	Cries to pain	3
	Disoriented conversation	Irritable	4
	Oriented	Coos, babbles	5
Best motor	No response	No response	1
	Decerebrate posturing	Decerebrate posturing	2
	Decorticate posturing	Decorticate posturing	3
	Withdraws to pain	Withdraws to pain	4
	Localizes pain	Withdraws to touch	5
	Obeys commands	Normal spontaneous movement	6
Total score			3-15

3. Importantly, SCI above the fourth cervical vertebrae results in paralysis of the respiratory muscles.
4. Children with refractory cardiopulmonary resuscitation following blunt cervical injury should be suspected of having atlanto-occipital dislocation.

V. Evaluation: Secondary survey

Inspection and palpation of the neck, scalp, and skull must be performed. A thorough general and neurologic examination completes the assessment after the initial resuscitative management has been instituted and while cardiorespiratory monitoring is maintained.

A. Neurologic examination

A detailed neurologic examination includes assessment of mental status, cranial nerves (CNs), fundi, motor function, tone, sensitivity, deep tendon reflexes, superficial reflexes, and cerebellar function. The motor and sensory levels of complete and partial neurologic deficits are important to identify when suspecting SCI.

1. Mental status: Alertness, orientation, attention, memory, language, and behavior
2. CNs (**Table 15-2**)
3. Pupils: Examine for size, symmetry, and reactivity to light (CNs III, IV, VI).

a. Unilateral dilation—no response to direct or consensual stimulation—of one pupil may indicate compression of CN III, and implies significant intracranial pathology and the possibility of impending herniation. Immediate therapy for herniation may be needed.

TABLE 15-2

CRANIAL NERVES: RELEVANCE TO EXAMINATION OF CHILDREN FOLLOWING TRAUMA (WITH POSSIBLE CLINICAL SIGNIFICANCE)

Cranial Nerves	Function	Feature Examined for Secondary Survey	Possible Significance in a Child with Trauma
CN I-Olfactory	Smell	Ability to smell	May indicate skull fracture at the level of cribriform plate
CN II-Optic	Vision	Visual acuity, visual fields, fundi	May indicate direct trauma to eye, optic tract, or primary visual cortex
CN III-Oculomotor	Pupillary reactivity to light. Eye movement Superior levator palpebrae	Measure in mm pupillary diameter and reactivity to light Adduction, downward and elevation Open palpebrae	Unilateral dilated pupil (>4mm) or fixed pupil signify nerve compression, implies increased ICP, impending uncal herniation, and brain stem injury Bilateral dilated or fixed pupils are consistent with very severe injury Toxic, metabolic causes, and direct ocular bulb injury must be ruled out
CN IV-Trochlear	Eye movement	Inward, downward and rotation	May indicate orbital fractures
CN V-Trigeminal	Facial sensation, corneal reflex and mastication	Facial sensation and corneal reflex	May indicate basal skull fracture
CN VI-Abducens	Eye movement	Abduction	May indicate basal skull fracture or increased ICP
CN VII-Facial	Facial expression and symmetry	Symmetry of facial expression	May indicate internal capsule, cortical brain damage, peripheral nerve injury from facial skin and bone laceration
CN VIII-Vestibulocochlear	Hearing and balance	Response to sound Balance	May indicate basal skull fracture
CN IX-Glossopharyngeal CN X-Vagus	Gag, cough, airway protective function	Swallow, gag reflex, voice	Important indicator of overall decreased cerebral function, brain stem dysfunction, depth of coma
CN XI-Accessory	Trapezius and sternomastoid movement	Raising shoulder and head rotation	May indicate brain stem dysfunction or peripheral injury
CN XII-Hypoglossal	Tongue movement	Protruding tongue	May indicate brain stem dysfunction or peripheral injury

ICP, Intracranial pressure.

15

   b. Bilateral dilation of pupils is ominous and is caused by bilateral CN III compression or severe ischemia.
   c. Toxic, metabolic, or direct injury to the eye must be excluded.
4. Extraocular movement: Absence or weakness of movement in any quadrant may indicate serious brain injury or orbital entrapment.
5. Oculocephalic reflexes—Doll's eyes (CNs III, IV, VI)
   a. Do not test with movement of the neck in suspected SCI.
   b. Hold eyelids open and briskly rotate head from side to side, holding briefly at endpoint. Normal response is conjugate eye deviation to opposite side.
   c. Briskly flex and extend the neck. Normal response is upward deviation on flexion, downward on extension.
6. Roving eyes
   a. Intact brain stem: Slow random horizontal deviations, conjugate or dysconjugate
   b. Depressed brain stem: Absent roving movement
7. Caloric responses for oculovestibular reflexes
   a. Inspect canals for blood, CSF, or a ruptured tympanic membrane before irrigating with ice water.
   b. Head should be 30 degrees above horizontal (unless child is hypotensive).
   c. Place small catheter (tubing from a 19- or 21-gauge butterfly intravenous [IV] set) in the external canal near the tympanic membrane.
   d. Slowly instill from 50 to 120 mL ice water.
   e. Observe at least 5 minutes; wait 5 minutes before irrigating opposite side.
      (1) Normal response: Nystagmus with slow component toward cold and fast component away from cold back to midline.
      (2) Oculocephalic reflexes can be present despite absent cold caloric responses in patients because of preexisting vestibular disease or certain drugs (e.g., ototoxic agents, barbiturates, phenytoin, tricyclic antidepressants, and neuromuscular blockers)
B. Cerebellum
   Coordination of voluntary movement and nystagmus are assessed.
C. Motor
   Strength, tone, and posture are assessed.
D. Sensation
   Pain, temperature, light touch, and two-point discrimination are assessed.
E. Reflexes
   Deep tendon reflexes and symmetry are assessed.

VI. Diagnostic imaging studies

Following the history and physical examination, imaging studies may be required to make the diagnosis. After minor trauma, radiographs may help to diagnose skull fracture, evaluate continuity of ventricular shunts, or identify foreign bodies.

Computed tomography (CT) scans should be obtained after the child has been stabilized and prior to transfer to the intensive care unit or to another hospital. Conscious but combative or agitated patients may require elective intubation and/or general anesthesia for safe immobilization. Vigilant comprehensive care and cardiorespiratory monitoring should be maintained throughout diagnostic imaging studies.

A. Criteria for noncontrast CT after trauma
   1. Age <1 year
   2. Decreased level of consciousness—GCS <15 on examination or history of loss of consciousness after injury
   3. Post traumatic seizure
   4. New focal neurologic deficit
   5. Clinical suspicion of skull fracture or penetrating injury
      a. Palpable scalp hematoma or skull depression
      b. CSF from nose or ear
      c. Blood in middle ear
      d. Battle sign (**Fig. 15-4**)
   6. Suspicion of nonaccidental injury
   7. Multiple trauma
   8. Dangerous falls or motor vehicle-related injury
B. Criteria for cervical spine radiography after trauma
   See Chapter 24.
   1. Nonverbal or GCS <15 at time of assessment
   2. Intoxicated
   3. Neurologic deficit or paresthesias of the extremities
   4. Midline cervical tenderness
   5. Painful distracting injury
   6. Unexplained hypotension
   7. If these children are younger than 9 years, anteroposterior and lateral cervical spine radiographs are obtained; if they are 9 years or older, anteroposterior, lateral, and open-mouth cervical spine radiographs are obtained.
   8. Quality open-mouth views are technically difficult to achieve in intubated patients, are not reliable in this setting, and should not delay the stabilization.
   9. CT cervical spine imaging at the vertebral level suspected to be injured can be considered if clinical or radiologic examination suggests injury or if plain radiographs cannot be clearly obtained.

15

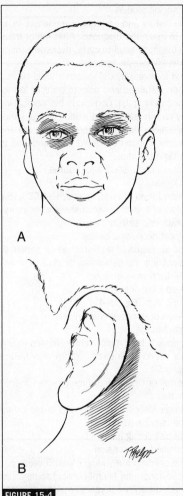

T. Phelps

FIGURE 15-4

Physical signs of basilar skull fracture.
A, Raccoon eyes, periorbital ecchymoses.
B, Battle sign, ecchymosis behind the ear.

VII. Head injuries defined using clinical and radiologic criteria
   A. Concussion
      1. A concussion is a term describing a transient loss of consciousness following trauma.
      2. There are no focal neurologic deficits on examination.

3. Occasionally, concussions are associated with amnesia, headache, dizziness, and nausea.
4. The length of post-traumatic amnesia is proportional to the severity of injury.
5. CT scanning is recommended to delineate any underlying brain injury.
6. Close observation is recommended in hospital or at home with a reliable caregiver; a planned medical follow-up assessment is necessary.

B. Skull fractures
1. Linear, nondepressed fractures
   a. No particular immediate treatment is required.
   b. Management is directed to underlying brain injury and to the treatment of nausea and vomiting.
   c. Consultation with a neurosurgeon is required only if the neurologic examination is abnormal.
2. Depressed skull fractures: Inner table of the skull is displaced by more than the thickness of the bone.
   a. Neurosurgical consultation
   b. Best diagnosed using bone windows of CT scan
   c. Management is primarily directed toward any underlying brain injury. Surgical débridement and repair and elevation of the depressed fragment are performed in the operating room.
3. Compound skull fractures: Direct communication exists between the scalp laceration and cerebral substance.
   a. Neurosurgical consultation
   b. These fractures require early operative intervention: Elevation of the fracture, débridement of the brain, and closure of the dura
   c. Antibiotics covering skin flora (cephalosporins) are usually administered.
4. Basilar skull fractures are diagnosed on physical examination and with CT imaging.
   a. Physical examination
      (1) Raccoon eyes: Circumscribed periorbital ecchymoses; caused by intraorbital bleeding from orbital roof fractures (see Fig. 15-4, *A*)
      (2) Battle sign: An area of ecchymosis behind the pinna; suggests a mastoid fracture (see Fig. 15-4, *B*)
      (3) CSF or bloody otorrhea or rhinorrhea
   b. Neurosurgical consultation
   c. Antibiotic prophylaxis is not usually recommended but should be discussed with the neurosurgeon.

15

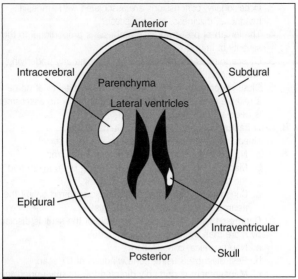

FIGURE 15-5

Reproduction of a CT scan image of the brain with various types of acute cerebral hematomas and their classical morphology showing hyperdense images: epidural (lenticular configuration from the adherence of dura to the skull); subdural (crescentic configuration); intraventricular (with the lateral ventricle); and intracerebral (intraparenchymal lesion).
CT, Computed tomography.

  C. Contusion

    1. An area of bruising or microscopic hemorrhage of the brain caused by trauma, either directly (coup) or indirectly (contre coup) diagnosed on CT scan.

    2. Close observation in hospital is recommended, governed by the clinical severity of the injury as assessed by the primary and secondary surveys.

  D. Hemorrhage or hematoma

    Intracranial hemorrhages require neurosurgical evaluation. These can occur between the skull and dura, between the dura and brain substance, in the ventricular system, or within the brain tissue itself (**Fig. 15-5**). These space-occupying lesions can be classified as epidural, subdural, intraventricular, or intracerebral hemorrhages, respectively; subarachnoid hemorrhages also occur in children. These lesions can be arterial or venous and often continue to expand, producing acute increases in ICP.

Extracranial hemorrhages in the soft tissue rarely require special treatment other than in the young infant, who may require monitoring for blood loss; however, in any child, their topography may indicate how the injury occurred and may suggest the site of underlying intracranial injury.

1. Acute epidural hemorrhage usually occurs from a tear in the middle meningeal artery.
   a. Such arterial tears are associated with linear skull fractures over the parietal or temporal bones, but occasionally may arise from a tear in the dural sinus. In children, 20% of epidural bleeds are venous in origin and may present after a lucid interval of 1 to 2 weeks.
   b. This injury can be rapidly fatal and requires immediate neurosurgical intervention.
   c. Secondary brain injury will occur if the hematoma is not quickly removed. If treated early, prognosis is usually good.
2. Acute subdural hematoma is usually caused by tearing of the bridging veins or cortical arteries.
   a. The onset of symptoms is slow.
   b. A skull fracture may be present.
   c. The underlying brain injury may often be severe, even if the hematoma is evacuated early.
   d. Mortality with this injury is high if not recognized early.
   e. A subdural hematoma will not reabsorb and requires neurosurgical removal.
3. Chronic subdural hematoma is most often associated with repeated injuries, such as abusive head trauma (shaken impact syndrome) or with intracranial shunt complications.
   a. Children commonly present with seizures.
   b. Management is directed to the underlying associated cause of acute brain injury.
4. Intracerebral hemorrhage or hematoma accompanying injury is usually small, petechial, multifocal, and cortical.
   a. It is common in contused brain, directly or contre coup, and may continue to bleed over 2 to 3 days.
   b. Significant intracerebral bleeding usually accompanies penetrating injuries.
   c. Late complications of these injuries depend on the location and size of the remaining defect and include seizure disorders, learning disabilities, and other alterations in higher brain function.
5. Intraventricular hemorrhage is defined by the presence of blood in cerebral ventricles.
   a. They are most often treated conservatively.
   b. Occasionally, large bilateral hemorrhages may require surgical drainage.

   c. Posthemorrhagic hydrocephalus may develop and require shunting.
  6. Subarachnoid hemorrhage occurs in children following trauma when cerebral cortical vessels bleed, most often along the falx or tentorium.
   a. Subarachnoid hemorrhage itself is not responsible for early severe neurologic deterioration; it can be associated with fever, headache, nuchal rigidity, and nausea and vomiting.
   b. Management is based on ensuring adequate hydration, analgesia, and close monitoring.
 E. Penetrating head injuries
  1. These injuries require immediate neurosurgical evaluation and intervention.
  2. Never attempt to remove a foreign body penetrating the head.
  3. These injuries require antibiotic prophylaxis (cephalosporins); antiseizure prophylaxis may be considered.
  4. TBI (or SCI) related to a gunshot wound most often leads to very profound injury.
 F. Diffuse cerebral injury
  1. Diffuse cerebral injury is the most common type of head injury in children and is found in both blunt and penetrating injuries.
  2. Usually, there is no associated skull fracture or intracranial hemorrhage.
  3. Neurologic examination reveals global depression of cerebral function.
  4. Diffuse cerebral injury may not be visible early and is underestimated by CT imaging.
  5. Treatment consists of nonoperative management (see later, Section XI).
VIII. Spinal cord injury
 Bony fragments or projectiles can cause the cord to be compressed, displaced, lacerated, or transected; distraction injuries from stretching can also lead to SCI (see Chapter 24).
 A. Anatomic characteristics of the pediatric spine
  1. Children <9 years are predisposed to injuries in the upper cervical region because of the disproportionately larger head, wedge-shaped vertebral bodies of the developing spine, increased ligamentous laxity, horizontally inclined facetted joints, and vascular supply.
  2. These characteristics explain the occurrence of spinal cord injury without radiographic abnormality.
  3. Location
   a. 70% involve the cervical spine.

TABLE 15-3

CHECKLIST FOR SECONDARY DETERIORATION IN LEVEL OF CONSCIOUSNESS

Causes	Checks
Hypoxia	☐ Adequacy of ventilation
	Oxygen delivery system (O_2 source)
	Endotracheal tube placement (auscultation and end-tidal CO_2), ventilation (chest expansion, exclude pneumothorax)
	☐ Arterial blood gas (measure PaO_2, and compare $PaCO_2$ with end-tidal CO_2 when suspecting fat embolism)
	☐ Chest radiograph
Ischemia	☐ Circulation/hypotension
	☐ Hematocrit/hemoglobin
	☐ Electrocardiogram (tachycardia, bradycardia)
Metabolic	☐ Blood glucose level
	☐ Serum electrolytes (Na, Ca)
	☐ Toxicology screen
Intracranial hematoma	☐ Reevaluate intracranial status
Seizures	☐ Unexplained physical signs or instability based on the signs noted, or convulsive movements evident

$PaCO_2$, Partial pressure of arterial carbon dioxide; *PaO_2*, partial pressure of arterial oxygen.

      b. In younger children, injuries occur most often between the first and fourth cervical vertebrae (C1-C4).

      c. Older children suffer from lower cervical spine injury from the fifth to the seventh cervical vertebrae (C5-C7).

      d. The most common SCIs in adolescents are lumbar spine injuries associated with abdominal trauma.

    B. Management

      1. External immobilization with the application of traction to restore alignment or to immobilize and allow healing of the injury

      2. Operative decompression of cervical spine injuries in children—uncommon and more often used for thoracolumbar injuries

      3. Medical management to maintain oxygenation and blood pressure (BP)

IX. Acute management and interventions

The priority in the management of children with TBI and/or SCI is complete and rapid physiologic resuscitation by anticipating, preventing, and treating hypoxia, respiratory acidosis, and hypotension (**Table 15-3**). Oxygenation, ventilation, and BP must be measured, monitored continuously, and maintained to ensure adequate blood flow and O_2 delivery, and prevent ischemia.

   • If GCS <9, immediately follow the algorithm for severe TBI (**Fig. 15-6**). Management is aimed at optimizing CPP and minimizing increased ICP.

15

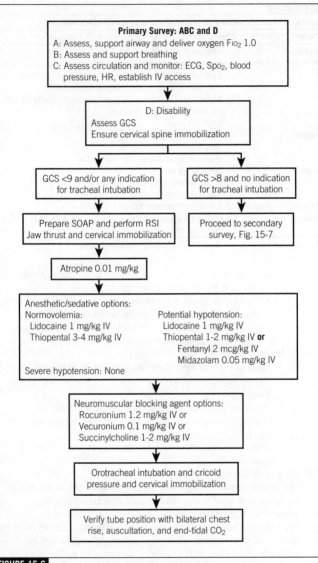

Primary Survey: ABC and D
A: Assess, support airway and deliver oxygen FIO₂ 1.0
B: Assess and support breathing
C: Assess circulation and monitor: ECG, SpO₂, blood pressure, HR, establish IV access

D: Disability
Assess GCS
Ensure cervical spine immobilization

GCS <9 and/or any indication for tracheal intubation

GCS >8 and no indication for tracheal intubation

Prepare SOAP and perform RSI Jaw thrust and cervical immobilization

Proceed to secondary survey, Fig. 15-7

Atropine 0.01 mg/kg

Anesthetic/sedative options:
Normovolemia:
 Lidocaine 1 mg/kg IV
 Thiopental 3-4 mg/kg IV

Potential hypotension:
 Lidocaine 1 mg/kg IV
 Thiopental 1-2 mg/kg IV **or**
 Fentanyl 2 mcg/kg IV
 Midazolam 0.05 mg/kg IV

Severe hypotension: None

Neuromuscular blocking agent options:
Rocuronium 1.2 mg/kg IV or
Vecuronium 0.1 mg/kg IV or
Succinylcholine 1-2 mg/kg IV

Orotracheal intubation and cricoid pressure and cervical immobilization

Verify tube position with bilateral chest rise, auscultation, and end-tidal CO₂

FIGURE 15-6

Primary survey with airway management for TBI and/or SCI.
ECG, Electrocardiogram; *FIO₂,* fraction of inspired oxygen; *GCS,* Glasgow Coma Scale; *HR,* heart rate; *IV,* intravenous; *RSI,* rapid sequence intubation; *SCI,* spinal cord injury; *SOAP,* **S**uction **O**xygen **A**irway equipment **P**harmacology; *SpO₂,* oxygen saturation by pulse oximetry; *TBI,* traumatic brain injury.

- If GCS >8, continue resuscitation interventions and diagnostic studies and treat specific injuries (**Fig. 15-7**).
A. Airway
    1. Oxygenation with fraction of inspired oxygen (FiO_2) 1.0 or 100% O_2 during resuscitation and transport
    2. During the initial airway evaluation, cervical spine and spinal immobilization should maintain the head and neck in neutral position, without applying traction to the neck.
    3. If airway interventions need to be initiated such as bag and mask ventilation or tracheal intubation, consider using two providers, one to manage the airway and one to stabilize the neck in a midline position.
    4. After stabilizing the airway and manually immobilizing the spine, a rigid cervical collar appropriately sized for age should be placed as an adjunct to cervical spine immobilization.
    5. If transport is planned after initial ABC stabilization, the child should be log-rolled onto a spine board with an additional layer of linen under the torso to keep the head and neck in neutral position, given the larger head size of the children, and to avoid neck flexion.
        a. Three anatomic points (thighs, pelvis, shoulders)
        b. Finally, the head should be secured to the board for transport without compromising oxygenation, ventilation, and monitoring of the child.
B. Indications for endotracheal intubation
    1. Upper airway obstruction from loss of pharyngeal muscle tone, inability to clear oral secretions, seizures, foreign body
    2. Loss of protective airway reflexes
    3. Inadequate gas exchange from inability to maintain PaO_2 >60 mm Hg or SaO_2 >93%, despite supplemental O_2, or from respiratory failure
    4. ICP elevation if suspicion of herniation syndrome or GCS <9: Hyperventilation is the fastest method available to lower elevated ICP.
        a. Lowering $PaCO_2$ to a range of 25 to 30 mm Hg decreases cerebral blood volume and ICP.
        b. Cerebral ischemia is the major risk associated with hypocapnia.
        c. For this reason, comatose head trauma patients with normal ICP should not receive prophylactic hyperventilation.
    5. Seizures or status epilepticus
    6. Decompensated shock
    7. During imaging or surgical procedures, to provide safe immobility, sedation, and analgesia

15

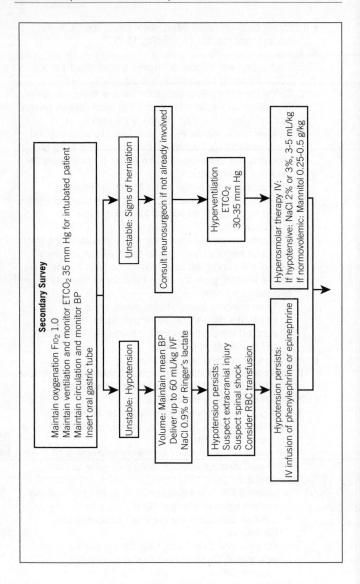

Secondary Survey
Maintain oxygenation Fio_2 1.0
Maintain ventilation and monitor $ETCO_2$ 35 mm Hg for intubated patient
Maintain circulation and monitor BP
Insert oral gastric tube

Unstable: Signs of herniation

Consult neurosurgeon if not already involved

Hyperventilation
$ETCO_2$
30-35 mm Hg

Hyperosmolar therapy IV:
If hypotensive: NaCl 2% or 3%, 3-5 mL/kg
If normovolemic: Mannitol 0.25-0.5 g/kg

Unstable: Hypotension

Volume: Maintain mean BP
Deliver up to 60 mL/kg IVF
NaCl 0.9% or Ringer's lactate

Hypotension persists:
Suspect extracranial injury
Suspect spinal shock
Consider RBC transfusion

Hypotension persists:
IV infusion of phenylephrine or epinephrine

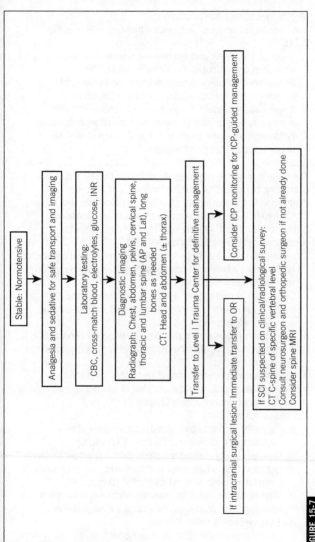

FIGURE 15-7

Secondary survey for TBI and/or SCI.

BP, Blood pressure; *CBC*, complete blood count; *CT*, computed tomography; *ETCO₂*, end-tidal CO₂; *FIO₂*, fraction of inspired oxygen; *ICP*, intracranial pressure; *INR*, international normalized ratio; *IV*, intravenous; *IVF*, intravenous fluid; *OR*, operating room; *RBC*, red blood cell; *SCI*, spinal cord injury; *TBI*, traumatic brain injury.

C. Medications to facilitate intubation
See Chapter 2 and rapid sequence intubation (RSI; see Fig. 2-11).
   1. Because the larynx and trachea are heavily innervated, intubation and tracheal suctioning increase ICP.
   2. Several medications are used to blunt the intracranial responses and cardiovascular reflexes to intubation.
   3. These patients have full stomachs and require RSI with preoxygenation, cricoid pressure, and spinal immobilization.
   4. Following successful intubation, the stomach should be decompressed using an orogastric tube.

D. Circulation
The brain and spinal cord tolerate ischemia poorly. The circulating blood volume, cardiac output, and BP must be maintained in the normal range. Acute hypovolemic shock (see Chapter 6) is treated with isotonic crystalloid salt solutions, colloid, and/or blood. Measuring BP and heart rate with continuous monitoring is mandatory.
   1. Hypoperfusion: Use Ringer's lactate (RL) or normal saline (NS; NaCl, 0.9%) solution. Fluids containing free water (e.g., D5W) may worsen brain edema.
   2. Once there is evidence of adequate perfusion (urine output >1 mL/kg/hr), maintenance IV fluid (IVF) should be administered with RL or NS
   3. Neurogenic shock is rare but may develop with cervical SCI; hypotension and relative bradycardia arise from disrupted sympathetic activity.
   4. Associated hypovolemia should be treated similarly to hypovolemic shock, with the addition of vasoactive medications such as phenylephrine (see Chapter 6).
   5. Volume resuscitation
      a. Rapid 20 mL/kg isotonic crystalloid solution; if no improvement, repeat up to a total of 60 mL/kg
      b. Consider giving packed red blood cells. Type-specific blood is almost as good as typed and crossed blood. If unavailable or no time, use trauma release blood (O negative).
      c. If no response, consider pneumothorax and other source of bleeding (e.g., abdomen, long bone fractures, pelvis).
      d. Start vasoactive medications.
         (1) Phenylephrine (1 to 10 mcg/kg/min) or
         (2) Norepinephrine (0.01 to 0.1 mcg/kg/min)
         (3) Epinephrine (0.01 to 0.1 mcg/kg/min)

X. Continued management following initial resuscitation
   A. Monitor CO_2
      1. Increased $Paco_2$ is a potent cerebral vasodilator.
         a. Increased $Paco_2$ will increase CBF, cerebral blood volume, and ICP.

      b. The use of hyperventilation to achieve hypocapnia is the fastest method available to decrease ICP.

  2. Decreasing $PaCO_2$ to 30 mm Hg decreases CBF and cerebral blood volume and should thereby decrease ICP.

      a. Prophylactic mild hyperventilation ($PaCO_2$ <35 mm Hg) should be avoided unless clinical signs of increasing ICP are present, such as fixed or dilated pupils or neurologic deterioration, indicating the need for urgent treatment.

      b. BP must be maintained in the normal range during hyperventilation.

  3. Continuous end-tidal CO_2 monitoring is necessary in intubated patients.

B. Hyperosmolar therapy

  1. Osmotic diuretics

      a. Mannitol (0.25 to 0.5 g/kg) is an osmotic agent that draws cerebral extracellular water across the blood-brain barrier into the vasculature. The net result is reduced volume of normal brain and change in intracranial compliance.

      b. Hypertonic saline: Hypertonic sodium chloride (2% to 3% or sodium acetate) can be given in doses of 3 to 5 mL/kg.

C. Anticonvulsants

  1. Following head injury, early post-traumatic seizures may result in considerable secondary deterioration.

  2. When present, these must be treated acutely.

  3. For severe TBI, fosphenytoin or levetiracetam (Keppra) may be given for 7 days.

  4. Prophylactic therapy is controversial.

D. Glucose

  1. The brain's two critical needs are O_2 and glucose.

  2. Normoglycemia is essential.

  3. Either hypoglycemia or hyperglycemia will worsen brain injury and must be prevented.

E. Temperature

  1. Normothermia should be maintained and hyperthermia aggressively treated with antipyretics (acetaminophen, 15 mg/kg by rectum) and external cooling.

  2. There are insufficient data to recommend hypothermia therapy.

F. Analgesia

  1. There are no generally accepted specific recommendations for the type of sedative or analgesic in children with severe TBI and/or SCI.

  2. However, pain related to extracranial injuries can be judiciously treated with analgesic agents (e.g., morphine, fentanyl) while closely considering the respiratory and cardiovascular effects of the drug and dosage.

15

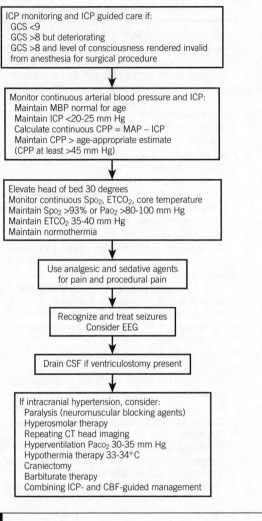

ICP monitoring and ICP guided care if:
GCS <9
GCS >8 but deteriorating
GCS >8 and level of consciousness rendered invalid
from anesthesia for surgical procedure

Monitor continuous arterial blood pressure and ICP:
Maintain MBP normal for age
Maintain ICP <20-25 mm Hg
Calculate continuous CPP = MAP – ICP
Maintain CPP > age-appropriate estimate
(CPP at least >45 mm Hg)

Elevate head of bed 30 degrees
Monitor continuous SpO_2, $ETCO_2$, core temperature
Maintain SpO_2 >93% or PaO_2 >80-100 mm Hg
Maintain $ETCO_2$ 35-40 mm Hg
Maintain normothermia

Use analgesic and sedative agents
for pain and procedural pain

Recognize and treat seizures
Consider EEG

Drain CSF if ventriculostomy present

If intracranial hypertension, consider:
Paralysis (neuromuscular blocking agents)
Hyperosmolar therapy
Repeating CT head imaging
Hyperventilation $PaCO_2$ 30-35 mm Hg
Hypothermia therapy 33-34° C
Craniectomy
Barbiturate therapy
Combining ICP- and CBF-guided management

FIGURE 15-8

ICP-guided management for TBI.

CBF, Cerebral blood flow; *CPP,* cerebral perfusion pressure; *CSF,* cerebrospinal fluid; *CT,* computed tomography; *EEG,* electroencephlograph; *ETCO$_2$,* end-tidal carbon dioxide; *GCS,* Glasgow Coma Scale; *ICP,* intracranial pressure; *MAP,* mean arterial pressure; *MBP,* mean blood pressure; *PaCO$_2$,* partial pressure of arterial carbon dioxide; *PaO$_2$,* partial pressure of arterial oxygen; *SpO$_2$,* oxygen saturation by pulse oximetry; *TBI,* traumatic brain injury.

G. Corticosteroids

There is no clear evidence of the beneficial effects of steroids in TBI or SCI.

XI. Intracranial pressure monitoring

The use of ICP monitoring in children with GCS <9 is appropriate to guide further management. The presence of open fontanels and sutures does not preclude the development of increased ICP or the need to measure and use ICP monitoring. Physicians may choose to use ICP monitoring in children with GCS >8 in situations in which the patient's status is deteriorating or if the use of sedation, anesthesia, or neuromuscular blockade will obscure valid clinical neurologic assessments, such as during an early orthopedic or intra-abdominal operation, or if close monitoring of an impending deterioration from an intracranial space-occupying lesion is necessary.

A. Specific goals of therapy for ICP-monitored guided management (**Fig. 15-8**)

1. Maintain ICP <20 mm Hg.
2. Maintain CPP >45 to 70 mm Hg; adjust for expected normal BP for age.
3. Consider using a ventriculostomy for draining CSF to control increased ICP.

Chapter 16

Nontraumatic Stupor and Coma

Steven Haun, MD,
Myron Yaster, MD,
and David G. Nichols, MD, MBA

I. Overview
   A. Consciousness
      Defined as a state of arousal in which the patient is aware of self and environment
   B. Classification
      1. Lethargy is a state of unresponsiveness from which the patient can be aroused by minimal stimulation.
      2. Stupor is a state of unresponsiveness from which the patient can be aroused by vigorous stimulation. The stuporous patient will lapse back into the unresponsive state when the stimulus is withdrawn or lessened.
      3. Coma is a state of unresponsiveness from which the patient cannot be aroused.
   C. Altered states of consciousness
      1. Result from many disease processes (**Box 16-1**)
      2. In the acute care setting, the clinician must remember that any acute alteration of consciousness represents significant neurologic dysfunction and must be regarded as a life-threatening emergency.
II. Pathophysiology
   A. Conscious behavior
      This requires intact function of the brain stem reticular activating system and both cerebral hemispheres.
   B. Stupor *or* coma
      1. Results from dysfunction or destruction of the ascending reticular activating system or both cerebral hemispheres
      2. Unilateral injury or dysfunction of the cerebral hemispheres will not cause stupor or coma unless the injury produces secondary effects (e.g., ischemia) on the contralateral hemisphere.
   C. Herniation
      1. Herniation is defined as the shift of brain tissue across regions within the skull, usually as a result of mass effect.

BOX 16-1

COMMON CAUSES OF COMA IN INFANTS AND CHILDREN

- Trauma
- Poisoning
- Hypernatremia
- Hyperammonemia
- Infection
- Hypercapnia
- Hypoglycemia
- Cerebrovascular disease
- Obstructive hydrocephalus
- Seizures and postictal states
- Hypoxic-ischemic brain injury
- Uremia
- Diabetic ketoacidosis
- Hypothermia

TABLE 16-1

SIGNS SUGGESTIVE OF IMPENDING HERNIATION

Respiratory Pattern	Pupillary Responses	Motor Response to Pain	Hemodynamic Responses
Cheyne-Stokes	Sluggish reaction to light	Asymmetric	Hypertension and bradycardia
Hyperventilation	Unequal pupils	Decorticate	Hypertension and tachycardia
Apneustic	Fixed pupils	Decerebrate	Hypotension
Ataxic	Dilated pupils	Motionless	—
Apnea	—	—	—

2. Some typical regions for herniation may involve central transtentorial, subfalcine, uncal, or cerebellar herniation.
3. Signs of impending herniation (see **Table 16-1**)

III. Management
   A. Coma management goals
      1. Prevent secondary hypoxic-ischemic brain injury.
      2. Prevent herniation.
      3. Diagnose and treat (if possible) the underlying cause of coma.
   B. Classification of causes of coma
      This simple classification scheme establishes priorities for diagnosis and treatment and provides the framework for management.
      1. Immediately treatable coma
         a. Hypoglycemia (see Chapter 10)
         b. Diabetic ketoacidosis or nonketotic hyperosmolar coma (see Chapter 10)
         c. Meningitis (see Chapter 19)
         d. Seizures (see Chapter 18)
         e. Opioid, benzodiazepine, or cyanide poisoning (see Chapter 17)
         f. Hyponatremia, hypernatremia
         g. Hypocalcemia or hypercalcemia, hypophosphatemia, hypomagnesemia
         h. Hyperammonemia
         i. Thyroid disorders (hyperthyroidism and hypothyroidism)

16

2. Potentially treatable coma
   a. Inborn errors of metabolism (e.g., urea cycle disorders, organic acid disorders)
   b. Reye syndrome–like illness (e.g., influenza A and B, varicella zoster, adenovirus, Epstein Barr virus)
   c. Hepatic encephalopathy
   d. Renal failure
   e. Thiamine (vitamin B_1) deficiency
3. Rapidly progressive intracranial lesions
   a. Trauma
   b. Cerebrovascular disease
   c. Infection
   d. Brain tumor
   e. Hydrocephalus
4. Stable coma
   a. All other causes of coma
   b. Stable only if the patient is receiving adequate cardiorespiratory support

C. Management
   1. Emergency stabilization
   2. Diagnostic workup
   3. Definitive treatment

D. Emergency stabilization: ABCs
   1. This phase begins on arrival of the patient and continues during the diagnostic workup and definitive treatment phases.
   2. Two goals of this phase of management
      a. Prevent secondary hypoxic-ischemic brain injury.
      b. Prevent herniation.
   3. Establish an adequate airway and ensure adequate oxygenation and ventilation (see Chapter 2).
      a. In all comatose patients, immobilize the cervical spine until spinal injury has been ruled out.
      b. Provide 100% oxygen.
      c. Jaw thrust or triple jaw maneuver to relieve airway obstruction (see Chapter 2)
      d. Indications for intubation (**Box 16-2**)
   4. Establish venous access and ensure an adequate blood pressure (see Chapters 5 and 6). If the patient is hypotensive or poorly perfused, administer isotonic (or hypertonic; see later) fluids and vasopressors as necessary to maintain normal blood pressure and perfusion.
      a. If the patient is normotensive, administer isotonic fluids at a maintenance rate.
      b. Obtain blood for rapid glucose determination and obtain initial laboratory studies.

BOX 16-2

INDICATIONS FOR INTUBATION OF THE COMATOSE CHILD

- Inability to maintain patent airway
- Glasgow Coma Scale ≤8 (see Table 16-1)
- Absent cough
- Absent gag
- Hypoxemia
- Hypoventilation
- Impending herniation (hyperventilation treatment)

---

   c. Administer 25% dextrose, 2.0 mL/kg IV, for hypoglycemia.

   d. If the history suggests an inborn error of metabolism (e.g., sudden vomiting, coma, seizures, or cardiac arrest after minor illness or decreased oral intake in an infant), administer 10% dextrose with 0.45% or 0.9% saline at maintenance rates pending consultation with a metabolic disease specialist.

   e. If patient has fever and meningismus, antibiotics should be administered after obtaining a blood culture (see Chapter 19).

   f. Although opioid overdose is rare in children, 0.01 to 0.1 mg/kg of naloxone may be administered at this time (see Chapter 17).

5. Perform emergent neurologic examination to assess for impending herniation.

   a. Level of consciousness: Use Glasgow Coma Scale (**Table 16-2**).

   b. Pupillary response to light

6. Signs suggestive of impending herniation (**Fig. 16-1**)

   a. Asymmetric motor response to pain

   b. Decorticate or decerebrate responses to pain

   c. Cranial nerve palsies (especially unilateral or bilateral fixed pupils)

   d. Cushing's triad (irregular respiration, hypertension, and bradycardia)

   e. Other abnormalities of vital signs (e.g., tachycardia, hypertension, or hypotension)

7. Treat impending herniation

   a. Hyperventilation is the primary mode of emergency therapy.

     (1) Titrate to signs of impending herniation (e.g., a fixed and dilated pupil becomes smaller and reacts to light during hyperventilation).

     (2) Hyperventilation should be used as an acute short-term measure to treat impending herniation.

16

TABLE 16-2

GLASGOW COMA SCALE

Response	Adults and Children	Infants	Points
Eye opening	No response	No response	1
	To pain	To pain	2
	To voice	To voice	3
	Spontaneous	Spontaneous	4
Verbal	No response	No response	1
	Incomprehensible	Moans to pain	2
	Inappropriate words	Cries to pain	3
	Disoriented conversation	Irritable	4
		Coos, babbles	5
Motor	No response	No response	1
	Decerebrate posturing	Decerebrate posturing	2
	Decorticate posturing	Decorticate posturing	3
	Withdraws to pain	Withdraws to pain	4
	Localizes pain	Withdraws to touch	5
	Obeys commands	Normal spontaneous movement	6
Total score			3-15

---

        (3) Hyperventilation outside the setting of impending herniation is not recommended because it reduces cerebral blood flow and thus may produce cerebral ischemia.

    b. Osmotherapy should be initiated without delay.

        (1) 3% NaCl, 2-5 mL/kg, may be used to restore intravascular volume and reduce intracranial pressure (ICP).

        (2) Mannitol, 0.25 g/kg, may be used to reduce ICP provided intravascular volume is adequate and blood pressure is stable.

    c. Maintain normothermia and avoid hyperthermia, keep head midline, and elevate head of bed 15 to 30 degrees.

    d. Obtain neurosurgical consultation.

    e. Obtain an emergent computed tomography (CT) scan to rule out a mass lesion.

E. Diagnostic workup

    1. This phase begins on arrival of the patient but becomes a major priority only after the patient has been stabilized and immediately life-threatening causes of coma and rapidly progressive intracranial lesions have been appropriately treated.

    2. If the clinician thinks that the patient is *not* at risk of impending herniation, a history and physical examination may be performed while preparations are being made for CT and/or magnetic resonance imaging.

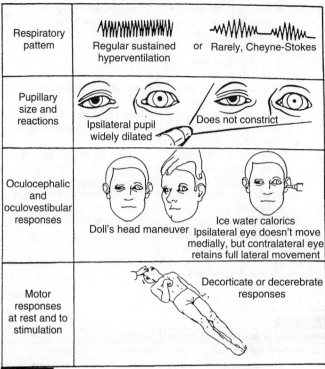

Respiratory pattern	Regular sustained hyperventilation or Rarely, Cheyne-Stokes
Pupillary size and reactions	Ipsilateral pupil widely dilated Does not constrict
Oculocephalic and oculovestibular responses	Doll's head maneuver Ice water calorics Ipsilateral eye doesn't move medially, but contralateral eye retains full lateral movement
Motor responses at rest and to stimulation	Decorticate or decerebrate responses

FIGURE 16-1

Signs of impending herniation. *(From Plum F, Posner JP. The diagnosis of stupor and coma. 3rd ed. Philadelphia: FA Davis; 1982, pp. 104, 111.)*

3. A CT scan will determine whether a mass lesion is present. If present, neurosurgical consultation should be obtained immediately.
   a. If no mass lesion is identified, the clinician can proceed with an exhaustive workup to determine the cause of the coma (stable coma).
   b. A detailed physical examination should be the first step in this process.
4. Initial laboratory evaluation should include the following:
   a. Arterial blood gas and carboxyhemoglobin levels
   b. Complete blood count
   c. Electrolyte levels (sodium, potassium, chloride, bicarbonate)
   d. Osmolality

16

e. Creatinine, glucose, calcium, magnesium, phosphate, ammonia, blood urea nitrogen, and lactate levels

f. Coagulation studies

g. Blood culture

h. Toxicology screen

i. Urinalysis and urine culture

5. Obtain urine and measure acetone, ketoacid, electrolyte, urea, and creatinine levels.

6. A lumbar puncture may be performed only after the patient has been stabilized, the head CT scan shows no mass lesions, and there are no other contraindications.

7. Some contraindications to lumbar puncture include intracranial mass lesion or brain swelling on CT scan, focal neurologic deficit, coagulopathy, or infection at site of puncture.

8. Obtain electroencephalogram to rule out nonconvulsive status epilepticus.

9. History and physical examination will guide the clinician for further diagnostic studies.

IV. Obstructed ventricular shunts

A child with a malfunctioning ventricular shunt is evaluated according to the scheme in **Table 16-3.**

TABLE 16-3

MANAGEMENT OF OBSTRUCTED VENTRICULAR SHUNTS

Status of Patient	Status of Shunt	Probable Diagnosis	Solution
Normal	Pumps freely, fills freely	Functional shunt	Routine follow-up
	Pumps freely, fills slowly	Partial obstruction, ventricular end • Plugged with choroid plexus or ependyma • Ventricle collapses on shunt tip	Close follow-up
Normal	Pumps with difficulty or not at all	Obstructed distal end; probable diagnosis: compensated hydrocephalus	Close follow-up
Symptomatic	Pumps freely, fills freely	Disconnection in shunt system Cyst around peritoneal end Symptoms may not be shunt related	Repair shunt Revise distal end Diagnostic tests
Symptomatic	Pumps freely, refills slowly or not at all	Obstructed ventricular end	Revise shunt emergently; aspirate fluid from shunt
Symptomatic	Pumps poorly or not at all	Distal obstruction resulting from growth of patient, kinking of tubing, clot, adhesions	Revise shunt emergently; aspirate fluid from shunt

A. Shunt obstruction with mild symptoms
   1. Signs and symptoms
      a. Headache
      b. Vomiting
      c. Change in mental status
      d. Seizures are a rare presentation of shunt malfunction.
   2. Treatment
      a. Secure airway, breathing, circulation (ABCs).
      b. Urgent neurosurgical consultation
      c. Plain films of shunt—shunt series
      d. Head CT scan
B. Shunt obstruction with impending herniation
   See Table 16-3.
   1. Observe ABCs. Consider intubation, hyperventilation, and osmotherapy.
   2. Emergent neurosurgical consultation: If a neurosurgeon is not immediately available and the condition is deemed immediately life-threatening, proceed with shunt aspiration (**Fig. 16-2,** *A*).
   3. Aspiration of cerebrospinal fluid (CSF) from the proximal shunt chamber (see Fig. 16-2, *B*)
      a. Wash skin with 2% chlorhexidine or iodine-alcohol (Duraprep) solution.
      b. Insert 25-gauge butterfly needle attached to a stopcock and 10-mL syringe into the proximal shunt chamber; remove sufficient fluid to relieve symptoms.
      c. Send CSF sample for Gram stain, cell count, glucose, protein, and culture.
   4. If proximal end of shunt is obstructed, aspirating the shunt chamber may not decrease ICP.
      a. A neurosurgeon must emergently revise the shunt.
      b. If a neurosurgeon is unavailable and the patient shows signs of herniation, CSF can be aspirated from the lateral ventricle by direct aspiration (see Fig. 16-2, *C*).

16

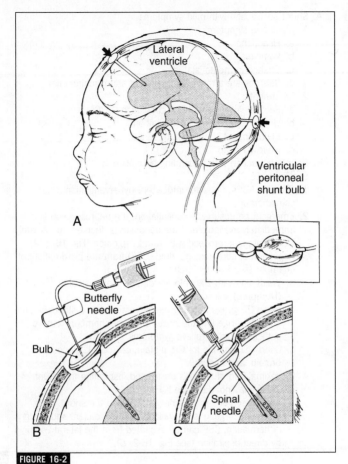

FIGURE 16-2

A, Aspiration of an obstructed ventricular shunt through either **B,** the proximal shunt chamber, or **C,** directly into the lateral ventricle.

Chapter 17

Drug Intoxication

Jennifer Schuette, MD,
Enrico M. Ligniti, MSCP, PharmD,
and Charles L. Schleien, MD, MBA

I. Overview
   A. Incidence
      1. Five million poison exposures occur annually in the United States.
      2. Up to 10% of all emergency department visits are for poisoning.
      3. More than 50% of such exposures occur in children younger than 6 years.
   B. Causes
      1. 85% to 90% of all cases are the result of unintentional ingestions (i.e., substance found in the home).
      2. In older children (~10% to 15% of all pediatric cases), intoxication is generally considered intentional.
      3. Single agent intoxication is more typical in young children; multi-agent overdose should always be considered in the adolescent.
      4. Munchausen syndrome by proxy and child abuse should also be considered in a child younger than 1 year. Child abuse or neglect should also be considered in children who present with recurrent poisonings or history of trauma.
   C. General approach
      1. There is no substitute for clinical judgment and expertise.
      2. The physician should discuss with a clinical toxicologist the appropriateness of each intervention and custom tailor these to patient-specific parameters.
      3. The regional poison center is the best resource for up-to-date management recommendations.
II. Diagnosis of poisoning
   A. Most common pediatric exposures
      1. Analgesics
      2. Cosmetics
      3. Personal hygiene products
      4. Cleaning substances
      5. Topical agents
      6. Plants

17

BOX 17-1

GENERAL CLINICAL PRESENTATIONS SUGGESTIVE OF POISONING

- Acutely disturbed consciousness
- Abnormal behavior
- Arrhythmia
- Metabolic acidosis
- Respiratory distress
- Cyanosis
- Seizures
- Severe vomiting
- Diarrhea
- Shock
- Unusual odor
- Bradycardia, tachycardia

---

    7. Cough and cold preparations
    8. Foreign bodies
  B. Agents most commonly responsible for morbidity
    1. Carbon monoxide (CO)
    2. Analgesic agents
    3. Hydrocarbons
  C. Adolescents
    Adolescents have a greater incidence of toxic ingestion as a result of experimentation with illicit drugs and/or suicide attempts.
  D. General considerations
    Most important is the rapid and accurate clinical assessment of the patient (**Box 17-1**)
      A complete history and thorough laboratory testing may not be available before the necessary supportive measures should be initiated.
  E. Physical examination to help determine probable poison
    See **Table 17-1**.
  F. Toxidromes
    See **Table 17-2**.
    1. Definition: A group of signs and symptoms often associated with a particular type of poison
    2. Familiarity with common toxidromes is important to assist with potential recognition of the overdose agent.
  G. Initial laboratory testing
    See **Table 17-3**.
III. Resuscitation and stabilization
  A. Management
    1. Provide supportive care.
    2. Prevent further poison exposure (i.e., absorption).
    3. When necessary, administer antidotes and carry out poison elimination interventions.
  B. Initial management
    1. Ensure adequate airway, breathing, and circulation (ABCs).
    2. Check vital signs.
    3. Monitor cardiorespiratory signs.
    4. Perform rapid mental status and pupillary examination.

TABLE 17-1

CLINICAL CLUES TO THE DIAGNOSIS OF UNKNOWN POISONS

Parameter	Sign or Symptom	Suspected Poison
Odor	Bitter almond	Cyanide
	Acetone	Isopropyl alcohol, methanol, acetylsalicylic acid
	Pungent aromatic	Ethchlorvynol
	Oil of wintergreen	Methyl salicylate
	Garlic	Arsenic, phosphorus, thallium, organophosphates
	Alcohol	Ethanol, methanol
	Petroleum	Petroleum distillates
Skin	Cyanosis	Methemoglobinemia secondary to nitrates, nitrites, phenacetin, benzocaine
	Red flush	Carbon monoxide (CO), cyanide, boric acid, anticholinergics
	Sweating	Amphetamines, lysergic acid diethylamide (LSD), organophosphates, cocaine, barbiturates
	Dry	Anticholinergics
Mucous membranes	Dry	Anticholinergics
	Salivation	Organophosphates, carbamates
	Oral lesions	Corrosives, paraquat
	Lacrimation	Caustics, organophosphates, irritant gases
Temperature	Hypothermia	Benzodiazepines, barbiturates, ethanol, carbon monoxide, clonidine, phenothiazines, TCAs
	Hyperthermia	Anticholinergics, salicylates, phenothiazines, cocaine, TCAs, amphetamines, theophylline
Blood pressure	Hypertension	Sympathomimetics (especially phenylpropanolamine in over-the-counter cold remedies), organophosphates, amphetamine, phencyclidine (PCP), cocaine
	Hypotension	Antihypertensives, barbiturates, benzodiazepines, beta blockers, calcium channel blockers, clonidine, TCAs
Pulse rate	Bradycardia	Digitalis, benzodiazepines, barbiturates, beta blockers, ethchlorvynol, opioids
	Tachycardia	Anticholinergics, sympathomimetics, amphetamines, alcohol, aspirin, theophylline, cocaine, TCAs
	Arrhythmias	Anticholinergics, TCAs, organophosphates, digoxin, phenothiazines, beta blockers, CO, cyanide
Respirations	Depressed	Alcohol, opioids, barbiturates, benzodiazepines, TCAs, paralytic shellfish poisoning
	Tachypnea	Salicylates, amphetamines, CO
	Kussmaul's sign	Methanol, ethylene glycol, salicylates
	Wheezing	Organophosphates
	Pneumonia	Hydrocarbons
	Pulmonary Edema	Aspiration, salicylates, opioids, sympathomimetics

TCAs, Tricyclic antidepressants.

Continued

TABLE 17-1

TABLE 17-1

CLINICAL CLUES TO THE DIAGNOSIS OF UNKNOWN POISONS—cont'd

Parameter	Sign or Symptom	Suspected Poison
CNS	Seizures	Camphor, CO, cocaine, amphetamines, sympathomimetics, anticholinergics, salicylates, pesticides, organophosphates, lead, PCP, phenothiazines, isoniazid, lithium, strychnine, theophylline, TCAs
	Miosis	Opioids (except meperidine and diphenoxylate), phenothiazines, organophosphates (late reaction), benzodiazepines, barbiturates, mushrooms (muscarinic types), barbiturates (late reaction), PCP
	Mydriasis	Anticholinergics, sympathomimetics, cocaine, amphetamines, LSD, PCP, TCAs, methanol, glutethimide
	Blindness, optic atrophy	Methanol
	Fasciculation	Organophosphates
	Nystagmus	Phenytoin, barbiturates, carbamazepine, PCP, carbon monoxide, glutethimide, ethanol
	Hypertonia	Anticholinergics, strychnine, phenothiazines
	Myoclonus, rigidity	Anticholinergics, phenothiazines, haloperidol
	Delirium, psychosis	Anticholinergics, sympathomimetics, alcohol, phenothiazines, PCP, LSD, marijuana, cocaine, heroin, methaqualone, heavy metals
	Coma	Alcohol, anticholinergics, benzodiazepines, barbiturates, opioids, carbon monoxide, TCAs, salicylates, organophosphates
	Weakness, paralysis	Organophosphates, carbamates, heavy metals
GI system	Vomiting, diarrhea	Iron, phosphorus, heavy metals, lithium, mushrooms, fluoride, organophosphates

CNS, Central nervous system; *GI*, gastrointestinal.

5. Establish intravenous (IV) or intraosseous access.
6. Carry out seizure control prior to instituting diagnostic steps or specific antidotal therapy.
7. Contact the regional poison center as soon as the patient is stabilized to ensure that maximal effective therapy is provided.

C. Considerations for patients with altered mental status
   1. Check point of care glucose or administer glucose empirically (25% dextrose, 2 mL/kg IV)
   2. Naloxone (doses typically range from 10 to 100 mcg/kg IV; 2 mg maximum initial dose)
   3. Flumazenil if known benzodiazepine overdose in patients **without history of seizures** (0.01 mg/kg/dose IV; 0.2 mg maximum initial dose), with subsequent doses given every 1

TABLE 17-2

TOXIDROMES

Agent Involved	Clinical Manifestations
Anticholinergics (atropine, scopolamine, TCAs, antihistamines, mushrooms)	Agitation, hallucinations, coma, extrapyramidal movements, mydriasis, flushed, warm, dry skin, dry mouth, tachycardia, arrhythmias, hypotension, hypertension, decreased bowel sounds
Cholinergics (organophosphate and carbamate insecticides)	Salivation, lacrimation, urination, defecation, nausea, vomiting, sweating, bronchorrhea, rales and wheezes, weakness, paralysis, confusion, coma, muscle fasciculations, miosis
Opiates	Bradycardia, hypotension, pulmonary edema, slow respirations, seizures, hypothermia, coma, miosis
Sedative-hypnotics	Coma, hypothermia, slow respirations, hypotension, tachycardia.
TCAs	Coma, convulsions, arrhythmias, anticholinergic manifestations
Salicylates	Vomiting, hyperpnea, fever, lethargy, coma
Isoniazid	Seizures, coma, elevated anion gap acidosis
Iron	Shock, hyperglycemia, hemorrhagic diarrhea.
Phenothiazines	Hypotension, tachycardia, torsion of head and neck, oculogyric crisis, trismus, ataxia, anticholinergic manifestations
Sympathomimetics (amphetamines, phenylpropanolamine, ephedrine, caffeine, cocaine, aminophylline)	Tachycardia, arrhythmias, psychosis, hallucinations, delirium, nausea, vomiting, abdominal pain, piloerection
Alcohol, isopropanol, methanol, ethylene glycol, salicylates, paraldehyde, toluene	Elevated anion gap metabolic acidosis

TCAs, Tricyclic antidepressants.

TABLE 17-3

ROUTINE LABORATORY TESTS THAT CAN INDICATE POISONING

Test	Poison
Decreased hemoglobin saturation with normal or increased PO_2	Agents causing methemoglobinemia (nitrates, nitrites, benzocaine)
Elevated anion gap metabolic acidosis*	Methanol; ethanol, isopropyl alcohol ethylene glycol, salicylates, isoniazid, paraldehyde, toluene, iron, phenformin, carbon monoxide, cyanide
Elevated osmolar gap†	Ethanol, methanol, isopropyl alcohol, ethylene glycol
Hypoglycemia	Insulin, ethanol, isopropyl alcohol, isoniazid, phenformin, acetaminophen, salicylates, oral hypoglycemic agents
Hyperglycemia	Salicylates, isoniazid, organophosphates, iron
Hypocalcemia	Ethylene glycol, methanol
Urinalysis	Oxalic acid crystalluria: Ethylene glycol
	Ketonuria: Isopropyl alcohol, ethanol, salicylates

*Anion gap = $Na^+ - (Cl^- + HCO_3^-)$; normal value = 8-12 mEq/L.
†Osmolar gap = measured osmolality − calculated osmolality
Calculated osmolality = $(2 \times Na) + (BUN/2.8) + (Glucose/18)$

17

minute to a maximum of 0.05 mg/kg or 1 mg, whichever is less.
 D. Prevention of further drug absorption
   1. Surface decontamination of external poisons
     a. Skin: remove clothes, wash skin (e.g., for organophosphates)
     b. Eyes: copious irrigation (e.g., for liquid corrosives)
   2. Gastrointestinal (GI) tract decontamination: Consult a poison control center prior to intervention (**Table 17-4**).
 E. Hastening elimination of poisons from blood and tissues
    Consult a poison control center prior to intervention (**Table 17-5**).
 F. Antidotal therapy
   1. Only a small proportion of poisoned patients are amenable to antidotal therapy (**Table 17-6**).
   2. Antidotal therapy is urgent in only a few poisonings (e.g., CO, cyanide, organophosphate, opioid intoxication).
   3. Prior to antidote implementation, prescriber must discuss with a clinical toxicologist the appropriateness of each intervention and tailor therapy to patient-specific parameters.
IV. Specific poisonings
 A. Acetaminophen
   1. Acetaminophen is present in many over-the-counter analgesic and antipyretic compounds.
   2. A dose of >140 mg/kg is considered toxic in children and adults.
 B. Clinical manifestations
   1. First 12 to 24 hours: Either asymptomatic or develops nausea, anorexia, and vomiting
   2. Next 12 to 24 hours: Resolution of earlier GI symptoms
   3. After 72 hours
     a. Liver injury may develop with marked elevation of alanine aminotransferase (ALT) and aspartate aminotransferase (AST) levels, prolonged prothrombin time (PT) and partial thromboplastin time (PTT), and jaundice.
     b. Fulminant liver failure may occur but is not an inevitable occurrence
 C. Laboratory tests
   1. Measure serum acetaminophen level.
 D. Prediction of toxicity by interpretation of acetaminophen assays (based on nomogram)
   1. Probable toxicity
     a. When results of the plasma acetaminophen assay are available, refer to the nomogram (**Fig. 17-1**) to determine whether the plasma concentration is in the potentially toxic range.

Text continued on p. 286.

TABLE 17-4
GASTROINTESTINAL TRACT DECONTAMINATION

Technique	Indications	Precautions/Contraindications	Dosing Procedure	Concerns
Activated charcoal	Consider for all poison ingestions *unless* known caustic, hydrocarbon, or heavy metal. Effective for adsorbing and/or interrupting enterohepatic circulation of certain agents (e.g., phenytoin, carbamazepine, TCAs, meprobamate)	Altered mental status with loss of airway reflexes, known bowel obstruction, or perforation. Use caution with low-viscosity hydrocarbons. Avoid administering with ingestion of corrosive agents.	1 g/kg PO/NG (max, 60 gm/dose) within 1 hr of ingestion. Administer PO as a slurry in 72–240 mL of water; cola drink or fruit juice may be added to disguise taste; or administer via NG tube (after airway protection). Repeated doses also enhance drug elimination via GI dialysis.	Do not use large amounts of sorbitol in children (causes diarrhea and electrolyte imbalance). Abdominal cramps or constipation occur with aqueous preparation. Does not adsorb acids, bases, alcohols, iron and other heavy metals, cyanide, most solvents, and most water-insoluble compounds. Charcoal interferes with GI endoscopy.
Gastric lavage	Controversial (no longer recommended by American Academy of Clinical Toxicology) Consider for: (1) obtunded child in whom charcoal is ineffective, and (2) potentially lethal ingestions (e.g., cyanide, TCAs, iron, calcium channel blockers, beta blockers). Perform within 60 min of ingestion.	Altered mental status with unprotected airway Risk of hemorrhage (e.g., coagulopathy, varices) Ingestion of corrosive materials	Administer via 24–28 Fr orogastric tube *after endotracheal intubation for airway protection*; gravity instillation and drainage using tap water or normal saline	Tracheal aspiration, perforation of esophagus, laryngospasm, fluid and electrolyte shifts; do not perform with ingestion of caustic or corrosive agents; controversial with ingestion of petroleum distillates.

Continued

GI, Gastrointestinal; *NG,* nasogastric; *PO,* orally; *TCAs,* tricyclic antidepressants.

17

TABLE 17-4

GASTROINTESTINAL TRACT DECONTAMINATION—cont'd

Technique	Indications	Precautions/Contraindications	Dosing Procedure	Concerns
Syrup of ipecac	Use in ambulatory setting is controversial (no longer recommended by AAP). Administer to decrease drug absorption by shortening GI transit time. Never use with ingestion of caustic or corrosive agents.	Infant <6 mo of age. Altered mental status with unprotected airway; bowel obstruction, perforation, ileus, bleeding; corrosive agents, alkali, acids, low viscosity hydrocarbons Pregnancy	<6 mo of age: Do not use 6-12 mo: 10 mL PO 1-12 yr: 30 mL PO; may repeat in 20 min if ineffective	Efficacy is controversial; may counteract the timeliness of charcoal because of protracted vomiting. Do not use with known ingestion of petroleum distillates, other caustic agents, and rapid coma-inducing drugs (e.g., TCAs, propoxyphene).
Whole bowel irrigation	Sustained release medications, heavy metals (As, Fe, Li, Hg, Zn) May be useful for foreign body ingestion (drug packs such as cocaine).	Altered mental status with unprotected airway; bowel obstruction, perforation, ileus, bleeding	PEG 3350 via NG tube as follows: 1-6 yr: 40 mL/kg/hr (max, 500 mL/hr) 6-12 yr: 1 L/hr >12 yr: 1-2 L/hr Administer until clear rectal effluent is present.	Fluid shifts and electrolyte changes, nausea and vomiting accompanied by abdominal cramping
Cathartics	Sorbitol may be an optional adjunct to charcoal, but its use is controversial. Administer to decrease drug absorption by shortening GI transit time.	Altered mental status with unprotected airway, known bowel obstruction, or perforation; electrolyte imbalance; use caution with magnesium cathartics in patients with renal failure.	Sorbitol (35%): 4.3 mL/kg PO/NG × 1 for children (max, 2 g/kg) given with charcoal Sorbitol (70%): 4.3 mL/kg PO/NG for adults Magnesium citrate: 4 mL/kg PO/NG (max, 300 mL/dose) given with charcoal	Nausea, vomiting, diarrhea, hypermagnesemia, hypernatremia Do not use with known ingestion of petroleum distillates, other caustic agents, and rapid coma-inducing drugs (e.g., TCAs, propoxyphene).
Endoscopy and surgical removal	Removal of concretions (pharmacobezoar), ruptured drug packs, precipitated heavy metals	Removal of intact drug packs—avoid potential for rupture.	Intervention	Aspiration and perforation
Dilution	Corrosive ingestions, but use is controversial	Retching patient	Administer 5 mL/kg tap water (max 180 mL)	Aspiration, vomiting, and repeated toxic exposure

AAP, American Academy of Pediatrics; *PEG 3350,* polyethylene glycol 3350.

TABLE 17-5

ENHANCED ELIMINATION FROM BLOOD AND TISSUES

Technique	Dosing Procedure	Concerns	Indications
Multidose aqueous activated charcoal	0.5-1 g/kg NG (max, 60 g/dose); may repeat every 2-6 hr; ensure that bowel sounds are present.	Nausea, vomiting, diarrhea, constipation, bowel obstruction, aspiration	Toxins undergoing enterohepatic recirculation: Carbamazepine, phenobarbital, theophylline, quinine, nadolol, dapsone, meprobamate, salicylates, valproate, sustained-release and enteric-coated preparations
Forced diuresis	Isotonic fluid (e.g., normal saline) at 500 mL/hr in adults; not recommended for children because of unacceptably high risk of complications	Fluid overload, pulmonary edema, cerebral edema, acid-base and electrolyte disturbances, drug-induced SIADH	Barium, bromides, chromium, cisplatin, iodide, fluoride, calcium, lithium, potassium
Urinary alkalinization	Initial: 1-2 mEq/kg sodium bicarbonate IV bolus (max, 100 mEq/dose), then D5W plus 50-150 mEq NaHCO$_3$/L at 2-3× maintenance IV fluid Goal: Urine flow = 3 mL/kg/hr and urinary pH ≅ 7.5	Fluid overload, pulmonary edema, cerebral edema, ionized hypocalcemia, hypernatremia, hyperosmolarity, hypokalemia, metabolic alkalosis; contraindicated in cerebral and pulmonary edema and in renal failure	Chlorpropamide, barbiturates, methotrexate, fluoride, salicylates, sulfonamides
Peritoneal dialysis	Usually not beneficial in overdose situations (mesenteric blood flow cannot be adjusted); controversial in small children	Infections and possible bleeding	Limited effectiveness in removal of alcohols, glycols, barbiturates, bromide, ethchlorvynol, inorganic mercury, lithium, salicylates, theophylline
Hemodialysis	Use with poison with molecular weight <500 Da, low plasma protein binding, high water solubility, low endogenous clearance, small volume of distribution	Hypotension, bleeding, central venous access complications	Barbiturates, bromides, chloral hydrate, alcohols, lithium, procainamide, theophylline, salicylates, atenolol, sotalol
Hemoperfusion	Requires toxin to be bound by activated charcoal	Charcoal embolization, hypocalcemia, hypoglycemia, thrombocytopenia, leukopenia, bleeding	Barbiturates, meprobamate, glutethimide, phenytoin, carbamazepine, valproate, theophylline, disopyramide, procainamide, methotrexate
Hemofiltration (CVVH)	Continuous mode	Bleeding complications, clotting of filter	Aminoglycosides (renal failure), vancomycin, metal chelate complexes, procainamide
Exchange transfusion	2-3× volume exchanges usually performed	Transfusion reactions, ionized hypocalcemia	Arsenic, sodium chlorate, methemoglobinemia, sulfhemoglobinemia; may be useful in neonates

CVVH, Continuous veno-venous hemofiltration; *SIADH,* syndrome of inappropriate antidiuretic hormone hypersecretion.

TABLE 17-6
SPECIFIC INTOXICATIONS AND THEIR ANTIDOTES

Poison	Antidote	Indications	Antidote Dose
Acetaminophen	N-Acetylcysteine (Mucomyst)	Give 1st dose based on clinical suspicion. Give subsequent doses based on serum acetaminophen level in probable hepatotoxic range (see Fig. 17-1). Benefit seen principally in patients treated within the first 8-10 hr after the overdose.	**Oral:** 140 mg/kg, followed by 17 doses of 70 mg/kg every 4 hr; repeat dose if emesis occurs within 1 hr of administration. Therapy should continue until all doses are given, even though acetaminophen plasma level has dropped below the toxic range. **IV:** Loading dose, 150 mg/kg over 60 min, followed by two additional infusions. **Initial maintenance dose:** 50 mg/kg infused over 4 hr, followed by 2nd maintenance dose of 100 mg/kg infused over 16 hr. **Total dosage:** 300 mg/kg administered over 21 hr
Anticholinergics	Physostigmine	For management of anticholinergic syndrome; supraventricular tachycardia with hemodynamic compromise; severe agitation.	**Child:** 0.01-0.03 mg/kg/dose IV push over 3-5 min every 20 min to desired effect (max 0.5 mg/dose; 2 mg total) **Adult:** 1 mg slow IV push over 3-5 min every 20 min (max 4 mg total)
Beta blockers	Atropine Glucagon	Bradycardia Bradycardia	0.02 mg/kg IV (min 0.1 mg; max 1 mg); may repeat **Child:** 50-150 mcg/kg IV bolus over 1 min, followed by continuous IV infusion of 0.07 mg/kg/hr **Adult:** 5-10 mg IV over 1-2 min, then 1-5 mg/hr titrated to max of 10 mg/hr IV infusion
	Isoproterenol ± dopamine ± epinephrine	Bradycardia	Titrate all infusions to restore heart rate. Isoproterenol: Continuous IV infusion, 0.05-0.5 mcg/kg/min, plus dopamine, 5 mcg/kg/min, titrated to BP; epinephrine: 0.2-2 mcg/kg/min if severe hypotension
Benzodiazepine	Flumazenil	Coma	**Initial dose:** 0.01 mg/kg/dose rapid IV push (max, 0.2 mg/dose) over 30-60 sec; may repeat every 1 min as needed to total max dose of 0.05 mg/kg or 1 mg, whichever is less. NOTE: Flumazenil associated with increased risk of seizures.

Calcium channel blocker	Calcium replacement	Bradycardia Arrhythmia	Calcium gluconate (peripheral access) **Child:** 100 mg/kg slow IV push **Adult:** 3-12 g slow IV push Calcium chloride (central line) **Child:** IV 20 mg/kg (0.2 mL/kg) over 5 min; may repeat up to four × **Adult:** 1-2 g (10-20 mL) IV over 5 min; repeat up to four ×
Carbon monoxide (CO)	Oxygen ± hyperbaric chamber	Smoke inhalation	100% oxygen; consider hyperbaric oxygenation for CO levels >20%-25% plus coma
Cholinesterase inhibitors (organophosphates)	Atropine	Profuse secretions (nose, mouth, airway, GI tract) Weakness Respiratory failure	**Child:** 0.05 mg/kg IV/IM (min, 0.1 mg; max, 0.5 mg); may double dose every 3-5 min until bronchorrhea resolved. **Adult:** 1-5 mg IV/IM; double every 3-5 min until bronchorrhea resolved.
Cyanide	Amyl nitrite ampules	**Consistent history:** House fire; sodium nitroprusside infusion (prolonged, high dose); dietary—pits, seeds of bitter almond, apricot, plum, peach, pear, apple	First: **Amyl nitrite**, one ampule by inhalation for 15 sec every 3 min until IV access obtained **Followed by sodium nitrite**
	Sodium nitrite, 3% IV solution	**Symptoms:** CNS—headache, confusion, seizure, coma; cardiac—tachycardia, hypertension → bradycardia, hypotension; respiratory—tachypnea → bradypnea; GI—vomiting, abdominal pain; skin—flushed (cherry red)	**Child:** 0.33 mL/kg IV, max, 10 mL, no faster than 2.5 mL/min; may repeat 50% of dose in 30 min; monitor methemoglobin level. **Adult:** 10 mL (300 mg) IV over 2-5 min **Followed by sodium thiosulfate**
	Sodium thiosulfate, 25% IV solution	**Laboratory findings:** Elevated mixed venous Sao$_2$ (>85%), metabolic acidosis	**Child <25 kg:** 1.65 mL/kg IV, max, 50 mL, over 10-30 min; may repeat 50% of dose in 30 min; monitor methemoglobin level **Adult and child >25 kg:** 50 mL (12.5 g) IV over 10-30 min, monitor methemoglobin level

Continued

CNS, Central nervous system; *GI,* gastrointestinal; *IM,* intramuscular; *IV,* intravenous.

TABLE 17-6
SPECIFIC INTOXICATIONS AND THEIR ANTIDOTES—cont'd

Poison	Antidote	Indications	Antidote Dose
Digitalis	Specific Fab antibodies, digoxin immune Fab (Digibind)	Treatment of potentially life-threatening digoxin intoxication (cardioactive steroids) in carefully selected patients; use when life-threatening ventricular arrhythmias secondary to digoxin, acute digoxin ingestion (i.e., >10 mg in adults or >4 mg in children), hyperkalemia (serum potassium >5 mEq/liter) in setting of digoxin toxicity	**Determine total body load (TBL).** TBL (in mg) = serum digoxin concentration (ng/mL) × 5.6 × (body weight in kg)/1000 If overdose <6 hr, give X vials = TBL/0.8 If overdose >6 hr, X vials = TBL/0.6 *or* **Empirical dosing:** Adult acute: 10–20 vials Chronic: 3–6 vials Child: 1–2 vials; reconstitute vial with 4 mL sterile water; then dilute in normal saline (NS) to 1 mg/mL and administer IV via 0.22-μm filter over 15–30 min. May give IV push in cardiac arrest setting. **NOTE:** Nondigoxin cardioactive glycosides (herbs, plants)—use empirical dose only
Ethylene glycol	Ethanol, 10% in D5W ± hemodialysis (HD)	Osmolar gap and metabolic acidosis regardless of ethylene glycol level; serum level >20 ng/dL regardless of symptomatology	**Loading dose:** 8–10 mL/kg IV (max, 200 mL) of 10% ethanol over 30 min, then **Continuous IV infusion:** 0.8–2 mL/kg/hr IV infusion (titrate to serum ethanol level = 100–150 mg/dL) **Consider increasing infusion rate by 2–3× during HD**
	Fomepizole (Antizol) ± HD	May be superior to ethanol therapy	**Loading dose:** 15 mg/kg IV over 30 min, then 10 mg/kg/dose IV every 12 hr × four doses, then 15 mg/kg IV every 12 hr until ethylene glycol concentration <20 mg/dL (if needed) **Consider administering 10 mg/kg/dose IV every 4 hr during HD**

Heparin	Protamine sulfate	Heparin administration and bleeding risk; rapid heparin reversal desired	1 mg neutralizes ≈ 90-115 units of heparin **Initial protamine dose:** Time since IV heparin dose <30 min, use 1 mg/100 units of heparin; 30-60 min, use 0.5-0.75 mg/100 units of heparin; 60-120 min, use 0.375-0.5 mg/100 units of heparin; >120 min, use 0.25-0.375 mg/100 units of heparin If subcutaneous (SC) heparin, use protamine 1-1.5 mg/100 units of heparin; give portion of dose (i.e., 25-50 mg) IV, then infuse remainder over next 8-16 hr. Always infuse protamine slowly to avoid hypotension.
Iron	Deferoxamine	Hematemesis, melena, hypovolemic shock; serum iron >350 mcg/dL or serum iron >TIBC; postdeferoxamine challenge test	Initiate continuous IV infusion at 5 mg/kg/hr and titrate to 15 mg/kg/hr (max, 6000-8000 mg/day), dilute to 10 mg/mL. May also be given IM at 50 mg/kg/dose every 6 hr, max, 6000-8000 mg/day. Generally given until iron level <300 mcg/dL.
Isoniazid	Pyridoxine (vitamin B₆)	Seizure, psychosis, nausea, vomiting, anemia, peripheral neuropathy; correction of GABA deficiency	For known isoniazid dose, administer equivalent amount of IV pyridoxine. If supplies are limited or the dose unknown, administer pyridoxine, 5 g IV over 10 min; may repeat every 5-20 min as needed. Max cumulative dose is 20 g in children, 40 g in adults.

Continued

GABA, γ-aminobutyric acid; *TIBC,* total iron-binding capacity.

17

TABLE 17-6
SPECIFIC INTOXICATIONS AND THEIR ANTIDOTES—cont'd

Poison	Antidote	Indications	Antidote Dose
Lead (notify public health authorities)	Dimercaprol (BAL—British antilewisite) in peanut oil	Blood lead level >45 mcg/dL; contraindicated in patients with known peanut allergy or renal dysfunction	**Encephalopathy:** 4 mg/kg deep IM every 4 hr; first dose administered ≈4 hr prior to EDTA **Nonencephalopathy:** 4 mg/kg IM followed by 3-4 mg/kg/dose IM every 4 hr for 2-7 days
	Calcium disodium EDTA	In acute poisoning with encephalopathy or lead level >70 mcg/dL	**Encephalopathy:** 40-70 mg/kg/day as continuous IV infusion NOTE: Administer BAL 4 hr prior to first dose of EDTA. **Nonencephalopathy:** 25-50 mg/kg/day as continuous IV infusion
	2,3-Dimercaptosuccinic acid (DMSA) succimer (only oral treatment approved for lead chelation in children); chemically similar to BAL and produces a lead diuresis comparable to that seen with calcium sodium EDTA without depletion of other metals.		**Child and adult:** 10 mg/kg orally every 8 hr for 5 days, then every 12 hr on days 6-14; may repeat after 2-wk drug-free period
	D-Penicillamine: Not currently FDA-approved for lead intoxication but has been used with success when intolerant to DMSA		15-30 mg/kg/day PO divided q6-8h; max, 1.5 g/day; start at 25% of dose and titrate over 2-3 wk

Low-molecular-weight heparin (LMWH)	Protamine sulfate	LMWH administration with bleeding risk; rapid heparin reversal desired.	1 mg of protamine neutralizes = 1 mg of LMWH dose given <4 hr; administer 1 mg of protamine/1 mg LMWH. May repeat with 0.5 mg protamine/1 mg LMWH if aPTT still prolonged 2-4 hr after first dose.
Mercury	Dimercaprol in peanut oil	Refer to manufacturer's recommendations specific to mercury toxicity	2.5-6 mg/kg/dose IM q4-6h × 10 days
	DMSA succimer		See lead section
Methanol	Ethanol		For dosage, see ethylene glycol section
Methemoglobinemia-producing agents (nitrites, nitrates, phenacetin, phenazopyridine)	Methylene blue, 1% solution	Symptomatic poisoning: methemoglobin level >30%-40%; follow each dose with fluid flush	Initial dose: 1-2 mg/kg IV (0.1-0.2 mL/kg of 1% solution) over 5-10 min; may repeat in 1 hr; max dose = 7 mg/kg. Contraindicated in methemoglobinemia secondary to sodium nitrite administration for cyanide poisoning.
Methotrexate	Folinic acid (leucovorin)	Because of calcium content, do not administer IV solutions at a rate >60 mg/min; can be administered IM, IV push, or IV infusion (15 min to 2 hr).	100 mg/m^2 infused IV over 15-30 min every 3-6 hr for several days, or until methotrexate serum concentration <1 × 10^8 M in absence of any signs suggesting bone marrow toxicity
Narcotics (opiates)	Naloxone	Obtundation, respiratory depression; titrate dosing upward to reversal while avoiding opioid withdrawal.	Adult: 0.4 mg IV (max, 2 mg) Child: 0.01 mg/kg IV, IM, SC (max, 2 mg); repeat every 30-60 sec to clinical response desired. May require 10× initial dose if no response and findings are consistent with narcotic overdose.

Continued

aPTT, Activated partial thromboplastin time; *EDTA,* ethylenediamine tetra acetic acid; *FDA,* U.S. Food and Drug Administration; *PO,* orally; *SC,* subcutaneous.

17

TABLE 17-6

SPECIFIC INTOXICATIONS AND THEIR ANTIDOTES—cont'd

Poison	Antidote	Indications	Antidote Dose
Oral hypoglycemic agents	Glucagon	Hypoglycemia	**Child:** Glucagon, 50-150 mcg/kg IV bolus over 1 min, followed by continuous IV infusion, 0.07 mg/kg/hr **Adult:** 5-10 mg IV bolus, then continuous infusion of 1-5 mg/hr titrated to max of 10 mg/hr
Organophosphate insecticides	Atropine	Cholinergic crisis	**Initial dose:** **Child:** 0.05 mg/kg/dose IV (max, 2 mg/dose); may repeat every 3-5 min until excess secretions are resolved. **Adult:** 0.5-2 mg IV; may repeat every 3-5 min until sweat and secretions are clear.
	Pralidoxime (Protopam, 2-PAM)	Fasciculation and weakness	**Only after atropine:** **Child:** 20-50 mg/kg (max, 1-2 g) infused IV over 30-60 min, then 10-20 mg/kg/hr (max, 500 mg/hr) for patients still manifesting symptoms **Adult:** 1-2 g infused IV over 30-60 min, then up to 500 mg/hr by infusion for patients still manifesting symptoms

Phenothiazines	Diphenhydramine	Symptomatic intoxication: Dystonia, oculogyric crisis	0.5–1.0 mg/kg IV or IM (max, 50 mg)
Sulfonylureas	Octreotide (dextrose should be administered in conjuction with octreotide)	Interventions for sulfonylurea-induced **hypoglycemia**; additional symptomatic, metabolic, hemodynamic support may be required.	**Initial dose:** **Child:** 1–2 mcg/kg/dose SC or IV initially, then repeat dose (max, 50 mcg) SC, IV every 12 hr until euglycemia is sustained without dextrose infusion **Adult:** 50–100 mcg SC/IV, then 50 mcg every 12 hr until euglycemia is sustained without dextrose infusion
	Glucagon		**Child:** 50 mcg/kg IV, IM, SC bolus (max, 2 mg/dose) **Adult:** 1–2 mg IV, IM, SC bolus
	Diazoxide		Consult poison control center.
Tricyclic antidepressants (e.g., imipramine, clomipramine, desipramine, amitriptyline, nortriptyline)	Sodium bicarbonate 8.4% (1 mEq/mL)	Hypotension, tachycardia, prolonged QT interval Additional symptomatic, metabolic, hemodynamic support may be required.	**Initial dose:** **Child:** 1–2 mEq/kg IV bolus (max, 100 mEq/dose), followed by IV infusion to maintain blood pH of 7.45–7.55 **Adult:** 50–100 mEq IV bolus, then IV infusion to maintain blood pH of 7.45–7.55 and $Pco_2 \cong 30$ mm Hg
Valproic acid–induced hyperammonemia	Levocarnitine	Hyperammonemia; elevated AST, ALT levels Additional symptomatic, metabolic, hemodynamic support may be required.	**Initial dose:** 100 mg/kg (max, 6 g) infused over 30 min, then 15 mg/kg infused over 30 min every 4 hr. In less severe cases, 100 mg/kg/day PO qid (max 3 g/24 hr)

ALT, Alanine aminotransferase; *AST,* aspartate aminotransferase.

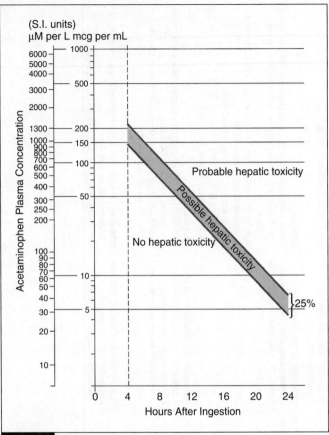

FIGURE 17-1

Rumack-Matthew nomogram: Plasma or serum acetaminophen concentration versus
time post–acetaminophen ingestion. *(From Rumack BH, Hess AJ (eds). Poisindex.
Denver: Micromedix; 1995.)*

  b. Values above the line connecting 200 mcg/mL at 4 hours
     with 50 mcg/mL at 12 hours (probable line) are associated
     with a probability of hepatic toxicity if an antidote is not
     administered.
  2. Possible toxicity
     a. If the predetoxification plasma level is above the line
        connecting 150 mcg/mL at 4 hours with 37.5 mcg/mL at

12 hours (possible line), continue with maintenance doses of acetylcysteine.

b. It is better to err on the safe side; thus this line, defining possible toxicity, is plotted 25% below the line defining probable toxicity.

3. Low-probability toxicity

   a. If the predetoxification plasma level is below the line connecting 150 mcg/mL at 4 hours with 37.5 mcg/mL at 12 hours, there is minimal risk of hepatic toxicity.

   b. The acetylcysteine treatment may be discontinued.

E. Management

1. Gastrointestinal decontamination (Table 17-4).

2. Administer activated charcoal if <4 hours have elapsed since overdose.

3. Administer the antidote *N*-acetylcysteine (NAC) up to 24 hours after ingestion if serum acetaminophen level is in the possible or probable hepatotoxic range.

4. NAC has been shown to reduce extent of liver injury following acetaminophen overdose by maintaining or restoring glutathione levels or by acting as an alternative substrate for the reactive metabolite.

5. See Table 17-6 for NAC dosing.

6. If levels are unavailable, treat as if toxicity is possible. Stop therapy if levels are reported subsequently as nontoxic.

V. Anticholinergics

A. Specific drugs with anticholinergic properties

1. Antihistamines

2. Belladonna alkaloids

3. Phenothiazines

4. Butyrophenones

5. Tricyclic antidepressants (TCAs)

6. Gastrointestinal and genitourinary antispasmodics

7. Antiparkinsonian drugs

8. Cold remedies and sleep aids

B. Clinical manifestations

1. "**Hot** as a hare, **Blind** as a bat, **Dry** as a bone, **Red** as a beet, **Mad** as a hatter."

2. Peripheral anticholinergic effects

   a. Tachycardia

   b. Hypertension

   c. Dry mucous membranes

   d. Flushed dry skin

   e. Fever

   f. Mydriasis

   g. Blurred vision

h. Constipation
i. Urinary retention
3. Central anticholinergic effects
a. Confusion
b. Memory loss
c. Agitation
d. Movement disorder
e. Hallucinations
f. Convulsions
g. Coma
C. Laboratory tests
1. Urine toxicology screen can detect anticholinergic compounds.
D. Management
1. GI decontamination (Table 17-4)
2. Administer the antidote physostigmine, a short-acting, nonspecific cholinesterase inhibitor that antagonizes peripheral muscarinic blockade and central anticholinergic effects for the following:
a. Severe hallucinations and agitation
b. Seizures unresponsive to conventional anticonvulsants
c. Coma (use as diagnostic test)
3. Administer antidote edrophonium for anticholinergic-induced supraventricular arrhythmias with hemodynamic compromise.
4. Edrophonium and physostigmine are contraindicated in anticholinergic-induced ventricular arrhythmias.
VI. Salicylates
A. Preparations
1. Aspirin or acetylsalicylic acid is available alone or in combination in many over-the-counter preparations.
2. Alternative salicylate preparations include methyl salicylate (wintergreen oil) and salicylic acid (a keratolytic).
B. Pathophysiology
1. Systemic illness caused by disturbed oxidative phosphorylation
2. Alterations in carbohydrate, protein, and lipid metabolism
3. Direct stimulation of medullary respiratory centers
C. Manifestations
See **Box 17-2** and **Table 17-7**.
D. Prediction of toxicity
1. Ingested dose can predict the severity of acute intoxication (**Table 17-8**).

BOX 17-2

LABORATORY FINDINGS IN SALICYLATE TOXICITY
- Mixed metabolic acidosis/respiratory alkalosis
- Hypokalemia

TABLE 17-7

CLINICAL MANIFESTATIONS OF SALICYLATE TOXICITY

Common	Uncommon
Fever	Respiratory depression
Sweating	Noncardiogenic pulmonary edema
Nausea, vomiting	SIADH
Coagulopathy, bleeding	Hemolysis
Dehydration	Renal failure
Hyperpnea	Hepatotoxicity
Tinnitus	Cerebral edema
Seizures	
Coma	

SIADH, Syndrome of inappropriate antidiuretic hormone hypersecretion.

TABLE 17-8

PREDICTION OF ACUTE SALICYLATE TOXICITY

Ingested Dose (mg/kg)	Potential Severity of Toxicity
<150	Toxicity not expected
150-300	Mild to moderate
300-500	Severe
>500	Potentially lethal

    2. Serum salicylate level may be helpful in predicting severity of intoxication.

       a. In acute overdose, measure serum salicylate level 6 hours after ingestion.

       b. The nomogram (**Fig. 17-2**) can be used to help predict the severity of intoxication based on serum salicylate levels at various intervals following ingestion; however, a patient's clinical presentation should also be used to guide therapy, especially in cases of chronic exposure where the nomogram is felt to be unreliable.

    3. Clinical manifestations reflect the severity of acute and chronic salicylate intoxication (**Table 17-9**).

  E. Management

    1. GI decontamination (Table 17-4)

    2. General supportive care

       a. Antidote therapy (Table 17-6)

       b. Treat acidosis with IV $NaHCO_3$.

       c. Monitor electrolyte, glucose, and calcium levels and replace if necessary.

       d. Administer vitamin K, 0.5 to 2 mg IV for clinical bleeding.

       e. Decrease fever with external cooling.

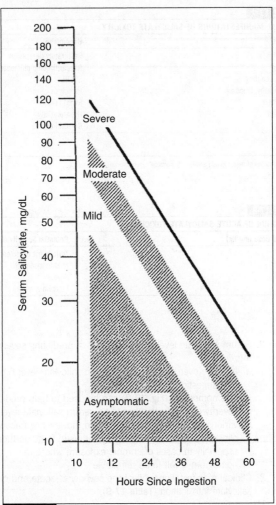

FIGURE 17-2

Nomogram for estimating the severity of salicylate poisoning using serum salicylate levels. *(From Temple AR. Acute and chronic effects of aspirin toxicity and their treatment. Arch Intern Med 1981;141:366.)*

TABLE 17-9

SEVERITY AND SYMPTOMS OF ASPIRIN INTOXICATION

Severity Category	Symptoms
Asymptomatic	None
Mild	Mild to moderate hyperpnea, possible lethargy
Moderate	Severe hyperpnea, prominent neurologic disturbances (marked lethargy and/or excitability) without seizures or coma
Severe	Severe hyperpnea, coma, sometimes with seizures

   f. Perform dialysis: Hemodialysis is more efficient than peritoneal dialysis. Indications for dialysis include the following:
      (1) Severe intoxication (using Done nomogram, dose ingested, or clinical findings)
      (2) Severe acidosis unresponsive to $NaHCO_3$
      (3) Renal failure
      (4) Pulmonary edema
      (5) Severe central nervous system (CNS) manifestations

VII. Iron
   A. Severity of intoxication
      1. Directly related to amount of elemental iron ingested
      2. Iron content of ferrous gluconate, sulfate, and fumarate—12%, 20.7%, and 33.75%, respectively
   B. Clinical manifestations
      1. GI stage (first 6 hours): Nausea, vomiting, hemorrhagic diarrhea, abdominal pain, hematemesis, and hypovolemia
      2. Relative stability stage (6 to 12 hours): Temporary recovery and deceptive quiescence
      3. Shock stage
         a. Shock
         b. Metabolic acidosis
         c. Hyperglycemia
         d. Hemorrhagic diathesis
         e. CNS depression progressing to coma and death
      4. Hepatoxicity stage
         a. Hepatoxicity
         b. Jaundice
         c. Coagulopathy and hypoglycemia
         d. GI scarring with pyloric, gastric, or intestinal stenosis at 4 to 6 weeks after ingestion
   C. Laboratory tests
      1. Measure serum iron and total iron-binding capacity (TIBC) 2 to 4 hours after ingestion.
         a. After 6 hours, iron has been rapidly cleared from serum by the liver.

17

INGESTED IRON LOAD AND TOXICITY

Potential Severity	Amount Iron Ingested (mg/kg)
Insignificant	<20
Moderate	20-60
Potentially lethal	>200

TABLE 17-11

SERUM IRON LEVEL AND TOXICITY

Iron Level (mcg/dL)	Potential Severity
<100	Insignificant
100-300	Minimal
300-350	Moderate
500-1000	Severe
>1000	Potentially lethal

      b. Thus, low iron levels can be measured in a potentially
        lethally intoxicated patient.
   2. Ancillary laboratory tests with moderate or severe ingestion
     should include complete blood count (CBC), glucose,
     electrolytes, AST, ALT, blood urea nitrogen (BUN) levels,
     arterial blood gases, PT, and PTT.
   3. Obtain radiographs of the abdomen after emesis or lavage to
     detect residual pill fragments.
  D. Prediction of toxicity
   1. Dose of elemental iron ingested (**Table 17-10**)
   2. Signs and symptoms of significant iron poisoning are typically
     associated with the following:
     a. Elevated anion gap metabolic acidosis
     b. White blood cell count >15,000/mm^3
     c. Glucose concentration >150 mg/dL
     d. Abdominal radiograph demonstrating radiopaque pills
   3. Serum iron level (**Table 17-11**)
     a. The normal serum iron level range is 50 to 100 mcg/dL.
     b. Serum level in excess of TIBC is diagnostic of iron
       intoxication; normal TIBC is 250 to 400 mcg/dL.
   4. Deferoxamine challenge test
     a. Use when serum iron determination is not readily available
       in moderately symptomatic patients.
     b. Method
       (1) Administer deferoxamine, 40 mg/kg IM once or 15 mg/
         kg/hr IV for 1 hour.
       (2) The appearance of vin rose–colored urine indicates the
         presence of free iron in excess of the iron-binding
         capacity and the need for continued chelation therapy.

(3) However, urine does not always change color, despite a serum iron level that exceeds TIBC.
E. Management
   1. Supportive care: Fluid resuscitation and $NaHCO_3$ administration
   2. GI decontamination (Table 17-4)
   3. When postemesis abdominal radiograph reveals radiopaque material, perform gastric lavage. The use of $NaHCO_3$ or deferoxamine-containing lavage solutions is controversial.
   4. Indications for chelation therapy
      a. Symptomatic patient: GI symptoms and lethargy, tachypnea, hypoperfusion, and tachycardia
      b. Serum iron level >350 mcg/dL (Table 17-11) or positive deferoxamine challenge test
      c. Antidote therapy (Table 17-6)
VIII. Alcohols: Ethanol, methanol, isopropanol, and ethylene glycol
   A. Basic epidemiology
      1. Ethanol is the most commonly used mood-altering drug.
      2. In children, ingestion of the other three alcohols is generally accidental; occasionally they are ingested as ethanol substitutes.
   B. Clinical manifestations
      1. Ethanol
         a. CNS depression, slurred speech, muscular incoordination, coma
         b. Respiratory depression
         c. Hypoglycemia (in children)
         d. Alcohol breath odor
      2. Methanol
         a. Initial phase of mild inebriation, then asymptomatic from 6 to 24 hours afterward
         b. Subsequent headaches, vomiting, CNS depression, visual disturbances with retinal edema
         c. Metabolic acidosis
         d. Formaldehyde odor on breath
      3. Isopropanol
         a. Clinical features resemble those of ethanol ingestion with predominant CNS depression, including confusion, nystagmus, and coma.
         b. GI symptoms: Abdominal pain, vomiting, and hematemesis
         c. Acetone breath odor
      4. Ethylene glycol
         a. Phase 1: CNS depression, confusion, nausea, and vomiting; no breath odor.
         b. Phase 2: Cardiorespiratory failure
         c. Phase 3: Renal failure

17

TABLE 17-12

LABORATORY FINDINGS IN PATIENTS INTOXICATED WITH ALCOHOL

Finding	Type of Alcohol			
	Ethanol	Methanol	Isopropranol	Ethylene glycol
Osmolar gap	Present	Present	Present	Present
Metabolic acidosis (increased anion gap)	Mild to moderate (e.g., adults with chronic abuse)	Severe	None to mild	Severe
Ketosis	Alcoholic ketoacidosis (e.g., adults with chronic abuse)	None	Marked	None
Other laboratory findings	↓ Glucose	↑ Amylase ↓ Ca^{2+}	↓ Glucose	↑ BUN ↑ Creatinine ↓ Na^+

BUN, Blood urea nitrogen.

    C. Laboratory tests
       1. Laboratory test results assist in the correct diagnosis of intoxication by the alcohols (**Table 17-12**).
         a. Blood levels of alcohols
           (1) Use gas chromatography because enzymatic method using alcohol dehydrogenase will not distinguish among these alcohols.
           (2) This is important because early antidotal therapy is crucial with ethylene glycol and methanol intoxication.
         b. Additional blood tests: Arterial blood gas, glucose, electrolytes, BUN, creatinine, ionized calcium, anion gap, osmolar gap
         c. Urinalysis
           (1) Ketones
           (2) Oxalate crystals
    D. Management
       1. GI contamination (Table 17-4)
       2. Treat metabolic acidosis with $NaHCO_3$ (methanol, ethylene glycol poisoning).
       3. Antidote therapy (Table 17-6)
       4. Consider hemodialysis for any of the following:
         a. Methanol and ethylene glycol serum levels >50 mg/dL
         b. Severe metabolic acidosis resistant to $NaHCO_3$ therapy
         c. Renal failure in ethylene glycol poisoning
  IX. Organophosphate and carbamate insecticides
    A. Clinical manifestations (**Table 17-13**)
       1. These are potent acetylcholinesterase inhibitors that are rapidly absorbed from the GI tract and skin.

TABLE 17-13

ORGANOPHOSPHATE AND CARBAMATE POISONING

Anatomic Site	Manifestations
CNS	Headache, lethargy, restlessness, dizziness, confusion, coma, seizures, respiratory depression
Nicotinic effects	
Skeletal muscle	Cramps, fasciculations, weakness, paralysis
Sympathetic ganglia	Tachycardia, hypertension, arrhythmias, pallor, mydriasis
Muscarinic effects	
Cardiac	Bradycardia, hypotension, heart block, arrhythmias
Respiratory	Bronchorrhea, wheezing, respiratory distress
GI	Cramps, vomiting, nausea, diarrhea, tenesmus, abdominal pain
Salivary glands	Excess salivation
Sweat glands	Sweating
Eyes	Miosis, lacrimation, blurred vision
Bladder	Incontinence
Miscellaneous	Garlic odor, fever

GI, Gastrointestinal.

   2. Mnemonic **SLUDGE: S**alivation, **L**acrimation, **U**rination, **D**efecation, **G**astrointestinal symptoms, and **E**mesis
  B. Laboratory tests
    1. Red blood cell cholinesterase and serum pseudocholinesterase levels
    2. Arterial blood gas
    3. Chest radiography
    4. Electrocardiography
    5. Toxicologic examination of urine for metabolic byproducts of organophosphates (e.g., *p*-nitrophenol)
  C. Management
    1. Organophosphate poisoning
     a. Skin decontamination
     b. GI decontamination (Table 17-4)
     c. Antidote therapy (Table 17-6)
    2. Carbamate poisoning
     a. Pathophysiology differs from organophosphate poisoning.
      (1) Carbamates only inactivate cholinesterase temporarily.
      (2) Penetrate CNS poorly
      (3) Clinical manifestations resemble those of organophosphate poisoning but are of short duration and lack the signs and symptoms of CNS involvement.
     b. Treatment: Atropine; pralidoxime administration not necessary.

X. Tricyclic antidepressants
  A. Types of TCAs
    1. Tertiary: Amitriptyline, imipramine, doxepin
    2. Secondary: Nortriptyline, desipramine, protriptyline amines
    3. Tetracyclics: Mirtazapine, Maprotiline and amoxapine resemble the TCAs toxicologically.
  B. Mechanisms of toxicity
    1. Central and peripheral anticholinergic actions
    2. Decreased reuptake of norepinephrine in adrenergic nerve endings enhances catecholamine action in the CNS and peripheral nerve tissues.
    3. Quinidine-like myocardial depressant effect
  C. Clinical manifestations
    1. CNS effects
      a. Drowsiness
      b. Lethargy
      c. Delirium
      d. Agitation
      e. Hallucinations
      f. Respiratory depression
      g. Coma
      h. Movement disorders (e.g., twitching, myoclonic jerks, pyramidal tract signs, choreoathetosis)
    2. Peripheral anticholinergic effects
      a. Dry mucous membranes
      b. Flushed warm skin without sweating
      c. Mydriasis
      d. Blurred vision
      e. Urinary retention
      f. Ileus
    3. Cardiovascular effects
      a. Hypotension
      b. Arrhythmias
        (1) Caused by three pharmacologic mechanisms
          (a) Blockage of norepinephrine reuptake
          (b) Anticholinergic effects
          (c) Quinidine-like myocardial depressant effects
        (2) Results in the following:
          (a) QT prolongation
          (b) Second- and third-degree block
          (c) Right bundle branch block
          (d) Nonspecific intraventricular delay pattern
          (e) Tachyarrhythmias, including supraventricular and ventricular tachycardias (ventricular fibrillation and premature ventricular beats)

D. Laboratory tests
   TCAs can be detected in blood and urine but serum levels have no particular implications for therapy.
E. Prediction of toxicity
   1. Ingested dose of 10-20 mg/kg of most TCAs results in moderate to severe toxicity
   2. Prolonged QRS interval >100 milliseconds in the limb leads (reflection of quinidine-like myocardial depressant effect) correlates with the severity of TCA intoxication and with a serum level >1000 mg/mL.
F. Management
   1. GI decontamination (Table 17-4)
   2. Repeat charcoal administration every 4 hours to interrupt enterohepatic circulation.
   3. Antidote therapy (Table 17-6)
      a. Physostigmine reverses CNS and peripheral anticholinergic symptoms but is usually unnecessary.
      b. Seizures are best controlled with lorazepam, 0.05 to 0.1 mg/kg/dose (max dose, 2 mg/dose), IV push. Physostigmine may be used for resistant seizures. Coma *per se* is not an indication for physostigmine.
   4. Cardiovascular effects
      a. Hypotension
         (1) Administer fluids.
         (2) Administer vasoactive drugs. Use direct acting α-adrenergic agents (e.g., neosynephrine and norepinephrine) rather than catecholamine precursor drugs (e.g., dopamine).
      b. Ventricular arrhythmias
         (1) Alkalinize (pH, 7.45 to 7.55) with $NaHCO_3$ or hyperventilation
         (2) If alkalinization fails, administer lidocaine or phenytoin as second-line therapy.
         (3) Hypertonic saline can be considered in patients not responding to the above interventions.
         (4) Avoid quinidine, procainamide, and disopyramide.
         (5) Propranolol can be used for supraventricular tachycardia.
         (6) Physostigmine is not effective in treating TCA-induced arrhythmias.
      c. Heart block (second- and third-degree)
         (1) Alkalinization
         (2) β-Agonist chronotropes (e.g., epinephrine)
         (3) Ventricular pacing
         (4) Physostigmine and phenytoin are contraindicated.

17

XI. Opioids
  A. Clinical manifestations of toxicity
    1. CNS
      a. Coma (all opioids)
      b. Seizures (particularly propoxyphene)
      c. Miosis
    2. Cardiovascular
      a. Hypotension (aggravated by hypoxia)
      b. Arrhythmias
        (1) Uncommon
        (2) Atrial fibrillation, particularly with heroin overdose
        (3) Prolonged QRS, particularly with propoxyphene overdose
    3. Pulmonary
      a. Respiratory depression (all opioids)
      b. Pulmonary edema (noncardiogenic etiology)
    4. GI
      a. Ileus
      b. Nausea
  B. Laboratory tests
    1. Toxicology screen (urine for qualitative detection of opioids)
    2. Blood gas determination
  C. Management
    1. Resuscitation and stabilization (ABCs)
    2. GI decontamination (Table 17-4)
    3. Antidote therapy: Naloxone (Table 17-6)
XII. Hydrocarbons
  A. General considerations
    1. Categories
      a. Petroleum distillates—kerosene, lighter fluid, gasoline, additives in household cleaners and polishes
      b. Pine oil distillates—turpentine
    2. Toxicity
      a. Caused primarily by pulmonary aspiration rather than systemic absorption
      b. The risk of aspiration is higher with low-viscosity, highly volatile compounds (e.g., gasoline, kerosene, mineral seed oil) than with low-viscosity oils (e.g., lubrication oil, petrolatum, paraffin) because of low surface tension that permits spread into lungs.
      c. Toxic additives that include heavy metals, pesticides, toluene, and camphor produce additional toxicity.
  B. Clinical manifestations
    1. Respiratory
      a. Cough, respiratory distress, dyspnea, cyanosis, hemoptysis, wheezes, rales, fever (associated with aspiration pneumonia)

       b. Symptoms are secondary to aspiration, and usually present within 6 hours if aspiration has occurred

  2. CNS
    a. CNS depression, somnolence
    b. Uncommon; may be secondary to hypoxia or to additional toxicity from additives

  3. GI
    a. Nausea
    b. Vomiting
    c. Abdominal pain
    d. Diarrhea

  4. Hematologic
    a. Hemolysis
    b. Methemoglobinemia occurs with gasoline ingestion (from red cell membrane damage).

C. Laboratory evaluation
  1. Chest radiograph: Signs of aspiration
  2. CBC and blood gas
  3. Tests to identify poisoning from toxic additives to petroleum distillates (e.g., aniline, nitrobenzene [methemoglobin], organophosphates, heavy metals)

D. Treatment
  1. Resuscitation and stabilization (ABCs)
  2. GI decontamination
    a. See Table 17-4.
    b. Indications for emesis or lavage are controversial and not universally accepted.
      (1) Emesis or lavage is not indicated for ingestion of commonly ingested hydrocarbons that do not contain toxic additives.
      (2) Induce emesis or lavage with the ingestion of toxic additives (e.g., camphor, pesticides, aniline, toluene, nitrobenzene, chlorinated hydrocarbons, xylene, alpha benzene).

XIII. Caustics
  A. Household caustic agents
    1. Drain, toilet, oven cleaners
    2. Clinitest tablets
    3. Laundry and dishwasher detergents
    4. Disc batteries
  B. Clinical manifestations
    1. Oral burns: Swelling, pain, dysphagia, drooling
    2. Esophageal burns, particularly after ingestion of caustic liquids
  C. Management
    1. Keep NPO (nothing by mouth).
    2. GI decontamination is **contraindicated.**

17

3. Charcoal absorbs caustic agents but may interfere with subsequent endoscopy and/or cause emesis.
4. Perform esophagoscopy within 12 hours after ingestion to identify extent of esophageal burns.

XIV. Cocaine
   A. Basic principles
      1. May affect children of all ages
      2. Infants and young children may become intoxicated by passive inhalation of crack cocaine smoke, ingestion of contaminated breast milk of drug-abusing mothers, and casual accidental ingestion.
      3. Frequent drug of abuse by adolescents
   B. Mechanisms of toxicity
      Cocaine prevents presynaptic reuptake of catecholamines at adrenergic nerve endings, potentiating the sympathetic response.
   C. Clinical manifestations
      1. Cardiovascular
         a. Myocardial ischemia or infarction
            (1) Chest pain
         b. Arrhythmias
            (1) Most common: Sinus tachycardia; also supraventricular tachycardia and ventricular tachycardia
            (2) Palpitations
            (3) Cardiovascular collapse
         c. Hypertension (headache, palpitations)
         d. Cardiomyopathy (arrhythmias, heart failure)
      2. Neurologic
         a. Patterns
            (1) Ischemic stroke
            (2) Intracerebral hemorrhage
            (3) Subarachnoid hemorrhage
         b. Signs and symptoms
            (1) Altered mental status (including agitation)
            (2) Headache
            (3) Seizures
            (4) Syncope
            (5) Focal neurologic signs, including mydriasis, hyperreflexia
            (6) Behavioral symptoms: Euphoria, anxiety, panic, agitation, suicidal and/or homicidal behaviors
            (7) Autonomic manifestations: Hyperthermia, bradycardia or tachycardia, hypertension or hypotension
      3. Respiratory
         a. Pneumothorax
         b. Pneumomediastinum (from Valsalva maneuver during crack cocaine smoke inhalation)

TABLE 17-14	
TREATMENT OF ACUTE COCAINE INTOXICATION	
Clinical Manifestation	**Treatment**
Agitation	Diazepam
Seizures	Diazepam for status epilepticus; single seizures usually do not require therapy; phenytoin loading for seizures unresponsive to diazepam
Hyperthermia	Cooling blanket, antipyretics
Hypertension	Diazepam for agitation, nitroprusside, phentolamine, or labetalol
Arrhythmias	
Supraventricular tachycardia	Diazepam for agitation; then labetalol, or propranolol, or esmolol, or verapamil
Ventricular tachycardia	Labetalol or calcium channel blocker
Myocardial ischemia	Nitroglycerin, calcium channel blockers or beta blockers*, diuretics
Rhabdomyolysis	Alkalinize urine with $NaHCO_3$

*Use beta blockers cautiously because they may aggravate hypertension by leaving α-agonist action of cocaine unopposed.

       (1) Respiratory distress, tachypnea
       (2) Chest pain
    4. Gastrointestinal
      a. Hemorrhage or ischemia
        (1) GI hemorrhage
        (2) Bowel perforation (newborns)
        (3) Liver dysfunction
      b. Renal
        (1) Rhabdomyolysis
        (2) Renal failure
  D. Laboratory tests
    1. Cocaine is rapidly metabolized by cholinesterases and disappears from the blood within hours.
    2. The metabolites benzoylecgonine and ecgonine methyl ester persist longer in the urine where they are usually qualitatively detected.
  E. Management
    1. Resuscitation and stabilization (ABCs)
    2. GI decontamination (if cocaine was ingested): Activated charcoal and cathartics
    3. Treatment of specific clinical manifestations of intoxication (**Table 17-14**)

17

Chapter 18

Status Epilepticus
Jennifer G. Duncan, MD

I. Overview
   A. Definitions
      1. Status epilepticus (SE) is a single continuous seizure or repetitive seizures lasting longer than 30 minutes without recovery of consciousness.
      2. Seizures lasting longer than 5 minutes may produce neuronal damage, and have a high probability of lasting longer than 30 minutes. Therefore, treatment should commence for any seizure that has already lasted 5 minutes or longer.
      3. Nonconvulsive SE: A child with altered mental status and/or cranial nerve deficits may have nonconvulsive SE. Definitive diagnosis of nonconvulsive SE requires an electroencephalogram (EEG).
   B. Classification
      1. Generalized convulsive SE (grand mal)
         a. Tonic-clonic
         b. Clonic
         c. Myoclonic (e.g., after cardiac arrest)
      2. **Generalized nonconvulsive** SE (also called petit mal or absence seizures and manifested by staring spells)
      3. **Complex partial** SE (manifested as *focal* motor, sensory, autonomic, or cognitive symptoms with decreased consciousness)
      4. **Simple partial** SE (*focal* motor or sensory symptoms without loss of consciousness)
   C. Epidemiology and causes
      1. The cause is unknown in half of cases; the other half has acute or chronic central nervous system (CNS) disorders.
         a. Idiopathic without fever—approximately 25% of cases
         b. Fever-related—approximately 25% of cases
         c. Related to underlying chronic CNS insult (congenital, birth injury) and epilepsy often with inadequate anticonvulsant levels—approximately 25% of cases
         d. Related to acute CNS insult (e.g., meningitis, encephalitis, brain tumor, cerebrovascular insult) or acute metabolic derangement (e.g., hypoglycemia, hyponatremia, hypocalcemia, or toxins)—approximately 25% of cases

2. Most prevalent age group in children: Younger than 3 years

II. Pathophysiology

A. Direct CNS injury

1. Initial increased autonomic activity to maintain cerebral perfusion
2. Increased cerebral blood flow and cerebral metabolic demand
3. With prolonged seizures, there may be hypotension, decreased cerebral perfusion, decreased availability of substrate for brain metabolism, resulting in lactic acidosis, cellular hypoxia, and ultimately neuronal death.
4. Intracranial pressure may increase.

B. Systemic stress

1. Hypoxemia secondary to the following:

   a. Hypoventilation (often exacerbated by benzodiazepine or barbiturate anticonvulsant therapy)
   b. Pharyngeal hypotonia and upper airway obstruction
   c. Loss of airway reflexes
   d. Excessive secretions
   e. Increased oxygen (O_2) consumption

2. Hyperglycemia initially (secondary to catecholamine release) followed by hypoglycemia (secondary to substrate consumption)
3. Hypertension followed by hypotension
4. Tachycardia
5. Hyperthermia
6. Rhabdomyolysis leading to hyperkalemia

III. Management

An aggressive and organized approach to acute management is necessary to prevent or minimize morbidity and mortality from SE. Management is divided conceptually into three phases, which overlap in practice: (1) emergency stabilization; (2) anticonvulsant therapy; and (3) diagnostic workup.

A. Emergency stabilization (ABCs)

The primary goal of this phase is to prevent secondary hypoxic-ischemic brain injury.

1. Respiration: Establish an adequate airway and ensure adequate oxygenation and ventilation (see Chapter 2).

   a. 100% O_2
   b. Jaw thrust or triple jaw maneuver (see Chapter 2) if upper airway is obstructed. Consider nasal airway if upper airway obstruction recurs once jaw maneuvers are relaxed.
   c. Suction the mouth and pharynx.
   d. Bag and mask ventilation with cricoid pressure if patient is cyanotic or ventilating inadequately (in preparation for intubation)

2. Intubation and assisted ventilation

   a. Most SE patients do not require intubation.

b. High risk of respiratory failure necessitating intubation if SE persists despite more than two doses of benzodiazepine or phenobarbital administration.

c. Common indications for intubation include the following:

(1) Apnea or hypoventilation after multiple doses of anticonvulsant

(2) O_2 saturation <90% despite face mask O_2 and triple jaw maneuver

d. Thiopental or propofol are excellent anesthetic choices for a rapid sequence induction in the SE patient; ketamine is contraindicated because it lowers seizure threshold.

e. A short-acting (e.g., succinylcholine, mivacurium) or intermediate-acting (e.g., rocuronium, vecuronium) muscle relaxant is used to facilitate intubation.

(1) Longer-acting muscle relaxants will obliterate the neurologic examination for a prolonged period of time.

(2) Although rare, rhabdomyolysis and hyperkalemia may complicate SE and contraindicate succinylcholine.

f. See Chapter 2 for a full description of rapid sequence induction techniques.

3. Circulation

a. Establish venous (or intraosseous [IO]) access.

b. Perform serum glucose determination stat (Chemstrip or Dextrostick) on blood from venipuncture (see later).

c. Do not delay anticonvulsant therapy because of lack of intravenous (IV) or IO access.

d. Intramuscular (IM) or buccal midazolam and rectal (PR) diazepam are anticonvulsant options (see later).

e. Most SE patients are normotensive or mildly hypertensive on presentation and should receive 5% dextrose–normal saline (or normal saline) at maintenance rates pending laboratory results.

f. If the patient is hypotensive or poorly perfused, administer normal saline 20 mL/kg stat; may repeat twice if no improvement.

g. If hypotension or poor perfusion persist, start dopamine infusion and consider sepsis or meningitis, very prolonged SE (hours), anticonvulsant effects, or uncal herniation as causes.

h. Continuously monitor electrocardiogram, pulse oximetry, and blood pressure, and reassess the patient's cardiorespiratory status during and after administration of anesthetics and anticonvulsants.

i. Respiratory depression and hypotension are common side effects of anticonvulsants.

4. Metabolic management
   a. Obtain blood for rapid glucose determination (Chemstrip) and initial laboratory studies; hypoglycemia could be the cause of SE.
   b. Administer 25% dextrose, 2.0 mL/kg IV, if glucose is low (<60 mg/dL).
   c. Consider administering naloxone, 0.1 mg/kg, pyridoxine 50 to 100 mg, and/or thiamine, 100 mg, to unresponsive patients.
5. Fever management
   a. Control fever with acetaminophen, 10 to 15 mg/kg PR, cool compresses, or cooling blanket.
   b. Fever commonly triggers seizures, but may also be a result of excessive muscle activity during SE.
   c. Simple febrile seizures occur in children 6 months to 5 years of age.
   d. These are usually brief, generalized seizures and rarely last more than 20 minutes.
   e. Hyperthermia may exacerbate neuronal damage especially if seizures are prolonged.
6. Historical clues to guide management: Questioning the parents about these may provide important clues to management.
   a. Missed anticonvulsant dose(s)
      (1) Does the patient have a known seizure disorder and was an anticonvulsant dose missed?
      (2) If yes, then consider administering the missed anticonvulsant dose rather than proceeding with the standard SE protocol that follows.
   b. Hypoglycemia secondary to insulin overdose or inborn error of metabolism
      (1) Is there a history of diabetes mellitus treated with insulin or a history of vomiting or recent dietary change in an infant, suggesting the possibility of an inborn error of metabolism?
      (2) In these cases, glucose therapy alone is generally sufficient to correct SE unless secondary neurologic injury has already occurred.
   c. Hyponatremia
      (1) Is there a history of excessive water intake, vomiting, or diarrhea, which may have precipitated hyponatremia?
      (2) SE will not resolve until hyponatremia has been treated (see Chapter 8).
   d. Hypocalcemia
      (1) Are there signs or symptoms of hypovitaminosis D (growth retardation, hypotonia, muscle wasting, osteomalacia on radiograph), DiGeorge syndrome

18

(frequent infections, history of congenital heart disease), pancreatitis (abdominal pain, fever), or congenital or acquired hypoparathyroidism (family history of hypoparathyroidism, history of neck surgery)?

(2) SE will not resolve until hypocalcemia has been corrected.

(3) Serum calcium level should be measured in all patients with SE.

B. Anticonvulsant therapy
   1. Goals of therapy
      a. Rapid termination of seizure activity (usually achieved by benzodiazepines)
      b. Prevention of seizure recurrence and secondary injury (usually achieved by hydantoins or barbiturates)
      c. Avoidance of anticonvulsant-induced respiratory depression, if possible
   2. Route of administration
      a. The IV or IO route is preferred if establishing access does not delay in therapy.
      b. Midazolam, lorazepam, and fosphenytoin are effective via IM route. Diazepam is *contraindicated* via IM route.
      c. Midazolam, lorazepam, and diazepam are effective PR.
      d. Midazolam and lorazepam are effective intranasally, but require an atomizer for drug delivery.
      e. Buccal midazolam is effective.
   3. Benzodiazepines: Potent and rapidly acting agents, widely used for acute control of seizures
      a. Lorazepam
         (1) *Currently the preferred first-line IV drug to treat SE* because of the greater probability of rapid seizure control, longer duration of action, and lower incidence of respiratory depression compared to diazepam.
         (2) Dose: 0.05 to 0.1 mg/kg IV; may repeat once. However, if more than two doses are required, prepare for intubation and ventilatory support.
         (3) Onset of action: Within 2 minutes after IV administration
         (4) Duration of seizure control: 4 to 6 hours
         (5) Formulation: Includes propylene glycol, which may cause lactic acidosis and hyperosmolality after prolonged continuous IV infusion
      b. Midazolam
         (1) Dose: 0.15 mg/kg IV; may repeat q5min
         (2) Onset of action: Seizure control usually within 1 to 2 minutes after IV administration
         (3) Duration of seizure control: 1 to 2 hours

        (4) Alternative routes
- (a) Buccal midazolam, ~0.3 to 0.5 mg/kg (of the IV preparation) placed on the buccal mucosa between the gum and cheek using a syringe attached to a small IV cannula
- (b) Excess secretions should be suctioned from the buccal area before attempting buccal midazolam therapy.
- (c) *Buccal midazolam appears to be more effective than PR diazepam and is the best alternative when there is no IV access.*

  c. Diazepam
- (1) The oldest benzodiazepine—the gold standard for acute anticonvulsant therapy
- (2) Dose: 0.1 to 0.3 mg/kg IV
- (3) Onset of action: Seizure control in <60 seconds
- (4) Duration of seizure control: Less than 20 minutes (because of rapid redistribution from CNS to fat)
- (5) Alternative routes:
  - (a) PR diazepam gel (Diastat), 0.2 to 0.5 mg/kg
  - (b) The prepackaged gel formulation can be given in increments of 2.5, 10, and 20 mg.
  - (c) The dose is age-dependent (0.5 mg/kg for ages 2 to 5 years, 0.3 mg/kg for ages 6 to 11 years, and 0.2 mg/kg for those older than 11 years).
  - (d) *The prepackaging and easy storage make PR diazepam a useful alternative for families and prehospital providers.*

4. Hydantoins (phenytoin or fosphenytoin): Long-acting agents, recommended as second-line medication if seizures do not terminate with benzodiazepines

  a. Phenytoin
- (1) Reaches peak brain levels within 15 minutes of administration
- (2) Requires slow infusion (<50 mg/min for adults or 0.5 to 1 mg/kg/min for infants and children) to avoid bradycardia, hypotension, and local tissue reactions (venous thrombosis, edema, necrosis); these adverse effects are caused by the propylene glycol solvent for phenytoin.
- (3) *It has largely been replaced as an emergency IV anticonvulsant in the United States by fosphenytoin because of the latter's better safety profile.*

18

b. Fosphenytoin
   (1) Enzymatically converted to phenytoin
   (2) Should be ordered as "mg of phenytoin equivalent" (PE); each vial contains 75 mg/mL fosphenytoin, equivalent to 50 mg/mL phenytoin.
   (3) Can be infused more rapidly (3 mg/kg/min or 150 mg/min in adults)
   (4) Does not carry risk of extravasation
   (5) Lower incidence of hypotension and arrhythmia
   (6) Can be administered intramuscularly with rapid and complete absorption
   (7) Loading dose: 15 to 20 mg/kg PE IV.
   (8) Maintenance dose: 4 to 8 mg/kg PE/day divided bid or tid
   (9) Onset of action: Seizure control in 15 minutes after IV dose, 30 min after IM dose
   (10) Duration of seizure control: 12 to 24 hours
   (11) Start maintenance dose 12 hours after loading dose.

5. Phenobarbital (barbiturate)
   a. Potent, long-acting antiepileptic agent
   b. High doses are required for acute seizure termination, increasing risks of side effects.
   c. Side effects: Prolonged sedation, respiratory depression, hypotension
   d. Administration of benzodiazepines prior to loading with phenobarbital significantly increases the risk of respiratory depression and may necessitate intubation.
   e. The risk profile for phenobarbital makes it a third-line anticonvulsant after benzodiazepines and fosphenytoin have failed.
   f. Loading dose: 10 to 20 mg/kg IV slowly (over 10 to 20 minutes)
   g. Maintenance dose: 3 to 5 mg/kg/day divided or bid
   h. Onset of action: Seizure control in 30 minutes
   i. Duration of seizure control: 24 hours
   j. Start maintenance dose 12 hours after loading dose.

6. Valproate
   a. Available in IV and oral forms
   b. Indications for IV valproate during SE: Patients already taking oral valproic acid, prolonged complex partial seizures, SE refractory to lorazepam and fosphenytoin
   c. Loading dose: 30 mg/kg IV slowly (over 10 to 15 minutes)
   d. Maintenance infusion: 1 to 4 mg/kg/hr
   e. Pharmacokinetics: Inadequate data in children

      f. Dosing is dependent on drug level for patients with prior exposure to valproate.

      g. May be better tolerated in hemodynamically unstable patients.

      h. Major adverse reactions are hepatotoxicity and pancreatitis, especially in children younger than 2 years.

C. Treatment strategy

    1. There are only limited data to guide an evidence-based treatment algorithm.

    2. IV lorazepam will control SE in up to 76% of patients and is the preferred first-line therapy.

    3. In the absence of IV access, buccal midazolam is more effective than PR diazepam (56% versus 27% success rate), but PR diazepam is more likely to be available in the home or for prehospital providers.

    4. Fosphenytoin may be effective in some patients who were refractory to benzodiazepines and offers prolonged anticonvulsant activity after benzodiazepine effects have dissipated.

    5. One study has suggested that valproate may terminate seizures in 78% of cases after failure of other anticonvulsants; however, the risk of hepatotoxicity from valproate is increased in children younger than 2 years, suggesting that phenobarbital may be the safer choice in infants.

    6. Based on these limited data, we offer the algorithm in **Figure 18-1** to achieve the goals of rapid seizure termination, prevention of seizure recurrence, and avoidance of respiratory depression.

D. General anesthesia

    1. If seizures do not respond to aggressive administration of benzodiazepines, hydantoins, phenobarbital, and valproate, then a continuous infusion of a benzodiazepine (midazolam) or barbiturate (pentobarbital, thiopental) is available to control seizures.

    2. Patients will require intubation and ventilatory support and must be monitored **in an intensive care unit setting,** preferably with continuous monitoring of the EEG.

    3. Infusions are adjusted with a goal of burst suppression on continuous electroencephalography.

    4. We do *not* recommend the use of prolonged propofol infusion to control SE in children because of the risk of propofol infusion syndrome, characterized by severe metabolic acidosis, rhabdomyolysis, and death.

18

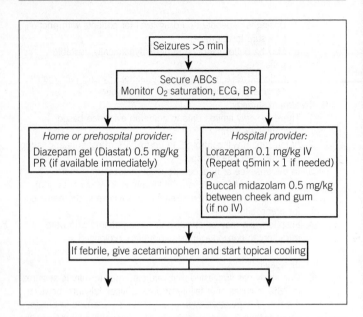

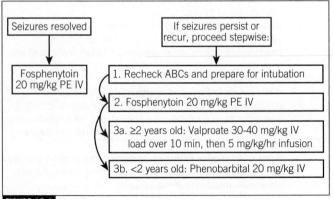

FIGURE 18-1

Treatment algorithm for prolonged seizures and status epilepticus (SE). Note the stepwise approach for refractory SE. Only proceed to the next step if SE persists. The anticonvulsant choice for step 3 depends on the patient's age.

ABCs, Airway, breathing, circulation; *BP,* blood pressure; *ECG,* electrocardiogram; *IV,* intravenous; *O_2,* oxygen; *PE,* phenytoin equivalent; *PR,* by rectum.

IV. Diagnostic workup
  A. Goals
     1. Diagnose the underlying disease process and initiate definitive treatment.
     2. Perform an exhaustive history and physical examination after the patient has been stabilized and seizures controlled.
  B. Laboratory evaluation
     1. Inadequate anticonvulsant levels represent the most common laboratory explanation for SE. All patients receiving anticonvulsants chronically should have drug levels checked when presenting with SE.
     2. Complete blood count, electrolytes, glucose, calcium, magnesium, phosphate, blood urea nitrate, creatinine, liver function tests, urinalysis, toxicology screen, ammonia, blood gas, metabolic screen for inborn error of metabolism (infants)
     3. Microbiology cultures if the presentation suggests infection
        a. Any febrile patient with SE should have cultures obtained and antibiotics started pending culture results.
        b. Lumbar puncture (LP) indications and contraindications are summarized in **Box 18-1.**
        c. Do not attempt LP unless the cardiorespiratory status has been stabilized.

BOX 18-1

INDICATIONS AND CONTRAINDICATIONS TO LUMBAR PUNCTURE IN STATUS EPILEPTICUS

INDICATIONS

- Meningeal signs (stiff neck)
- Febrile child <18 mo
- Immunocompromised host
- First episode of SE

CONTRAINDICATIONS

- Coagulopathy, thrombocytopenia
- Cardiopulmonary instability
- Evidence of increased intracranial pressure
- Focal seizure or neurologic deficit (unless computed tomography scan is normal)
- Infection at site of needle insertion

18

BOX 18-2

INDICATIONS FOR EMERGENCY HEAD COMPUTED TOMOGRAPHY* IN STATUS EPILEPTICUS

- Head trauma
- Focal neurologic deficit
- Examination findings suggestive of increased intracranial pressure
- New focal seizure activity
- First episode of SE

*With no IV contrast.

C. Imaging studies
   1. Computed tomography (without IV contrast) of the brain indications (**Box 18-2**). The patient must be stabilized before computed tomography scan.
   2. Magnetic resonance imaging is indicated if the cause of the seizure remains unknown after the diagnostic evaluation (see earlier).

Chapter 19

Meningitis and Sepsis

Lisa Saiman, MD, MPH,
and David G. Nichols, MD, MBA

I. Overview

Despite advances in effective vaccines, antimicrobial therapy, and supportive care, meningitis and sepsis syndromes continue to cause significant morbidity and mortality in children. Bacterial pathogens generally have more acute and fulminant presentations, whereas viruses, mycobacteria, or fungi usually have more subacute and/or chronic presentations. However, nonbacterial pathogens can be deadly in neonates or immunocompromised children. The central nervous system (CNS) and systemic response to infection is mediated by the inflammatory cytokines and is manifested as a systemic inflammatory response syndrome (SIRS).

II. Definitions*

A. Systemic inflammatory response syndrome

This is defined as the presence of two of the four following criteria, one of which must be abnormal temperature or leukocyte count:

1. Core temperature: >38.5° C or <36° C
2. Tachycardia: Persistent, unexplained heart rate elevation >2 standard deviations (SD) above normal for age; for infants younger than 1 year, the occurrence of bradycardia (heart rate <10% for age)
3. Tachypnea (respiratory rate >2 SD for age)
4. Leukocyte count elevated or depressed for age, or more than 10% immature neutrophils

B. Infection

1. A proven infection from any pathogen requires positive culture, tissue stain, or polymerase chain reaction (PCR) assay.
2. A clinical syndrome with suspected infection; the probable cause is based on physical examination (e.g., petechial or purpuric rash), imaging (e.g., perforated viscus, pneumonia), or laboratory test results (e.g., white cells in normally sterile fluid).

19

*Modified from Goldstein B, Giroir B, Randolph A. International Pediatric Sepsis Consensus Conference: Definitions for sepsis and organ dysfunction in pediatrics. Pediatr Crit Care Med 2005;6:2-8.

C. Sepsis

This is defined as SIRS with a suspected or proven infection.

D. Severe sepsis

This is defined as sepsis with one of the following:

1. Cardiovascular dysfunction
2. Acute respiratory distress syndrome (ARDS)

   or
3. Two or more other organ dysfunctions

E. Septic shock

Sepsis and cardiovascular organ dysfunction are defined as one of the following despite the administration of isotonic fluid (≥40 mL/kg in 1 hour):

1. Hypotension

   or
2. Need for vasoactive drugs to maintain normal blood pressure

   or
3. Two or more of the following:
   a. Unexplained acidosis (base deficit >5.0 mEq/L)
   b. Increased arterial lactate (>2× normal)
   c. Oliguria (urine output <0.5 mL/kg/hr)
   d. Prolonged capillary refill (>5 seconds)
   e. Core to peripheral temperature gap >3° C

F. Meningitis

Meningitis is defined as the inflammation of the meninges caused by invasion of the CNS by a bacterial, viral, fungal, or mycobacterial pathogen.

III. Initial evaluation and resuscitation

A. Assess and stabilize airway, breathing, and circulation

Septic shock requires a goal-directed and time-dependent therapeutic protocol for best results, as shown in Figure 6-1 (see Chapters 2, 6, and 7).

B. Make provisional diagnosis

A provisional diagnosis can be made, but create a differential diagnosis and continue to reassess.

C. History

Important elements of the history are detailed in **Table 19-1**.

D. Physical examination

Signs and symptoms are shown in **Table 19-2**.

E. Neonates

1. May have subtle findings from history and physical examination
2. A lower threshold is required for performing a sepsis workup on infants younger than 2 months.
3. Peripartum history may help predict the newborn at increased risk of infection (**Box 19-1**).

TABLE 19-1

IMPORTANT ELEMENTS OF PATIENT HISTORY TO OBTAIN IN DIAGNOSIS OF MENINGITIS AND SEPSIS

Element	Comment	Example of Pathogen
Birth history	Prematurity, hospitalization, maternal infections, maternal antibiotics, maternal dietary history	Resistant gram-positive or gram-negative organisms, Listeria, herpes simplex virus
Immunization status	Review immunizations to determine if appropriate for age	H. influenzae B, S. pneumoniae
Asplenia	Sickle cell disease	S. pneumoniae
Known exposures	Ill contacts	N. meningitides, enterovirus, Mycobacterium tuberculosis
Dietary history	Eating inadequately cooked hamburger meat	E. coli, hemolytic-uremic syndrome
Symptoms	Antecedent pharyngitis	Group A streptococcus
Recent foreign travel	Endemic regions	Tuberculosis, malaria
Menses history	Tampon use, menses	S. aureus, toxic shock syndrome
Animal or insect bite	Camping history, endemic area, mosquito bite	Rocky Mountain spotted fever, Lyme disease, West Nile virus

TABLE 19-2

PHYSICAL FINDINGS SUGGESTIVE OF MENINGITIS AND/OR SEPSIS

Age <3 mo	Age >3 mo
Fever (may be absent)	Fever*
Hypothermia	Dehydration
Dehydration	Severe headache*
Lethargy	Chills*
Irritability	Photophobia*
High-pitched cry	Change in mental status
Bulging or sunken fontanelle	Irritability
Seizures	Somnolence
Hypotonia	High-pitched cry
Irregular respirations	Ataxia
Respiratory distress/apnea	Seizures
Cardiovascular collapse	Meningismus*
Vomiting	Tachypnea
Jaundice	Cardiovascular collapse
Abdominal distention	Vomiting,* anorexia
Jitteriness (hypoglycemia)	Rash, purpura
	Arthritis, arthralgia
	Buccal or periorbital cellulitis

*Classic meningitis in older children and adolescents.

19

BOX 19-1

RISK FACTORS FOR EARLY ONSET NEONATAL MENINGITIS AND SEPSIS

Prolonged rupture of membranes (>18-24 hr)
Positive maternal GBS culture
Previous sibling with invasive disease caused by GBS
Multiple gestations*
Maternal fever
Chorioamnionitis
Prematurity
5-min Apgar <6
Male gender*
Maternal dietary history, including unpasteurized dairy products
Maternal illness (e.g., vomiting, diarrhea)

GBS, Group B streptococci.
*Not demonstrated by all studies for GBS.

F. Choose appropriate empirical antimicrobial therapy
See **Table 19-3.**
1. For the unstable patient, administer immediately.
   a. All efforts should be made to obtain blood cultures prior to initiating antimicrobial therapy, but **do not wait** to administer antibiotics.
2. For the stable patient, obtain appropriate cultures and laboratory tests before antibiotic administration.
G. Treat shock
See Chapter 6.
H. Treat seizures
See Chapter 18.
I. Continue to reassess patient for complications.
IV. Lumbar puncture (LP) procedure
A. Preliminary computed tomography (CT) brain scan
1. Consider obtaining CT scan of the brain prior to LP to rule out cerebral edema or space-occupying lesion (abscess) before proceeding with LP.
2. Rarely, an LP can cause acute decompensation and possible brain herniation.
3. LP should be avoided in high-risk patients, but administration of antimicrobials should not be delayed if cerebrospinal fluid (CSF) cannot be safely obtained.
B. Opening pressure
After successful LP (**Fig. 19-1**), measure opening pressure to estimate intracranial pressure (ICP) (**Fig. 19-2**).
C. Collect CSF for laboratory analyses
1. Minimum evaluation should include cell count and type,
2. Gram stain and culture, and glucose and protein measurement can be carried out (**Tables 19-4** and **19-5**).

TABLE 19-3

EMPIRICAL INITIAL ANTIMICROBIAL THERAPY FOR SUSPECTED SEPSIS*

Age	Antibiotic
Neonate (<30 days)	Ampicillin, 50-100 mg/kg IV q6h
	Acyclovir, 20 mg/kg IV q8h
	Vancomycin, 15-20 mg/kg IV q6-12h†
	Cefotaxime, 50 mg/kg IV q8-12h
	Gentamicin, 2.5 mg/kg IV q8-12h
>1 mo, previously well child	Vancomycin, 15 mg/kg IV q6-8h†
	Cefotaxime, 50 mg/kg IV q6h, or ceftriaxone, 100 mg/kg IV q12h (max 4 gm per day)
Suspected urinary source	Gentamicin, 2.5 mg/kg IV q8h‡
Suspected intra-abdominal focus	Metronidazole, 30 mg/kg IV q6h, or clindamycin, 5-10 mg/kg IV q6h
Immunocompromised host or suspected *Pseudomonas* infection (e.g., cystic fibrosis, tracheostomy)	Cefepime, 50 mg/kg IV q8h, or ceftazidime, 50 mg/kg IV q8h
	Gentamicin, 2.5 mg/kg IV q8h‡
	Vancomycin, 15 mg/kg IV q6-8h†
Central line or ventriculoperitoneal shunt	Cefepime, 50 mg/kg IV q8h
	Vancomycin, 20 mg/kg IV q6-8h†

IV, Intravenous.

*Culture results and serum antibiotic levels should guide subsequent therapy.

†After the initial dose, subsequent vancomycin dosing intervals should always be guided by measurement of serum vancomycin levels (peak and trough).

‡Gentamicin usage should be guided by knowledge of local resistance patterns and the history of the patient's prior pathogens.

    D. Additional CSF testing
        1. Depends on the clinical circumstances
        2. Examples include:
            a. PCR assay for herpes simplex virus in a septic-appearing neonate or older child with changes in mental status or seizures
            b. PCR assay for enteroviruses in a child presenting in the summer months with a lymphocytic pleocytosis in the CSF
        3. Extra CSF can be stored in the laboratory for future testing after consultation with an infectious disease consultant.
        4. Routine use of bacterial antigen tests has not been shown to be helpful in clinical management, nor is it cost-effective.
 V. Contraindications or relative contraindications to performing an LP (see Box 18-1)
    A. Airway incompetence prior to intubation
    B. Respiratory failure
    C. Hemodynamic instability
    D. Bleeding diathesis
    E. Likelihood of increased ICP

19

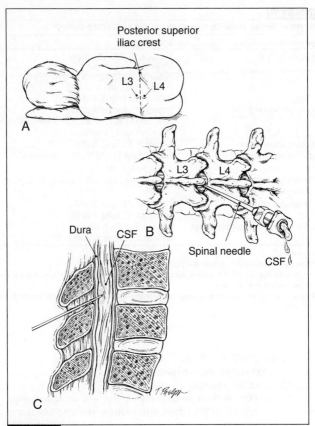

FIGURE 19-1

Performing a lumbar puncture. The patient is positioned in the lateral decubitus or seated position. **A,** The L2-3 or L3-4 interspace is chosen; the patient's legs and, less commonly, the hips are flexed to open the interspaces maximally. It is not necessary to flex the neck with good hip flexion. Using strict aseptic technique, including wearing mask, gown, and sterile gloves, prepare and drape the back. Infiltrate the skin, subcutaneous tissue, and superficial ligaments with local anesthetic. **B,** Insert the spinal needle into the prepared space. The approach should be in the midline and perpendicular to the patient's spinal axis. Deviations from the perpendicular plane result in needle tip placement lateral to the midline, not into the subarachnoid space. Needle lengths range from 1.5 inches for neonates to 3.5 inches for adults. **C,** A 22-gauge needle is a good size for collection of CSF and measurement of opening pressure.

CSF, Cerebrospinal fluid.

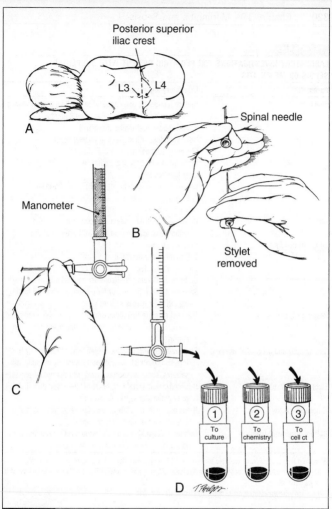

FIGURE 19-2

A, B, Measurement of opening pressure. The opening pressure is measured
immediately after obtaining CSF flow. This is most easily done by connecting the
manometer and stopcock to a short, flexible piece of tubing. This tubing is
connected directly to the spinal needle (all pieces of the system must be sterile).
The stopcock is turned so that CSF travels up the manometer. Allow the flow to
continue until it stops and the level varies with respirations. This is when the
patient's opening pressure is measured, in mm or cm H_2O. Normal intracranial
pressure is <10-15 mm Hg or 136-204 mm H_2O. The conversion of cm H_2O to
mm Hg is 10 cm H_2O to 7.5 mm Hg. **C,** After obtaining the opening pressure, turn
the stopcock so that CSF from the manometer flows into collection tubes. **D,** Turn
the stopcock again so CSF drips from the patient into the collection tubes. Note that
an accurate opening pressure can be obtained only in a quiet, noncrying child.
CSF, Cerebrospinal fluid.

TABLE 19-4

LABORATORY INVESTIGATIONS FOR PEDIATRIC PATIENT WITH SUSPECTED SEPSIS OR MENINGITIS

Parameter	Laboratory Analyses
Blood*	Culture (peripheral and central if in-dwelling central venous catheter is present; anaerobic blood cultures if intra-abdominal source suspected)
	CBC, including differential and platelet count
	Glucose (also compare with CSF glucose)
	Electrolytes with BUN and creatinine
	Liver function tests
	Coagulation profile including PT, PTT, INR, fibrinogen, D-dimer
	C-reactive protein
Urine*	Urinalysis for blood, protein, leukocyte esterase, and microscopic examination for WBC bacteria culture
Cerebrospinal fluid	Opening pressure
	Cell count and differential
	Glucose and protein
	Cultures and Gram stain (consider nonbacterial pathogens)
	Save extra CSF in laboratory for possible specialized testing, e.g., PCR for herpes simplex virus.
Respiratory tract	Tracheal aspirate for culture and Gram stain when indicated; nasopharyngeal washings for viral pathogens (PCR and culture)
Radiography and diagnostic imaging	Chest radiography, if signs or symptoms of respiratory tract infection; head CT scan, if focal neurologic examination, seizures, coma, suspected increased intracranial pressure
Electrocardiography	If hemodynamic instability, heart failure, respiratory distress, or symptoms of sepsis are present
Echocardiography	If hemodynamic instability, heart failure, respiratory distress, or symptoms of sepsis are present
Culture of relevant tissue	Culture relevant skin and soft tissue sites if cellulitis, fasciitis, or menses or tampon use is present.

BUN, Blood urea nitrogen; *CBC*, complete blood count; *CSF*, cerebrospinal fluid; *CT*, computed tomography; *INR*, international normalized ratio; *PCR*, polymerase chain reaction; *PT*, prothrombin time; *PTT*, partial thromboplastin time; *WBC*, white blood cell.

*Serum and urine osmolality if initial chemistry studies are abnormal.

VI. Causes of meningitis and sepsis
  A. Overview
    1. Causes vary with chronologic age and risk factors, including previous hospitalization in a neonatal intensive care unit.
    2. Common pathogens in different age groups are listed in **Table 19-6**.
    3. Less common pathogens are listed in **Table 19-7.**
  B. Neonatal sepsis and meningitis
    1. Bacterial pathogens
      a. The rate of early-onset group B streptococcal infections has decreased because of widespread use of peripartum chemoprophylaxis in many countries.

TABLE 19-5

CEREBROSPINAL FLUID FINDINGS

Patient	WBC (mm³)	Cell Type	Glucose	Protein
Normal child	<5	Mono	>60% serum level	<40 mg/dL
Normal neonate	<30	<60% PMN	>50% serum level	<100 mg/dL
Bacterial meningitis	>1000 (1000-5000)	PMN	<50% serum level	Elevated
Viral meningitis	<1000	PMN—early Lymphocytes—later	Normal-minimally low	Moderately elevated
Tubercular meningitis	50-500	Lymphocytes	Low	Very elevated
Fungal meningitis	100	Monocytes	Low	Elevated
Encephalitis	5-1000	PMN—early Mono—late	Normal	Normal-high
Brain abscess	Normal or 5-500	Variable—normal or PMNs	Normal	Normal-mildly elevated

Mono, Mononuclear leukocyte; *PMN,* polymorphonuclear leukocyte; *WBC,* white blood cell.

TABLE 19-6

COMMON BACTERIAL PATHOGENS IN MENINGITIS AND SEPSIS

Age Group/Source	Pathogen
Neonatal meningitis	
Community-acquired	GBS (subtype III); *Escherichia coli* (K1), enterococcal spp., *Listeria monocytogenes*
Hospital-acquired	Staphylococcal spp.; gram-negative bacilli (e.g., *Pseudomonas, Citrobacter* spp.)
Developing world	*E. coli, Salmonella* spp., *Klebsiella pneumoniae*
Infants, 1 to 3 mo	GBS, *E. coli* and *Klebsiella, Streptococcus pneumoniae, Neisseria meningitidis*
Infants >3 mo to children	*S. pneumoniae, N. meningitidis,* GAS, MRSA
Children >5 yr to adolescents	*S. pneumoniae, N. meningitidis* MRSA

GAS, Group A streptococci; *GBS,* group B streptococci; *MRSA,* methicillin-resistant *S. aureus.*

   b. Late-onset disease with group B streptococci (GBS) still occurs.
     (1) Risk factors are less well understood.
     (2) A history of prematurity, maternal anovaginal colonization with GBS, and race (African American) may be risk factors for late-onset disease.
   c. Enterococcal species may also cause early-onset sepsis and meningitis in neonates.
   d. *Escherichia coli* is a common cause of early-onset sepsis and meningitis in the newborn; other gram-negative enteric bacilli are less common causes of meningitis in neonates.
   e. *Listeria monocytogenes* is a well-described, although relatively uncommon, cause of newborn meningitis and sepsis.

19

TABLE 19-7	
LESS COMMON PATHOGENS ASSOCIATED WITH MENINGITIS	
Pathogen	**Diagnostic Test**
MYCOBACTERIA	
Mycobacterium tuberculosis	CSF culture and PCR, tuberculin skin test, chest radiography
VIRAL	
Enteroviruses (coxsackievirus, echovirus)	Culture of CSF, throat, rectum, PCR of CSF
Arboviruses	PCR or serology
West Nile virus	PCR and serology
Herpes simplex virus	PCR of CSF, culture of skin lesions and urine
Varicella-zoster virus	Biopsy, culture, PCR
Lymphocytic choriomeningitis	Serology, PCR
Epstein-Barr virus	Serology (IgM and IgG) and PCR of serum
Rabies	Biopsy of conjunctiva, brain, and skin
Adenovirus	Respiratory and gastrointestinal tract cultures and PCR of serum
SPIROCHETES	
Lyme disease	CSF antibodies—Western blot, PCR
Syphilis	VDRL, FTA-ABS, IgM
Leptospirosis	Culture—prolonged incubation, PCR
Rat bite fever (Streptobacillus moniliformus)	Cultures, blood or joint fluid
RICKETTSIAE	
Typhus (Rickettsia typhi)	Serology
Rocky Mountain spotted fever	Serology, PCR, cell culture
Ehrlichiosis	Culture, PCR, serology
FUNGI	
Candida albicans	Culture—Gram stain, India ink, or fluorescent stain, beta-D-glucan (Fungitell) assay
Cryptococcus neoformus	Cryptococcal antigen, CSF
PROTOZOA AND HELMINTHS	
Toxoplasmosis	CT scan, Wright-Giemsa stain, serum serology
Malaria	Peripheral smear of blood

CSF, Cerebrospinal fluid; *CT*, computed tomography; *FTA-ABS*, fluorescent treponemal antibody absorption; *IgG*, immunoglobulin G; *IgM*, immunoglobulin M; *PCR*, polymerase chain reaction; *VDRL*, venereal disease research laboratory.

---

   (1) It is associated with contaminated dairy products consumed by the mother prior to delivery.
   (2) Listeria might appear in outbreaks.
2. Herpes simplex virus (HSV)
   a. Presentation
      (1) Disseminated form in neonates can present with symptoms that mimic bacterial sepsis.
      (2) Additional signs and symptoms include focal seizures and skin vesicles.

    b. Diagnosis
- (1) Definitive diagnosis is made by viral culture or PCR assay of the vesicular lesions or CSF.
- (2) Tzanck smear and/or direct fluorescent antibody test are rapid screening tests, but have lower sensitivity and specificity.
- (3) Of patients with herpes simplex encephalitis, 50% may have red blood cells (median = 1000) in their CSF.
- (4) Characteristic electroencephalographic findings include focal spike and slow wave abnormalities present early in the process.
- (5) Serology is less helpful because of the presence of maternal antibodies.

    c. Treatment
- (1) High-dose acyclovir (60 mg/kg/day) is initiated when antibacterial agents are begun and while the diagnosis is being considered.
- (2) Hydration status should be maintained to avoid nephrotoxicity from acyclovir.

    d. Outcome: Disseminated HSV has very high morbidity and mortality rates.

3. Enteroviruses
    a. Enteroviruses cause meningitis generally during the summer months in temperate climates.
    b. Older children are usually clinically stable with enteroviral meningitis; infants can appear ill or septic.

C. Bacterial pathogens in older infants, children, and adolescents
1. *Streptococcus pneumonia*
    a. Most common cause of meningitis in older infants and young children
    b. More than 90 known serotypes, but most disease is caused by limited number of serotypes
    c. The protein-conjugated vaccine contains the seven most common serotypes associated with disease in the United States and has reduced the incidence of serious infections. Serotype replacement of these seven serotypes in some regions has lead to the development of a vaccine containing 13 serotypes.
- (1) Unfortunately, this pathogen has become multidrug resistant.
- (2) Therefore, empirical therapy is started with vancomycin, 15 mg/kg intravenous (IV) and ceftriaxone, 100 mg/kg IV, for suspected meningitis.

2. *Neisseria meningitides*
    a. Causes meningococcemia, which may have a particularly fulminant and fatal course in infants and children

b. The serotypes B, C, Y, and W-135 are responsible for most cases of severe illness in the developed world; serotype A is responsible for most epidemics. Vaccines are available for serotype A, C, Y, and W-135.

c. Meningitis and sepsis often accompany each other; meningitis alone has a better prognosis than sepsis.

d. The following features at presentation are associated with a poor prognosis:

(1) Leukopenia: <10,000 to 15,000 white blood cells/mm^3

(2) Thrombocytopenia: <100,000 platelets/mm^3

(3) Rapid onset of purpura: Presence of rash for less than 12 hours prior to admission

D. High-risk patients for sepsis and meningitis

1. Immunocompromised hosts are at risk for infection with the following:

a. Bacteria (staphylococcal species, gram-negative enteric bacilli, *Pseudomonas aeruginosa*, *S. pneumonia*)

b. Viruses (herpes zoster, cytomegalovirus, adenovirus)

c. Fungi and molds (*Candida* and *Aspergillus* spp.)

2. Neurosurgical procedures

Patients undergoing neurosurgical procedures (including CNS shunts) are at risk for meningitis caused most commonly by staphylococcal species, particularly *Staphylococcus epidermidis*, gram-negative bacilli, *Proprionobacterium acnes*.

E. Toxic shock syndrome (TSS)

In addition to the pathogens described, several pathogens that elaborate pyrogenic toxins can cause sepsis and septic shock. TSS should be considered in the differential diagnosis of any patient with fever and erythroderma or fever and hypotension. See **Table 19-8**.

TABLE 19-8

DEFINITION OF STREPTOCOCCAL TOXIC SHOCK SYNDROME

Case Definitions	Clinical Criteria
Clinical criteria	Hypotension or shock
Plus	*plus*
Definite case: Isolated from sterile body site	Two or more of the following:
Probable case: Isolated from nonsterile body site	• Renal insufficiency
	• DIC
	• Liver dysfunction
	• ARDS
	• Scarlatiniform rash
	• Soft tissue necrosis

ARDS, Acute respiratory distress syndrome; *DIC*, disseminated intravascular coagulation.

1. *S. aureus*: Staphylococcal TSS is divided into menstrual and nonmenstrual categories.
   a. Epidemiology of menstrual TSS
      (1) TSS was recognized initially in young, previously healthy women who used hyperabsorbent tampons and who developed fever, vomiting, diarrhea, myalgias, and an erythematous sunburn-like rash that progressed to desquamation, particularly on the hands and feet. Despite public health warnings, menstrual TSS still occurs.
   b. Epidemiology of nonmenstrual TSS: Nonmenstrual TSS in children usually follows cutaneous or subcutaneous tissue infections.
   c. Pathogenesis: Staphylococcal toxic shock syndrome is caused by the elaboration of several toxins that act as superantigens, including TSST-1 and TSST-2.
   d. Clinical features
      (1) Presentation includes fever, diffuse red macular rash involving the palms and soles, conjunctival and mucosal hyperemia, hypotension, and multiorgan system dysfunction.
      (2) Desquamation of the palms and soles occurs 1 to 2 weeks after onset of illness.
   e. Laboratory diagnosis
      (1) Based on clinical features
      (2) In most cases, *Staphylococcus* can also be isolated from cutaneous or mucosal sites suspicious for infection.
      (3) Specialized laboratories can then test the isolated *Staphylococcus* for exotoxin production.
      (4) Blood culture is usually sterile.
   f. Treatment
      (1) In addition to the supportive care for septic shock (see Fig. 6-1), antibiotic therapy for all types of TSS is designed to suppress exotoxin production (clindamycin) as well as kill bacteria.
      (2) Empirical therapy begins with clindamycin, 10 mg/kg IV q6h, and **either** vancomycin 10 mg/kg IV q6h **or** linezolid (10 mg/kg IV q8h under 12 yrs of age or 600 mg IV q12h over 12 yrs of age).
      (3) If supported by antibiotic sensitivity testing, vancomycin or linezolid may later be switched to oxacillin, 50 mg/kg IV q6h.

19

2. Group A streptococci (GAS)
   a. Epidemiology
      (1) Most patients with GAS TSS are immunocompetent and develop GAS TSS after viral infections (e.g., varicella zoster or influenza A) or minor trauma with bruising.
      (2) Other portals of GAS exotoxin entry may include pharynx or vagina.
      (3) In approximately 50% of cases, the portal to entry is unknown.
   b. Pathogenesis: The pathogenesis is the same as for staphylococcal TSS.
   c. Clinical features
      (1) Presentation is usually characterized by sudden onset of pain, fever, confusion, and hypotension.
      (2) Most patients have evidence of localized soft tissue infection, erythema, or ecchymoses.
   d. Laboratory diagnosis: GAS TSS is diagnosed based on isolation of GAS from a normally sterile site *plus* hypotension *plus* two or more of the following:
      (1) Elevated creatinine level
      (2) Coagulopathy
      (3) Elevated liver function test results
      (4) ARDS
      (5) Erythematosus macular rash
      (6) Soft tissue necrosis
   e. Treatment
      (1) See earlier, Section VI.
      (2) Empirical therapy begins with clindamycin, 10 mg/kg IV q6h, and **either** vancomycin 10 mg/kg q6h **or** linezolid (10 mg/kg IV q8h under 12 yrs of age or 600 mg IV q12h over 12 yrs of age).
      (3) Once GAS sensitive to penicillin G is identified, linezolid may be switched to penicillin G while clindamycin is continued.

VII. Antimicrobial management
   Antibiotic therapy is based on two concepts—choosing empirical therapy based on the known epidemiology of the common pathogens in a given host in a given setting (see Table 19-4) and modifying the therapy once a pathogen has been identified. Choosing an antibiotic is dependent on the following:
   A. Antimicrobial resistance pattern in hospital or community
   B. Pharmacokinetic properties: Penetration of the blood-brain barrier
   C. Efficacy
   D. Toxicity
   E. Cost, including cost of monitoring

VIII. Adjuvant therapies
  A. Use of corticosteroids
    1. Steroids are recommended for *Haemophilus influenzae*
       meningitis if the steroid dose can be given at the same time or
       before the first antibiotic dose; the use of corticosteroids for
       pneumococcal or meningococcal meningitis is less well
       studied, but many experts recommend the use of steroids.
    2. Dosage: Dexamethasone, 0.6 to 0.8 mg/kg/day IV in 4
       divided doses every 6 hours for the first 4 days of antibiotic
       treatment
    3. Should be given prior to the first dose of antimicrobials
    4. May reduce hearing loss in patients with meningitis
    5. Indicated for meningococcemia associated with adrenocortical
       insufficiency
       a. Dosage: Methylprednisolone, 30 mg/kg
       b. Followed by maintenance doses, 1 to 2 mg/kg/day
  B. Immunoglobulins
     There is little documented efficacy for the use of immunoglobulins
     in sepsis.
  C. Anticonvulsants
     See Chapter 18.
  D. Cardiovascular agents
     See Chapter 6.
  E. Stress ulcer prophylaxis
     The risk of stress ulcer is increased when steroids are used.
     Proton pump inhibitors, H2 blockers, or antacids should routinely
     be used to prevent stress ulcers.
  F. Syndrome of inappropriate antidiuretic hormone (SIADH)
     SIADH may be associated with meningitis. The diagnosis and
     management of SIADH are discussed in Chapter 8.
IX. Antibiotic prophylaxis
    Close contacts of patients with meningococcal or *H. influenzae* type
    B infection require antibiotic prophylaxis with rifampin, ceftriaxone,
    or ciprofloxacin.
  A. Meningococcal disease
    1. Antibiotics are indicated within 24 hours for all close contacts
       in the household, day care, and nursery school, or among
       health care workers who had close unprotected contact with
       the respiratory tract secretions of patients diagnosed with
       meningococcemia.
    2. Contacts are defined as persons who had contact with
       secretions within 7 days before symptoms appeared in the
       index case.
  B. *H. influenzae* infection
    1. Indicated for all nonimmunized contacts of patients with
       invasive *H. influenzae* type B infection

TABLE 19-9

COMPLICATIONS OF MENINGITIS AND SEPSIS

System	Meningitis	Sepsis
Respiratory	Apnea	Apnea
	Respiratory insufficiency	Respiratory insufficiency
	Aspiration	Aspiration
		ARDS
Cardiovascular		Myocardial insufficiency
		Myocardial ischemia
		Arrhythmias
		Shock
Neurologic	Coma	Coma
	Cerebral edema	Cerebral ischemia
	Cerebritis	
	Cerebral ischemia	
	Seizures	
	Hydrocephalus	
	Deafness	
	Ventriculitis	
Metabolic	SIADH	
Hematologic		Thrombocytopenia
		DIC
Other end-organ dysfunction		Hepatic insufficiency
		Renal insufficiency
Extremities		Arthritis
		Soft tissue necrosis

ARDS, Acute respiratory distress syndrome; *DIC*, disseminated intravascular coagulation; *SIADH*, syndrome of inappropriate antidiuretic hormone.

2. Rifampin dosage
   a. Meningococcemia: 10 mg/kg/day orally (PO) q12h for 2 days (max daily dose 600 mg)
   b. *H. influenzae*: 20 mg/kg PO q24h for 4 days
C. Meningococcal prophylaxis
   A single dose of ceftriaxone (125 mg intramuscular [IM] if <15 years of age or 250 mg IM if >15 years of age) or ciprofloxacin (20 mg/kg; max 500 mg)
X. Complications
   Numerous complications and long-term sequelae may result from meningitis and sepsis (**Table 19-9**).

Chapter 20

Pain Control and Sedation Management

Myron Yaster, MD

I. Overview

Even when their pain is obvious, children frequently receive no treatment or inadequate treatment for pain or painful procedures. The common wisdom that children neither respond to nor remember painful experiences to the same degree as adults is simply untrue. To achieve satisfactory procedural sedation, analgesia, and/or amnesia, various drugs, administered alone or in combination, can be safely given to children by various routes.

II. Pain assessment

A. Pain—a subjective experience

1. Pain can be defined operationally as what the patient says hurts, and exists when the patient says it does.

B. Measuring pain to treat it

1. To effectively treat pain, one must be able to measure it accurately.

2. In children older than 3 years, we use one of the following visual analogue scales (**Fig. 20-1**):

a. 10-cm line with a smiling face at one end and a distraught, crying face at the other (Fig. 20-1, *A*)

b. Six-face interval scale (revised) (Fig. 20-1, *B*)

c. 0 to 10 verbal scale, in which 0 is no pain and 10 is the worst pain imaginable

3. In infants and children who are unable to self-report, behavioral or observational pain scores are used. We use the FLACC (**f**ace, **l**egs, **a**ctivity, **c**ry, and **c**onsolability) scale (**Table 20-1**).

III. Opioid analgesics

At equianalgesic doses, all commonly used opioids produce similar degrees of euphoria, sedation, and side effects.

A. Risk factors when prescribing opioids or sedative/hypnotics

1. See **Box 20-1.**

2. Adverse cardiorespiratory effects depend on the following:

a. Dose

b. Rate of drug administration

c. Concomitant administration of other drugs

d. Patient's age and medical history

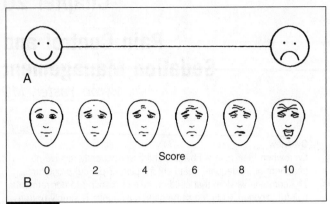

FIGURE 20-1

Pain assessment (visual analogue) scales. **A,** the 10-cm linear analogue scale and **B,** the Wong-Baker six-face interval scale (revised). The higher the score, the greater the child's pain.

TABLE 20-1

FLACC BEHAVIORAL PAIN ASSESSMENT SCALE

Category	Score* 0	1	2
Face	No particular expression or smile	Occasional grimace or frown, disinterested	Frequent to constant frown, clenched jaw, quivering chin
Legs	Normal position or relaxed	Uneasy, restless, tense	Kicking or legs drawn up
Activity	Lying quietly, normal position, moves easily	Squirming, shifting back and forth, tense	Arched, rigid, or jerking
Cry	No cry (awake or asleep)	Moans or whimpers, occasional complaint	Crying steadily, screams or sobs, frequent complaints
Consolability	Content, relaxed	Reassured by occasional touching, hugging, or being talked to; distractible	Difficult to console or comfort

*Each of the categories is scored 0-2, resulting in total score of 0-10.

    B. Opioid and sedative combinations
       1. The combination of an opioid and a sedative-hypnotic significantly increases the risk of respiratory depression.
       2. It is often necessary to reduce the doses of both medications below the usually recommended dosages for either medication when used alone.

BOX 20-1

MEDICAL CONDITIONS ASSOCIATED WITH INCREASED RISK OF CARDIORESPIRATORY COMPLICATIONS FOLLOWING OPIOID OR SEDATIVE ADMINISTRATION

- Infants <3 mo
- Premature infants <60 postconception wk
- History of apnea or disordered control of breathing
- Cardiorespiratory disease
- Hemodynamic instability
- Obtundation
- Airway compromise
- Renal or liver disease
- Neuromuscular disease
- Neurologic injury or chronic neurologic condition

---

   3. Opioid dosages must be individualized and administered by titration to effect, rather than by a fixed dosage schedule formulated by weight.
 C. Other common opioid-induced side effects
   1. Nausea, vomiting
   2. Sedation/mental clouding
   3. Constipation
   4. Pruritus
   5. Biliary tract spasm
   6. Urinary retention
   7. Cough suppression
   8. Chest wall rigidity (with high dose infusions of ultra short-acting opioids; see later)
 D. Choice of opioids
   See **Table 20-2.**
   1. Opioids are more similar than they are different.
   2. Although morphine remains the gold standard against which all other opioids are compared, fentanyl is the most commonly used opioid in the management of acute traumatic and procedure-related pain.
   3. The decision on which opioid to use is dependent on the following:
     a. Route of administration
     b. Onset time
     c. Duration of action
     d. Cost
     e. Receptor binding activity
     f. The nature and site of the pain entity
     g. Concurrent renal or liver disease

20

TABLE 20-2

COMMONLY USED OPIOIDS

Name/Route of Administration	Equipotent Dose (mg/kg)	Duration (hr)	Comments
Morphine		3-4	Vasodilator, avoid in shock
IV	0.1		Releases histamine
PO	0.3-0.5		Seizures at high doses and in newborn
			Sustained release oral form available
Fentanyl		0.5-1.5	Bradycardia
IV	0.001		Hypotension in the hypovolemic, critically ill
Transmucosal	0.015		patient
			Chest wall rigidity—treat with naloxone
			Ideal for short, painful procedures
Meperidine		3-4	Catastrophic interactions with monoamine
IV	1		oxidase inhibitors
PO	1.5-2		Toxic metabolite may cause seizures
			0.25 mg/kg used to treat shivering
			Negative inotrope; do not use in patients with
			poor myocardial function
Hydromorphone		3-4	May cause less sedation, nausea, and pruritus
IV	0.02		than morphine
PO	0.05-0.1		
Methadone		19	Very long-acting; first dose may last only 4 hours.
IV	0.1		Incomplete cross-tolerance: Patients tolerant
PO	0.1-0.2		to other opioids may be incompletely tolerant
			to methadone; hence, beware of overdose risk
			in opioid-tolerant patients.
Codeine		3-4	IV form not recommended.
PO	1.2		Must be metabolized by CYP2D6 to active form.
			Approximately 10% of the population cannot
			metabolize codeine into an active analgesic.
			Available combined with acetaminophen; drug
			titrated to opioid content; this may result in
			excessive acetaminophen (toxicity).
Oxycodone		3-4	Causes less nausea than codeine.
PO only	0.1		Sustained-release preparation available;
			sustained release-tablet must be swallowed
			whole.
			Large release of oxycodone if crushed or chewed
			Cannot be given through nasogastric tube.

IV, Intravenous; *PO*, orally.

E. Fentanyl
  1. Few cardiovascular effects in the healthy child; however, hypovolemic critically ill children may experience hypotension after fentanyl administration
  2. Short duration of action (<60 minutes) because of drug redistribution; excellent for short, painful procedures (1 to 3 mcg/kg)

3. Fentanyl is bound in the blood by α-1-acid glycoprotein. Because the newborn has low levels of this protein, levels of unbound or free drug will be higher than in older patients.
4. Chest wall and glottic **rigidity** occurs with high (>5 mcg/kg) bolus dosing or infusion, but rarely may occur even with low doses (1 to 2 mcg/kg).
5. Treat chest wall rigidity with either of the following:
    a. Naloxone, 0.001 to 0.01 mg/kg, *or*
    b. Neuromuscular blockade and controlled ventilation
        (1) Succinylcholine, 2 mg/kg, *or*
        (2) Rocuronium, 0.6 to 1 mg/kg, *or*
        (3) Vecuronium, 0.1 mg/kg,
6. Transmucosal (candy matrix, Actiq), transdermal (patch), or epidural route
    a. Transmucosal fentanyl (Actiq) can be used for painful procedures (burn débridement, fracture reduction, bone marrow aspiration)
    b. Transdermal patch
        (1) Contraindicated for the treatment of acute pain
        (2) Takes 2 to 4 hours before steady-state levels are reached
        (3) Will leave a depot in the subdermis for 24 hours after the patch is removed
7. High dose fentanyl (>10 mcg/kg)
    a. May lead to loss of consciousness (general anesthesia) and chest wall rigidity; reserved for use in the operating room
    b. Hemodynamic and endocrine responses to intubation and surgery are also obtunded.
IV. Opioid antagonists (naloxone)
    See **Table 20-3.**
    A. Overview
        1. Naloxone is potent and nonselective in its ability to antagonize opioid effects.
        2. Thus, it antagonizes respiratory depression, chest wall rigidity, sedation, and gastrointestinal effects, as well as analgesic effects.
        3. Exercise great caution in the use of antagonists in patients who are chronically tolerant to opioids or who are in severe pain.
        4. It is our practice to mechanically ventilate these patients as an alternative.
        5. In the nonarrest situation, begin with the lowest effective dose (0.001 mg/kg) and titrate up to effect.

TABLE 20-3	
INDICATIONS FOR NALOXONE USE	
Problem	**Dose (mg/kg)**
Itching, urinary retention	0.001-0.002
Biliary spasm	0.001-0.002
Respiratory depression in an opioid tolerant patient or a patient in severe pain	0.001 increased in a step-wise fashion (e.g., 0.002, 0.004, 0.006, etc.)
Overdose (apnea, arrest)	0.01-0.1
Newborn (maternal opioids)	0.01-1

B. Preparation
 1. Naloxone is supplied as a parenteral solution (1, 0.4, and 0.02 mg/mL).
 2. Administration routes: IV (intravenous), IM (intramuscular), intraosseous, or endotracheal
C. Duration of action
 1. The plasma elimination half-life of naloxone is 60 minutes, significantly shorter than many of the opioids that it is being used to antagonize.
 2. Patients may require repeat IV doses, IM (depot) injections, or continuous infusions.
 3. Monitor closely with pulse oximetry and observation for return of respiratory depression.
V. Patient-controlled analgesia
 A. Rationale
  1. Opioids prescribed for pain are often given in fixed doses (based on weight), at fixed time intervals (based on the drug's half-life of elimination), and as needed.
  2. Fixed dosing and time intervals in patients with sustained pain make little sense because of individual variations in pain perception and opioid metabolism.
  3. Rational pain management requires some form of titration to effect whenever an opioid is administered.
  4. On-demand analgesia or patient-controlled analgesia (PCA) devices have been developed to give patients some measure of control over their pain therapy.
  5. These devices are microprocessor-driven pumps with a button that the child presses to self-administer a small preset dose of an opioid.
 B. Indications for use
  1. Acute severe pain from medical conditions, such as sickle cell vaso-occlusive crisis and cancer pain
  2. Postoperative, postprocedure, post-traumatic, and burn pain
  3. Patients in whom preemptive pain treatment is advantageous to the care plan (e.g., prior to dressing changes)

4. A minimal constant blood plasma level can be delivered by constant infusion and is desirable in certain patients (e.g., terminal cancer pain, sickle cell vaso-occlusive crisis pain).

C. Patient selection criteria

1. Willingness on the part of the child, family, and/or nurse to use the PCA device appropriately

2. Child's and/or family's ability to understand and follow directions

3. No significant medical history necessitating restriction of opioids (see Table 20-2)

4. Age limitations

a. Children older than 4 years: Children who play handheld computer games can use IV PCA effectively and safely.

b. Children younger than 5 years (or developmentally or physically disabled)

(1) These patients should be assessed individually.

(2) The use of surrogates to push the PCA button, such as the patient's parent or nurse, is very controversial. We allow it in our practice.

D. Order requirements for PCA

1. Drug (**Table 20-4**): The most commonly used opioids are morphine, hydromorphone, and fentanyl.

2. Concentration of drug

3. Volume of drug to be dispensed

4. Basal or background rate: The use of a background infusion rate in IV PCA is controversial because it may increase the risk of overdosage and the incidence of side effects. We routinely use it in our practice.

5. Demand or bolus dose: The maximum number of demand doses that a patient may trigger per hour or per 4 hours is preprogrammed into the IV PCA pump.

6. Lockout period

a. Following the triggering of an IV PCA bolus, a timer in the pump prevents the administration of an additional bolus until a preset time period, the lockout period, has elapsed.

b. The lockout period ensures that the full effect of a dose is experienced by the patient before another demand dose may be administered.

TABLE 20-4				
INTRAVENOUS PATIENT-CONTROLLED ANALGESIA OPIOID INFUSION ORDERS				
Drug	Basal Rate (mcg/kg/hr)	Bolus Rate (mcg/kg/dose)	Lockout Period (min)	Maximum Dose/hr (mg/kg)
Morphine	10-30	10-30	6-10	0.1-0.15
Hydromorphone	3-5	3-5	6-10	0.015-0.02
Fentanyl	0.5-1	0.5-1	6-10	0.002-0.004

20

TABLE 20-5

MAXIMUM DOSAGE OF LOCAL ANESTHETIC AGENTS FOR PERIPHERAL NERVE OR SUBCUTANEOUS INFILTRATION

Drug	Concentration (%)	Dose (mg/kg)
Lidocaine (Xylocaine)	0.5-2	5-7*
Bupivacaine (Marcaine)	0.25-0.5	2-3*
Ropivacaine (Naropin)	0.2-0.5	2-3*
L-Bupivacaine (Chirocaine)	0.25-0.5	2-3*
Procaine (Novocaine)	0.5-2	10-15*
Prilocaine (Citanest)	1-2	5-7†

These are suggested safe upper limits for local anesthetic administration. Accidental intravenous or intra-arterial injection of even a fraction of these amounts may result in systemic toxicity.

*The higher dose is recommended only with the concomitant use of epinephrine, 1:200,000.

†Maximum dose, 600 mg. This drug is not recommended for children younger than 2 months because of decreased level of methemoglobin reductase and risk of methemoglobinemia.

VI. Local anesthetics

The administration of local anesthetics (regional blockade) is an effective, safe, and easy method of providing pain relief, particularly for procedure-related pain (e.g., IV catheter insertion, laceration repair, thoracostomy tube) and post-traumatic pain (e.g., fractures; **Table 20-5**)

A. Drug dosage and toxicity
   1. Determination of toxicity
      a. Total dose
      b. Speed of vascular uptake from deposition site
         (1) Toxicity occurs at lower doses if local anesthetics are directly injected intravascularly.
         (2) Little risk of toxicity if injected into relatively avascular areas such as fat
      c. Newborns are particularly vulnerable.
      d. Cocaine, alone or combined with other drugs (tetracaine-adrenaline-cocaine), is avoided because of its potential for toxicity and abuse.
   2. Toxic effects
      a. Mild: Tinnitus, light-headedness, visual and auditory disturbances, restlessness, muscle twitching
      b. Severe: Seizures, arrhythmias, coma, cardiovascular collapse, respiratory arrest
B. Eutectic mixture of local anesthetics
   1. Lidocaine, 2.5%, and prilocaine 2.5%, in cream
   2. Apply 60 to 90 minutes before the procedure.
   3. Requires a transparent watertight dressing

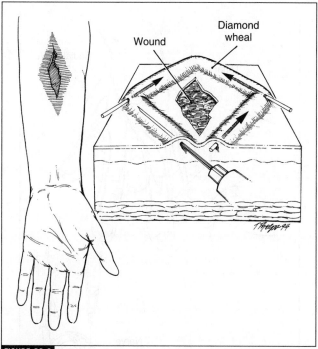

FIGURE 20-2

Subcutaneous infiltration of a laceration. A 25-gauge needle is inserted subcutaneously, and a local anesthetic is injected as the needle is advanced in a forward direction. A diamond-shaped field block surrounds the wound and produces analgesia.

    4. Used for superficial procedural pain (IV stick, arterial line or venous line placement, lumbar puncture)

    5. Safety in the newborn is not well established.

C. Subcutaneous infiltration

See **Figure 20-2.**

    1. To minimize the pain of injection, do the following:

      a. Use a small-gauge needle, 26- or 30-gauge (insulin).

      b. Add bicarbonate to the local anesthetic solution (9 mL lidocaine + 1 mL bicarbonate; 29 mL bupivacaine + 1 mL bicarbonate).

      c. Inject as the needle is being advanced.

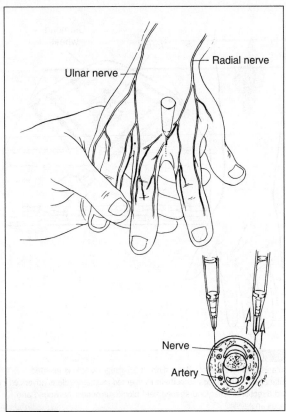

FIGURE 20-3

Digital nerve block. A 25-gauge needle is inserted perpendicularly
between the heads of the metacarpals (or metatarsals) on either side of
the digit; 1 to 3 mL of local anesthetic is injected continuously while
advancing the needle from the dorsal to the volar surface of the digit.

D. Peripheral nerve blocks

   See **Figures 20-3, 20-4,** and **20-5.**

   1. Use 25- or 26-gauge needles in children less than 20 kg; use
      22-gauge needles in all others.
   2. Add bicarbonate to decrease pain and hasten the onset of
      neural blockade.
   3. Add epinephrine to local anesthetics to increase the duration
      and intensity of the block. Never inject solutions with
      epinephrine into areas supplied by end arteries, such as the
      digits, ear pinna, penis, and nose.

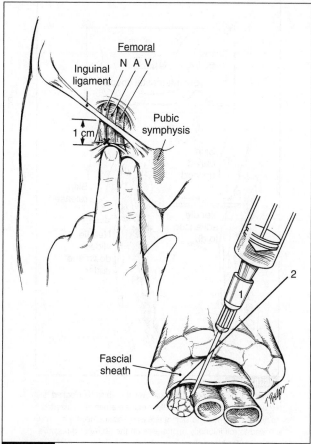

FIGURE 20-4

Femoral nerve block. The femoral artery is compressed against the underlying bone. A 22- or 25-gauge needle is inserted 1 to 1.5 cm laterally to the pulse of the femoral artery and 1 cm below the inguinal ligament. If blood is not aspirated during insertion of the needle, 2 to 3 mL of local anesthetic is injected as the needle is withdrawn. Three to five more fanlike injection sweeps are made away from the artery. 1. Initial angle for local anesthetic injection adjacent to femoral nerve. 2. Subsequent angle for fanlike injection sweeps.
A, Femoral artery; *N,* femoral nerve; *V,* femoral vein.

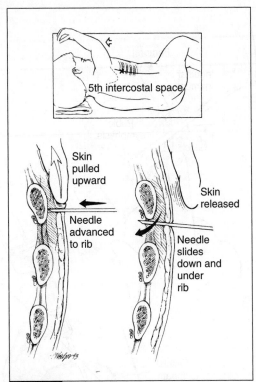

FIGURE 20-5

Intercostal nerve block. The skin over the rib to be blocked is rolled superiorly and the needle, held like a pencil, is inserted to contact the rib. The skin is released and the needle is allowed to roll inferiorly until it slips off the rib. After a negative aspiration for blood, 1 to 3 mL of local anesthetic is injected. Two ribs above and one below the painful site are blocked.

4. Increasing the concentration of local anesthetics increases the incidence of motor blockade and systemic toxicity. Use the lowest concentration available.

VII. Sedation

Sedation represents a continuum from simple alleviation of anxiety in a fully awake patient to the loss of consciousness and protective reflexes (**Fig. 20-6**). Regardless of the physician's initial intent, the

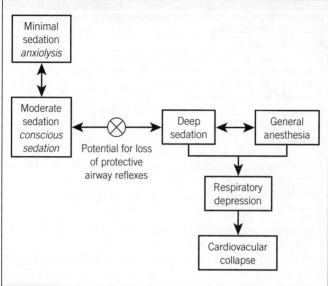

FIGURE 20-6

Sedation continuum.

level of sedation may uncontrollably and unpredictably progress from a loss of consciousness to general anesthesia. Thus, monitoring is essential whenever pharmacologic sedation is attempted (**Box 20-2**).

A. Minimal sedation (anxiolysis)
   1. One drug, low dose, no loss of consciousness
      a. Whenever a second drug family is added to a sedation regimen (e.g., an opioid to a benzodiazepine), by definition it becomes moderate sedation.
   2. Usually an anxiolytic (e.g., midazolam) or sedative drug in a low dose is given once.
   3. Not chloral hydrate

B. Moderate sedation
   This was formerly called *conscious sedation*. It is a medically controlled state of depressed consciousness.
   1. Sedatives or combinations of sedatives and analgesics titrated to produce an effect (anxiolysis, amnesia, immobility, sleep, analgesia)
   2. Patients retain the ability to maintain a patent airway independently.

BOX 20-2

EMERGENCY DRUGS AND EQUIPMENT REQUIRED FOR SEDATION AND LOCAL ANESTHETIC ADMINISTRATION

PERSONNEL FOR PROCEDURES

1. A credentialed practitioner performing the procedure
2. An assistant who is qualified (credentialed) to monitor and administer drugs, but who is not performing the procedure

EQUIPMENT FOR INTRAVENOUS ACCESS

1. Catheters (various sizes), fluid administration sets, infusion pumps
2. Fluids (D5W + salt (0.2%, 0.45%, 0.9% NaCl, Ringer's lactate)

EMERGENCY CART

1. Suction (large-bore device, e.g., Yankauer)
2. Oxygen and oxygen delivery system (passive and active systems for assisted ventilation, self-refilling, or Mapleson-type bag)

AIRWAY EQUIPMENT

1. Oral airways (various sizes)
2. Masks (various sizes)
3. Laryngoscope and appropriate size blades
4. Endotracheal tubes (various sizes)
5. Stylet

DRUGS

1. Antagonists: Naloxone, flumazenil
2. Epinephrine
3. Atropine
4. Bicarbonate
5. Antiarrhythmics (e.g., lidocaine or amiodarone)
6. Glucose
7. Anticonvulsants (e.g., midazolam, lorazepam, phenytoin)

MONITORING EQUIPMENT

This should be used for all children in whom consciousness may be impaired or lost.

1. Pulse oximeter
2. Blood pressure
3. Electrocardiography
4. Direct observation of adequacy of ventilation (capnography, direct visual observation, direct auscultation)

---

   3. Patients respond purposefully to verbal command or light touch (e.g., "Open your eyes").
   4. Chloral hydrate at low doses (<50 mg/kg)
 C. Deep sedation
   This is a medically controlled state of depressed consciousness; deep sedation and general anesthesia are almost the same.
   1. Protective reflexes may not be maintained.

      2. The patient may not retain the ability to maintain a patent airway independently.

      3. The patient will be unable to respond appropriately to physical stimulation or verbal command (e.g., "Open your eyes").

  D. General anesthesia

    General anesthesia will produce a medically controlled state of unconsciousness with the patient experiencing the following:

      1. Loss of protective reflexes

      2. Inability to maintain a patent airway independently

      3. Inability to respond appropriately to physical stimulation or verbal command (e.g., "Open your eyes")

  E. General anesthetic agents

    Even when given as a single agent, the following drugs automatically produce deep sedation or general anesthesia:

      1. Propofol

      2. Thiopental

      3. Ketamine

      4. Etomidate

      5. Methohexital

  F. Sedation requirements for procedures in children

      1. Painful procedures or nonpainful procedures requiring complete immobility cannot be realistically performed in a child (and many adults) who is minimally or moderately sedated.

      2. Thus, deep sedation is required for most pediatric procedures.

VIII. General principles of sedation

  The choice of the sedative will depend on the desired combination of analgesia, immobility, amnesia, or anxiolysis required for the procedure. The addition of an opioid to any sedative will significantly increase the potential for respiratory depression.

  A. Therapeutic goals

      1. Patient safety

      2. Minimal physical discomfort and pain

      3. Minimal psychological response to treatment

      4. Maximal potential for amnesia

      5. Behavior control and, when appropriate, immobility

      6. Adequate time for the physician to complete the procedure

      7. A return to a state of consciousness in which safe discharge is possible

  B. Common causes of sedation catastrophes

      1. Drug overdose

      2. Lack of appreciation of drug-drug interactions, drug pharmacokinetics, and pharmacodynamics

    3. Poor patient selection

    4. Lack of monitoring before, during, or after the procedure (premature discharge, drug given at home)

    5. Inadequate airway and cardiopulmonary resuscitation skills and equipment; failure to rescue

C. Monitoring

    1. Respiratory depression and upper airway obstruction are the most common causes of sedation catastrophes.

    2. Early detection and treatment are the goals of monitoring.

       a. Patients must be under continuous direct visual observation and/or auscultation for breath sounds.

       b. If not, capnography or capnometry is required.

    3. Cardiac arrest is a late manifestation of respiratory depression.

    4. The person performing the procedure cannot monitor the patient during the procedure. An assistant who is qualified to monitor, administer drugs, and resuscitate is required.

D. Documentation before the procedure

    1. Obtain written informed consent including risks, benefits, and alternatives.

    2. Obtain a history and physical examination.

       a. American Society of Anesthesiologists (ASA) physical status (PS) (**Table 20-6**): We recommend consultation with an anesthesiologist for patients who are ASA PS of 4.

       b. Airway examination (see Fig. 2-2; Chapter 2)

       c. Concomitant medical issues

       d. Weight in kilograms

TABLE 20-6

AMERICAN SOCIETY OF ANESTHESIOLOGISTS PHYSICAL STATUS CLASSIFICATION SYSTEM

ASA Class	Description
1	Healthy, no underlying organic disease
2	Mild or moderate systemic disease that does not interfere with daily routines (e.g., well-controlled asthma, essential hypertension)
3	Organic disease with definite functional impairment (e.g., severe steroid-dependent asthma, insulin-dependent diabetes, palliated or corrected congenital heart disease)
4	Severe disease that is life-threatening (e.g., head trauma with increased intracranial pressure)
5	Moribund patient, not expected to survive
E (suffix)	Physical status classification appended with an E connotes a procedure undertaken as an emergency (e.g., an otherwise healthy patient presenting for fracture reduction is classified as ASA PS 1E)

BOX 20-3

CREDENTIALS AND SKILLS REQUIRED BY HEALTH CARE PROFESSIONAL PROVIDING SEDATION FOR PROCEDURES

A registered nurse, nurse practitioner, physician assistant, physician, or dentist (credentialed to administer scheduled Class II BV drugs (e.g., opioids, sedatives)
    Training in the use of these drugs
    Training in monitoring unconscious patients
    Training in airway management and the use of resuscitation equipment—at a minimum, certification in basic life support (BLS) alone or in addition to the following:
• Advanced life support (ALS)
• Pediatric advanced life support (PALS)
• Advanced pediatric life support (APLS)
• Advanced trauma life support (ATLS)
    For deep sedation, no other responsibilities during the performance of the procedure other than administering drugs, monitoring vital signs, and keeping an ongoing record

---

 E. Aspiration risk and prophylaxis
     1. All trauma patients are at risk of aspirating gastric contents if they are sedated, regardless of their fasting status.
     2. Patients should not eat solids (including milk) for a minimum of 6 to 8 hours or clear liquids for a minimum of 2 hours before they are sedated and undergo a procedure.
     3. See aspiration prophylaxis in Chapter 2.
IX. Patient monitoring
    When administering potent analgesics or sedatives, the credentialed physician and nurse (**Box 20-3**) must anticipate, recognize, and be able to treat potentially life-threatening adverse drug effects.
    Compulsive monitoring is required during the administration of these drugs, during the performance of a procedure, and until the baseline state of consciousness returns.
X. Drugs used for sedation during procedures
    See **Table 20-7.**
    A. Analgesics
       All hypnotics, anxiolytics, and amnestics (except for ketamine) have minimal to no analgesic properties.
       1. For short procedures with minimal residual pain, IV (or transmucosal) fentanyl is the opioid of choice.
       2. Local anesthetics are crucial and are the first drugs to be used to minimize or prevent procedure pain.

Text continued on p. 348.

20

TABLE 20-7

COMMONLY USED SEDATIVES

Drug	Route of Administration	Dose(mg/kg)	Comments
Diazepam (Valium)	PO	0.2-0.5	Provides sedation, anxiolysis, and amnesia
	IV	0.05-0.2	
	IM	NR	No analgesic properties
			Painful on injection, poorly absorbed following IM injection
Midazolam (Versed)	PO	0.5	See diazepam; midazolam is 3-4 times more potent but slower in onset than diazepam
	IV	0.05-0.1	
	IM	0.05-0.15	
	Rectal	0.3-1	Painless on injection, well absorbed following IM injection, PO, or rectally.
			IV preparation can be given PO, but is very bitter; disguise with concentrated grape-flavored Kool-Aid or liquid acetaminophen.
Pentobarbital (Nembutal)	PO	2-6	Hypnotic
	IM	2-6	No analgesic properties
	Rectal	2-6	Maximum dose is 150 mg (any route)
			Ideal for diagnostic imaging
Promethazine (Phenergan)	IM, PO	0.5-1	Sedative
			Respiratory depressant
			Antiemetic
			Maximum dose: 25 mg
			Contraindicated for children <2 years
Chloral hydrate	PO	25-100	Hypnotic, no analgesic properties
	Rectal	25-100	Maximum dose: 2 g
			Respiratory depressant
			75-100 mg/kg required for immobility during radiologic procedure
Diphenhydramine (Benadryl)	IV, PO	1	Antihistamine (antipruritic)
			Antiemetic
			Often administered in combination with opioids
			Mildly sedating, weak hypnotic
			Maximum single dose: 50 mg
Meperidine (Demerol) *plus* Diazepam (Valium) *plus* Atropine	PO, IM	1.5	Effective PO or IM
		0.2	Must be given at least 30 minutes before procedure
		0.02	

| TABLE 20-7 |

COMMONLY USED SEDATIVES—cont'd

Drug	Route of Administration	Dose(mg/kg)	Comments
Morphine *plus* Scopolamine	IM, IV	0.1 0.01	Primarily used to minimize procedure-related pain for major procedures (e.g., cardiac catheterization, endoscopy) and as a premedication. Maximum scopolamine dose, 0.4 mg Scopolamine is a very potent amnestic, antisialagogue, and anticholinergic. Scopolamine is contraindicated in glaucoma, gastrointestinal, or genitourinary obstruction, and thyrotoxicosis. Scopolamine is antagonized by physostigmine. Scopolamine effects may last >24 hr unless antagonized.
Midazolam (Versed) *plus* Fentanyl	IV	0.05-0.2 0.001-0.003	*This combination is most commonly used.* See midazolam, fentanyl for specifics. Both drugs are short-acting and can be antagonized—flumazenil for midazolam, naloxone for fentanyl. Primarily used to minimize procedure-related pain; this combination can rapidly produce apnea and hypoxemia. Give fentanyl first, 1 mcg/kg every 2-3 min, to a max of 3 mcg/kg. Following the fentanyl, titrate midazolam, 0.05 mg/kg very slowly. The peak effect occurs 4-5 min after the bolus.
Propofol (Diprivan)	IV	Initially, 1-3 mg/kg, followed by continuous infusion of 100-200 mcg/kg/min	Used for general anesthesia, not sedation. No analgesic properties Painful as IV injection (prevent by adding lidocaine to the solution)
Ketamine	IV, IM	0.5-1	Used for general anesthesia, not sedation No significant respiratory depression Contraindicated in brain injury or seizures Produces a dissociative state with staring and minor movements Usually combined with midazolam (to prevent nightmares) and atropine (to prevent excess secretions)

IM, Intramuscular; *IV,* intravenous; *NR,* not recommended; *PO,* orally.

B. Sedatives, anxiolytics, and amnestics
1. Excellent adjuvants for painful procedures and the most popular in current practice are the benzodiazepines, particularly midazolam, which is given IV, orally, intranasally, or rectally.
2. Hypnotics are an excellent choice for nonpainful diagnostic imaging studies, such as magnetic resonance imaging or computed tomography scanning. Pentobarbital, 2 to 4 mg/kg IV or IM (maximum dose, 150 mg), is as effective as chloral hydrate, 50 to 100 mg/kg (maximum dose, 2 g).
3. Amnestics, such as benzodiazepines and scopolamine, are useful when analgesia and sedation cannot be adequately provided because of hemodynamic instability.

XI. Postprocedure documentation
Following a procedure with sedation, patients must be admitted to a postprocedure/postsedation care unit where they are monitored by a trained observer until they can be discharged home or to the hospital floor.

A. Emergence from sedation and recovery
1. Admission vital signs and level of consciousness
2. Report what transpired during the procedure, including drugs administered, nature of procedure, and preprocedure history.
3. Record vital signs at least every 15 minutes until discharge criteria are met.
4. Discharge criteria
   a. Return to presedation level of consciousness
   b. Normal vital signs
   c. Drinking *not* necessary
   d. Voiding *not* necessary
   e. Airway reflexes intact
5. Discharge instructions
   a. A responsible adult must accompany the patient.
   b. Written instructions must be understood.
   c. Emergency phone numbers
   d. Pain management
   e. Signature on discharge documentation
6. Follow-up phone call (24 hours)

Chapter 21

Thoracic Trauma

Charles N. Paidas, MD, MBA

I. Overview

Many thoracic injuries can be managed simply (thoracostomy tubes), but others require complex, definitive operative repair. Once the need for intervention is made, the pathophysiology of the injury will determine the critical decision of whether treatment is immediate in the emergency room, urgent (within 3 hours of arrival), or delayed.

II. Epidemiology

A. Blunt versus penetrating injury

1. Blunt trauma is the most common mechanism of childhood thoracic injury; motor vehicle crashes account for 90% of pediatric thoracic injuries.

2. Head injury is the leading cause of childhood deaths related to injury, and thoracic trauma ranks as the second leading cause of childhood injury mortality.

3. Most common injuries by age group

   a. Toddlers: Falls

   b. Prepubertal children: Pedestrian motor vehicle crashes

   c. Teenagers: Motor vehicle crashes

4. For blunt chest trauma, there is a high incidence (>50%) of associated systems' injuries—central nervous system > soft tissue and skeletal > abdominal.

5. **The lungs** are the most common chest organ injured, with pulmonary contusion the most common lung injury.

B. More common causes of fatal thoracic injury

1. Penetrating injuries (gunshot wounds)

2. Mass casualties

3. Suicides were historically infrequent in children but are increasing.

C. Mortality rates

1. Overall, pediatric mortality ranges from 7% to 15%; however, there is a 25% mortality in children younger than 6 years.

2. Deaths occur early in the hospital course (67%).

3. Of chest injuries, 85% can be managed acutely with nonoperative techniques and less than 15% will require thoracotomy.

III. Pathophysiology

The compliant chest wall in children allows energy transfer to intrathoracic structures, often without evidence of external chest wall injury. The mediastinum is also mobile and flexible. There is a low incidence of major vessel and tracheobronchial injury; however, cardiovascular and ventilatory compromise can rapidly occur with or without mediastinal shift. Aerophagia, gastric dilation, regurgitation, and reflex ileus are common events in the postinjury phase.

IV. Initial assessment and resuscitation

Thoracic injury may be diagnosed or suspected based on the history of the injury, physical assessment in the primary survey (abnormal chest auscultation, abnormal external surface chest examination, tachypnea, low systolic blood pressure [BP; age-specific], Glasgow Coma Scale [GCS] <15, and/or presence of a femur fracture). Once diagnosed or suspected, refer to the algorithm in **Figure 21-1,** based on the following priorities:

A. Definition of priorities in thoracic trauma
   1. Highest priority: **Life-threatening**
      a. Airway obstruction
      b. Tension pneumothorax
      c. Open pneumothorax
      d. Massive hemothorax
      e. Flail chest
      f. Cardiac tamponade
      g. Commotio cordis
   2. Second priority: Potentially life-threatening
      a. Tracheobronchial injury
      b. Pulmonary contusion
      c. Myocardial contusion
      d. Traumatic aortic rupture
      e. Traumatic diaphragmatic hernia
      f. Esophageal trauma
      g. Traumatic asphyxia
      h. Air embolism
   3. Third priority: Not life-threatening
      a. Simple pneumothorax
      b. Small hemothorax
      c. Rib fracture
      d. Chest wall contusion

V. Life-threatening chest injury
   A. Airway obstruction
      1. Definition and pathophysiology
         a. Thoracic trauma may be accompanied by airway obstruction from blood, mucus, emesis, teeth, or a foreign body.
         b. A high index of suspicion is required with a closed head injury and maxillofacial or laryngeal trauma.

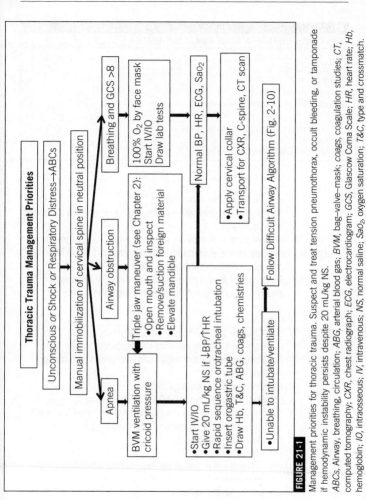

FIGURE 21-1

Management priorities for thoracic trauma. Suspect and treat tension pneumothorax, occult bleeding, or tamponade if hemodynamic instability persists despite 20 mL/kg NS.

ABCs, Airway, breathing, circulation; *ABG,* arterial blood gas; *BVM,* bag-valve–mask; *coags,* coagulation studies; *CT,* computed tomography; *CXR,* chest radiograph; *ECG,* electrocardiogram; *GCS,* Glasgow Coma Scale; *HR,* heart rate; *Hb,* hemoglobin; *IO,* intraosseous; *IV,* intravenous; *NS,* normal saline; *Sao₂,* oxygen saturation; *T&C,* type and crossmatch.

BOX 21-1

SIGNS AND SYMPTOMS IN ACUTE AIRWAY OBSTRUCTION

- Agitation, confusion
- Initial tachycardia
- Tachypnea
- Diaphoresis
- Ineffective respiratory movements
- Stridor
- Retraction (accessory muscle recruitment)
- Cyanosis
- Bradycardia with progressive hypoxia

---

2. History and physical examination
   a. The physical examination is the key to immediate diagnosis and treatment.
   b. Interference in ventilatory gas exchange and progressive hypoxia create a cascade of symptoms and signs in patients with traumatic airway obstruction (**Box 21-1**).
   c. Diagnosis of airway obstruction is made by examination, and radiographs are obtained only after the airway is secure.
3. Management
   a. See Chapter 2 for a detailed discussion of airway management, which includes the following steps:
      (1) Positioning, suctioning (clean secretions and foreign bodies)
      (2) Cervical spine immobilization
      (3) Supplemental oxygen (O_2) administration
   b. If the airway cannot be maintained safely (head injury with GCS <8, maxillofacial trauma), the following steps are required (see Fig. 21-1):
      (1) Intubation
      (2) Cervical spine immobilization during airway intervention
      (3) Mechanical ventilation
   c. Management of the difficult airway
      (1) See Chapter 2 and Figure 2-11.
      (2) Consider use of the laryngeal mask airway.
      (3) Needle cricothyrotomy may be required and is preferable to surgical cricothyrotomy in children younger than 12 years (see Figs. 2-20 and 2-21).
      (4) Emergency surgical cricothyrotomy or tracheostomy outside of the operating room is very hazardous in the child and is used when all other options have been exhausted.

BOX 21-2

SIGNS AND SYMPTOMS OF TENSION PNEUMOTHORAX

EARLY

- Dyspnea
- Tachypnea
- Unilateral chest wall movement
- Decreased breath sounds on affected side
- Hypertympany

LATE

- Tracheal deviation
- Mediastinal shift to contralateral side
- Profound respiratory distress
- Circulatory collapse
- Distended neck veins
- Cyanosis

   B. Tension pneumothorax
     1. Definition: Accumulation of air under pressure in the pleural space
     2. Pathophysiology
       a. Causes
         (1) The development of a tension pneumothorax entails a communication between air passages or lung parenchyma and the pleural space.
         (2) The injury results in a *closed system* such that air can enter the pleural space but cannot exit.
         (3) Most common cause is high airway pressure from mechanical ventilation.
         (4) Other causes include any blunt or penetrating force disrupting the tracheobronchial tree or lung parenchyma.
       b. Consequences
         (1) The expanding air space produces mediastinal shift with tracheal deviation, which can interfere with central venous return and lead to decreased cardiac output.
         (2) Profound respiratory distress and circulatory collapse result.
     3. History and physical examination (**Box 21-2**)
     4. Diagnostic tests
       a. The chest radiograph is diagnostic.
       b. However, the severely compromised patient will require thoracostomy before there is time to obtain a chest radiograph.

21

5. Immediate management
   a. Administer 100% O_2 and secure airway.
   b. Intubate if necessary.
   c. Perform needle thoracostomy in the midclavicular line at the second intercostal space (ICS).
      (1) Use a 22-gauge over-the-needle catheter in an infant and an 18-gauge over-the-needle catheter in an older child.
      (2) After sterile preparation of the skin, the catheter is advanced just beyond the rib superior margin of the rib into the pleural space; the needle is then removed and the catheter is advanced further.
      (3) The catheter is connected to a 20-mL syringe and three-way stopcock and air is evacuated.
6. Definitive management
   a. Access to the pleural space can be done using the Seldinger wire technique (**Fig. 21-2**), followed by insertion of a catheter chest tube.
   b. This is a quick, reliable, and easily performed method of chest tube insertion.
   c. An alternative method for chest tube insertion uses a cutdown and blunt dissection through the fifth ICS, just lateral to the nipple, at a point between the anterior and midaxillary lines.
   d. Regardless of the method of placement, once inserted, the chest tube is connected to an underwater seal and suction device (e.g., Pleurovac; **Fig. 21-3**).

C. Open pneumothorax (sucking chest wound)
   1. Definition
      a. There is a loss of a portion of the chest wall, with an opening greater than the diameter of the airway.
      b. This permits air to pass in and out through the defect with each breath.
   2. Pathophysiology
      a. The open pneumothorax is associated with penetrating trauma.
      b. Immediate equilibration of the intrathoracic and atmospheric pressures eliminates effective ventilation of the lung, with resultant hypoxia.
      c. Mediastinal shift can occur, leading to reduction in venous return.
   3. History and physical examination: Examination shows an obvious chest wall defect with air movement to and from the wound, along with signs and symptoms of acute respiratory distress.

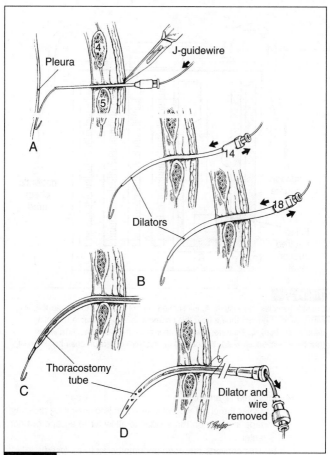

FIGURE 21-2

The Seldinger-wire technique for pigtail chest tube insertion at the fifth intercostal space between the anterior and midaxillary lines. After sterile preparation and 1% lidocaine infiltration, insert the needle attached to a syringe over the superior margin of the rib while gentle suction is applied. (**Never** insert a needle at the inferior margin of a rib, where it could damage the neurovascular bundle.) **A,** As soon as air is aspirated, remove the syringe and insert the J-tipped guidewire into the pleural space and then remove the needle. Enlarge the insertion site with a 3-mm incision adjacent to the wire using a no. 11 scalpel blade. **B,** Advance the dilator over the wire to enlarge the insertion track further. **C, D,** After removing the dilator, thread the pigtail catheter over the wire until all side holes are inside the chest. Secure the catheter with suture and sterile dressing.

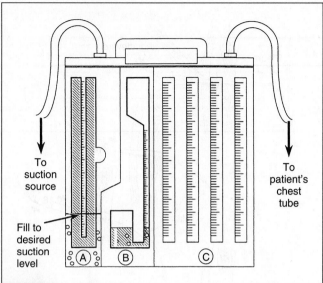

FIGURE 21-3

Chest tube collection system. **A,** Fill suction control chamber to desired level with sterile water. Connect tubing from this chamber to suction source (bubbling denotes suction). **B,** Fill water seal chamber to 0-cm level with sterile water (bubbling denotes air leak). **C,** Connect tubing from collection chamber to chest tube.

4. Initial management
    a. Cover the chest wound with a sterile overlapping dressing; tape in place on three sides to allow air to escape but not enter.
    b. This converts the *open* pneumothorax to a *closed* pneumothorax.
    c. Observe the patient closely for signs of tension pneumothorax, which may develop if the dressing becomes completely occlusive, preventing the escape of air.
5. Definitive management
    a. Tube thoracostomy in the fifth ICS, just lateral to the nipple, between the anterior and midaxillary line (see Fig. 21-2)
    b. There may be a need for exploratory thoracotomy if tracheobronchial injury exists.
D. Massive hemothorax
    1. Definition: Blood collection more than 20 mL/kg in the pleural cavity indicates the presence of a massive hemothorax.

2. Causes
   a. Massive hemothorax can occur in blunt and penetrating chest trauma.
   b. It is a known complication of subclavian or internal jugular vein cannulation.
3. Pathophysiology
   a. Ventilatory insufficiency and hypovolemic shock develop.
   b. Mediastinal shift exacerbates the cardiovascular compromise from hypovolemia.
4. History and physical examination
   a. Cardiorespiratory signs
      (1) Signs and symptoms are identical to those of tension pneumothorax.
      (2) Signs of respiratory distress usually precede evidence of poor perfusion.
      (3) Thus, hemothorax may be overlooked in the intubated and mechanically ventilated patient until significant blood loss has produced hypovolemic shock.
      (4) A high index of suspicion for hemothorax should be maintained in patients with a compatible history.
   b. Chest wall protuberance in infants
      (1) The compliant infant chest wall may protrude on the affected side in the face of a large hemothorax.
      (2) The subcostal region is particularly useful to detect this asymmetry.
5. Diagnostic tests: Chest radiography only confirms the clinical diagnosis.
6. Initial management
   a. Secure airway
   b. Ventilate, oxygenate
   c. Fluid (crystalloid and blood) resuscitation for volume restoration
   d. Tube thoracostomy (see Fig. 21-2) with the chest tube angled posteriorly
7. Definitive management: If blood loss continues (>2 to 4 mL/kg/hr × 4 hours or >10% of blood volume), definitive thoracotomy is necessary.
E. Flail chest
   1. Definition: Segment of chest wall lacks bony continuity with the remaining thoracic cage.
   2. Epidemiology
      a. The flail chest is associated with violent blunt trauma, multiple rib fractures, and underlying pulmonary parenchymal injury (contusion).
      b. Flail chest is unusual in infants and toddlers.
      c. The incidence increases with age.

21

3. Pathophysiology
   a. Ventilation-perfusion ($\dot{V}/\dot{Q}$) mismatch in the contused lung leads to hypoxia.
   b. Flail segment responds to changes in intrathoracic pressure rather than to the action of the respiratory muscles.
   c. During spontaneous breathing, the flail segment moves inward with the fall of intrathoracic pressure on inspiration.
   d. Conversely, the normal portions of the chest wall are pulled outward by the action of the respiratory muscles.
   e. Thus, there is paradoxical breathing.
   f. Children tolerate posterolateral flail segments poorly because this interferes significantly with diaphragmatic excursion.
4. History and physical examination
   a. Inspection
      (1) Flail chest is apparent on inspection and the paradoxical movement of the flail segment is pathognomonic.
      (2) Effective ventilation is not possible because of the uncoordinated movement of the thorax.
      (3) The patient develops signs of respiratory distress.
   b. Palpation
      (1) Paradoxical chest wall motion is also apparent on palpation of the chest wall.
      (2) Rib fractures and crepitus are frequently palpable.
5. Diagnostic tests
   a. Chest radiography reveals rib fractures and the pulmonary contusion.
   b. Arterial blood gas is used to confirm inadequate ventilation (partial pressure of carbon dioxide >40 mm Hg).
6. Management: Internal stabilization
   a. Accomplished with endotracheal intubation and mechanical ventilation with positive end-expiratory pressure (PEEP)
   b. The positive intrathoracic pressure throughout the respiratory cycle prevents inward motion of the flail segment during a spontaneous inspiration.
   c. The level of PEEP may have to be raised for large flail segments with severe underlying pulmonary contusions.
7. Intravenous (IV) fluid administration: After resuscitation, crystalloid administration is restricted because overhydration can worsen the pulmonary contusion.
8. Analgesia: Regional or opioid analgesia is needed to prevent splinting on the affected side.

F. Cardiac tamponade
1. Definition: Compression of the heart produced by accumulation of blood under pressure in the confined space of the pericardial sac
2. Causes
   a. Cardiac tamponade is more often the result of penetrating rather than blunt trauma.
   b. Tamponade may also occur after thoracic or cardiac surgery and as a complication of central venous line placement.
   c. Infectious pericarditis is the major nontraumatic cause of tamponade in children.
3. Pathophysiology
   a. The pressure in the pericardial space increases rapidly and exceeds intracardiac pressure.
   b. This results in decreased filling of the heart and decreased cardiac output.
   c. The rise in ventricular end-diastolic pressure produces systemic and pulmonary venous congestion.
   d. Right atrial, right ventricular, pulmonary artery diastolic, and pulmonary capillary wedge pressures are equalized.
4. History and physical examination
   a. Physical examination shows narrowed pulse pressure, muffled heart tones, and distended neck veins.
   b. The diagnosis should be strongly suspected in the presence of the following:
      (1) Rising central venous pressure
      (2) Lowered systolic BP initially, followed by lowered mean arterial pressure
      (3) Pulsus paradoxus: More than 10-mm Hg fall in systolic BP during inspiration
5. Ancillary tests
   a. Echocardiogram reveals an echogenic space between pericardium and epicardium.
   b. Chest radiograph shows widened cardiac and mediastinal shadows.
   c. Do *not* delay therapy in the symptomatic patient to obtain ancillary tests!
6. Management: **A**irway, **B**reathing, and **C**irculation (ABCs)—Standard resuscitative measures are used, including intubation and ventilation with 100% O_2, IV fluids, and blood administration.
7. Thoracotomy
   a. Procedure of choice for acute traumatic tamponade (or immediate postoperative tamponade).

21

    b. Pericardiocentesis may be used as a temporizing measure in case of the following:

        (1) The patient's tamponade is not caused by a penetrating cardiac wound.

        (2) Surgical personnel are not available for a thoracotomy.

    c. Penetrating wounds to the heart cannot be treated effectively with pericardiocentesis.

    d. Any ongoing hemorrhage into the pericardial sac requires thoracotomy to drain the pericardium and repair the bleeding site.

8. Pericardiocentesis (**Fig. 21-4**)

    a. Indications

        (1) All *medical* causes of tamponade (e.g., infection, inflammation)

        (2) Immediate subxiphoid pericardiocentesis if there is a compatible history, hypotension, systemic venous congestion, and pulsus paradoxus

    b. Preparation

        (1) A minimum of electrocardiogram (ECG), O_2 saturation, and BP monitoring is mandatory.

        (2) Sterile preparation (prep) is used for all patients.

        (3) If time permits, include sterile drapes and local anesthesia in the conscious patient.

        (4) Several manufacturers offer prepackaged pericardiocentesis kits with a 5- or 8-Fr pigtail catheter, dilator, guidewire, 18-gauge insertion needle, and sterile prep items.

        (5) If the prepackaged kit is unavailable, a standard 20-gauge (over-the-needle) IV catheter attached to a stopcock and syringe may be used for acute relief of tamponade in infants.

        (6) Older children receive a 6-inch, 16- or 18-gauge over-the-needle catheter.

    c. Procedure

        (1) After sterile prep and infiltration of 1% lidocaine local anesthetic, the needle attached to a syringe is inserted immediately adjacent to the xyphoid process and aimed toward the left scapula.

        (2) Ideally, the needle is advanced under echocardiographic guidance, with constant gentle suction applied.

        (3) As soon as blood or fluid is encountered, 10 to 20 mL may be aspirated to relieve immediate tamponade.

        (4) Then the syringe is removed and the J-tipped guidewire is inserted.

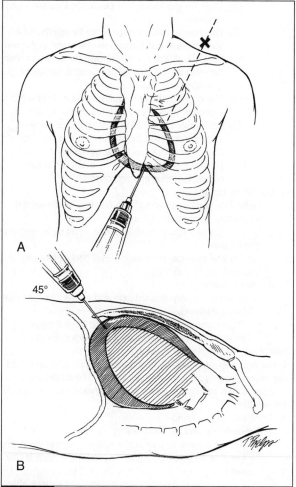

FIGURE 21-4

Pericardiocentesis. **A,** Insert a needle adjacent to the left side of the xiphoid process at a 45-degree angle and aim toward the left scapula. Aspirate as you advance the needle. **B,** If blood or fluid is encountered use Seldinger technique to replace needle with guidewire and catheter. Aspiration of as little as 10-20 mL should relieve tamponade.

        (5) Once the guidewire is in place, the insertion needle is removed.

        (6) The insertion site is augmented by inserting a no. 11 scalpel blade just through the skin next to the wire.

        (7) Next, the dilator is inserted over the wire and then removed so that the definitive pigtail catheter can be advanced over the wire.

        (8) The pigtail catheter is finally secured, connected to a collection device, and a sterile dressing applied.

        (9) Pericardial blood can be distinguished from intracardiac blood by its failure to clot because of the fibrinolytic properties of the pericardium.

       (10) Following pericardiocentesis, observe the patient closely for recurrent tamponade.

G. Commotio cordis
1. Definition: Ventricular arrhythmia (ventricular fibrillation) secondary to blunt chest trauma
2. Causes: Contact sports or child abuse resulting in severe blunt chest trauma
3. History and physical examination: Hallmark is blunt trauma and ventricular fibrillation.
4. Management
   a. Cardiopulmonary resuscitation and immediate defibrillation (see Chapter 5).
   b. This diagnosis is one of the reasons for automatic defibrillators being available at all sporting events.

VI. Potentially life-threatening chest injury
These are associated with damaged intrathoracic structures and are often missed during the primary survey. The diagnosis is obtained in the secondary survey after diagnostic and therapeutic intervention.

A. Tracheobronchial injury
1. Presentation and pathophysiology
   a. If blunt trauma injuries occur within 1 inch of the carina, the diagnosis can be subtle; penetrating trauma is more overt.
   b. Pneumothorax develops with a persistent air leak after chest tube placement.
   c. Tension pneumothorax with mediastinal shift may be present; in addition, there is partial upper airway obstruction.
   d. Approximately 50% of deaths from this injury occur within 1 hour.
2. History and physical examination
   a. History is important for making the diagnosis, particularly in patients with blunt trauma.

        b. External evidence of trauma may not be obvious.
        c. Signs include the following:
            (1) Labored breathing
            (2) Evidence of tension pneumothorax (see Box 21-2)
            (3) Hemoptysis
            (4) Subcutaneous emphysema
    3. Diagnostic tests
        a. The diagnosis is suggested by persistent air leak from the chest tube.
        b. Bronchoscopy usually confirms the diagnosis.
    4. Initial management
        a. Intubate to ensure adequate oxygenation and ventilation.
        b. Insert a chest tube; a second chest tube is often necessary to overcome a large air leak.
    5. Definitive management
        a. Patients without major anatomic distortion of the tracheobronchial tree will usually heal with just supportive care.
        b. Large paratracheal hematoma requires surgical intervention.
B. Pulmonary contusion
    1. Definition
        a. Blunt or penetrating forces to the chest produce laceration of lung tissue and interstitial hemorrhage.
        b. It is the most common parenchymal injury after thoracic trauma.
    2. Pathophysiology
        a. $\dot{V}/\dot{Q}$ mismatch results in hypoxia.
        b. The contusion may progress to acute respiratory distress syndrome (ARDS), with severe hypoxemia (see Chapter 3).
        c. Contusion may be complicated by aspiration of gastric contents, pneumothorax, or flail chest.
    3. History and physical examination: The initial physical examination may demonstrate hemoptysis, pleuritic pain, and labored breathing, or there may be only minimal signs.
    4. Diagnostic tests
        a. A high index of suspicion is necessary.
        b. Confirm the diagnosis by chest radiography, which reveals infiltrates in lung fields usually several hours after resuscitation has been completed.
    5. Management
        a. Standard ABCs resuscitation measures
        b. Supplemental O_2 by face mask may be sufficient in many cases.
        c. Avoid overhydration.

  d. Use intubation and mechanical ventilation with PEEP for patients with severe hypoxia (hypoxic on >50% O_2 by face mask).

  e. Atelectasis is treated with chest physiotherapy.

  f. Analgesia (see Chapter 20)

C. Myocardial contusion

  1. Definition: Consists of a cardiac muscle injury secondary to blunt traumatic forces

  2. Pathophysiology

  a. The lesion involves a disruption of myocardial blood flow, with subsequent myocardial ischemic injury.

  b. There exists a rare potential for infarction.

  3. History and physical examination

  a. History of injury is important because the physical examination can be unremarkable.

  b. Occasionally, there is visible evidence of sternal or chest wall contusion, or palpable rib fractures.

  c. Rarely, a new heart murmur can be identified.

  4. Diagnostic tests

  a. Abnormalities on the ECG (ST-T wave changes, premature atrial or ventricular contractions, other arrhythmias)

  b. Possible elevation of cardiac isoenzyme levels (e.g., troponin, creatine phosphokinase-MB)

  5. Management

  a. Ensure adequate airway and oxygenation.

  b. Continuously monitor cardiac function for ischemia and arrhythmias.

  c. Obtain follow-up ECGs.

  d. Obtain serial cardiac isoenzyme levels.

  e. Obtain a baseline echocardiogram if electrocardiographic and cardiac enzyme abnormalities are detected.

  f. In the absence of myocardial infarction, the risk for long-term cardiac disability is nil.

D. Traumatic aortic rupture

  1. Definition: A laceration of the aorta at or distal to the ligamentum arteriosum, just beyond the takeoff of the left subclavian artery

  2. Pathophysiology

  a. Tremendous force is associated with the mechanism of injury, causing a traumatic aortic rupture (e.g., deceleration from a high-speed motor vehicle or fall from a great height, as in a plane crash).

  b. Of these victims, 90% die in the field from exsanguination.

  c. Those who survive transport to a hospital have continuity of the aorta maintained by an intact adventitial layer.

BOX 21-3

DIAGNOSTIC SIGNS OF TRAUMATIC AORTIC RUPTURE

- Widened mediastinum
- Fracture of first and second ribs
- Obliteration of the aortic knob
- Deviation of the trachea to the right
- Presence of apical pleural cap (effusion)
- Depression of the left mainstem bronchus (140 degrees from the tracheal midline)
- Left pleural effusion
- Elevation and shift to the right of the right mainstem bronchus
- Obliteration of the aorticopulmonary window

---

      d. If untreated at initial presentation, the natural history of this injury involves secondary rupture, with intrapleural exsanguinations in the first week after injury.

      e. Alternatively, false aneurysms can rupture months or years following the injury.

   3. History and physical examination

      a. History of a motor vehicle accident or a fall from great height should suggest the diagnosis.

      b. Hypotension results from blood loss into the contained hematoma around the aorta.

   4. Diagnostic signs: See **Box 21-3.**

   5. Management

      a. Any patient with a compatible history and a widened mediastinum on a chest radiograph should undergo either angiography or computed tomography (CT) scan to rule out traumatic aortic rupture.

      b. The preferred imaging technique is dependent on institutional preference, associated injuries, and hemodynamic stability of the child.

      c. Once the diagnosis is confirmed, perform an immediate thoracotomy with resection of the injured area and direct repair, usually with a graft prosthesis or endovascular treatment in centers experienced in these procedures.

  E. Traumatic diaphragmatic hernia

   1. Definition

      a. Large radial tears in the left hemidiaphragm following *blunt* trauma, which allows immediate herniation of abdominal contents into the chest

      b. Penetrating trauma produces small tears and minimal herniation.

21

2. Pathophysiology
   a. Herniated abdominal contents may cause mediastinal shift and acute respiratory insufficiency.
   b. There is a 10% to 25% incidence of associated intra-abdominal injury.
3. History and physical examination
   a. Tachypnea
   b. Displaced heart impulse on cardiac examination
   c. Audible bowel sounds in the chest
4. Diagnostic tests
   a. Chest radiographs may be misinterpreted as left hemidiaphragm elevation, acute gastric distention, or subpulmonic hematoma.
   b. A definitive diagnosis is made by noting displacement of a nasogastric tube into an intrathoracic stomach.
5. Management
   a. ABCs
   b. If assisted ventilation is needed, the patient should be intubated rapidly because prolonged bag-mask ventilation will lead to gastric inflation and lung compression.
   c. Decompress the stomach with an orogastric or nasogastric tube to improve ventilation.
   d. Operative management: The acute traumatic diaphragmatic hernia should be repaired.

F. Esophageal trauma
1. Definition: Penetrating trauma (missiles or instrumentation) to the chest, or blunt trauma to the upper abdomen (crush), produces a perforation or linear tear in the esophagus.
2. Pathophysiology
   a. A linear tear in the lower left esophagus permits leakage of gastric contents into the mediastinum.
   b. There is early onset of mediastinitis and later rupture into the pleural space, producing empyema.
3. History and physical examination
   a. The clinical picture is identical to that of postemetic esophageal perforation, Boerhaave syndrome.
   b. Signs, often delayed, include the following:
      (1) Fever
      (2) Tachycardia
      (3) Pleural friction rub
      (4) Shock
      (5) Substernal or epigastric pain out of proportion to injury
4. Diagnostic tests
   a. Chest radiography reveals left mediastinal air.
   b. Gastrografin swallow demonstrates extravasation of dye into the mediastinum.

5. Management
   a. ABCs
   b. Contained leaks that result in dye going directly back into the esophagus can be observed in an otherwise asymptomatic child.
      (1) Nothing by mouth, antibiotics, and orogastric decompression
      (2) Mediastinal extravasation with pooling and air in the chest requires open thoracotomy.
   c. Operative management
      (1) Perform a thoracotomy with wide drainage of the pleural space and mediastinum to prevent empyema and mediastinal abscess formation.
      (2) If feasible, repair the esophageal tear with a patch.
      (3) If repair is not feasible, transect the stomach to allow diversion of the esophagus and proximal stomach.
      (4) Place a gastrostomy tube in the distal stomach segment for feeding.

G. Traumatic asphyxia
   1. Definition
      a. This is an unusual injury, which is more common in children because of their compliant chest wall.
      b. A crushing blunt force produces a compressive chest injury, which increases intrathoracic pressure.
      c. Increased intrathoracic pressure is transmitted through the superior vena cava and internal and external jugular veins.
      d. Cutaneous capillary pressure increases via a rise in external jugular pressure, and a sudden forceful rise in internal jugular pressure can cause swelling of the brain, deep tissues of the neck, and airway.
      e. The external jugular system has valves that cannot withstand any retrograde pressure, whereas a much higher pressure is required to exceed the competency of valves in the internal jugular system.
   2. History and physical examination
      a. Head, neck, upper torso cyanosis or petechial hemorrhages
      b. Cervical and facial edema
      c. Conjunctival, retinal hemorrhages
      d. Signs of respiratory distress
      e. CNS depression secondary to rapid increase in intracranial pressure
   3. Diagnostic tests: The diagnosis is made by physical examination.

21

4. Management
   a. ABCs: Intubation and mechanical ventilation for associated pulmonary contusion and ARDS
   b. Potential swelling of tongue or larynx may also require prophylactic intubation.
   c. CT scan of brain to rule out brain injury
   d. Consider intracranial pressure monitoring and therapy (see Chapter 15).

H. Air embolism
   1. Definition: A communication between the skin opening and a central vein, or between a bronchus and a pulmonary vein, leads to embolization of air to the heart.
   2. History and physical examination
      a. Usually, a history of penetrating trauma with exposed veins in the head or neck
      b. Mill wheel murmur
      c. Cardiovascular collapse may develop because of obstruction of the right ventricular outflow tract with air.
      d. Signs of respiratory distress may develop because embolic obstruction of the pulmonary vascular bed leads to pulmonary congestion and hemoptysis.
      e. Focal neurologic deficits may arise because of air embolization to the cerebral circulation if the patient has a patent foramen ovale or other intracardiac communication.
   3. Diagnostic tests
      a. The diagnosis is usually made by history and physical examination.
      b. In the monitored patient, air embolism is suggested by a sudden fall in the end-tidal carbon dioxide tension or by a change in pitch of a Doppler ultrasound detector on the chest over the heart.
      c. Transthoracic or esophageal echocardiography can identify air in the coronary arteries or within the ventricles.
   4. Management
      a. ABCs
      b. Ventilate patient with 100% O_2.
      c. Cover open wounds with saline-soaked pads.
      d. Immediately position the patient in the Trendelenburg position, with the left side down.
      e. If a right atrial catheter is in place, attempt aspiration of air.
      f. Additional conservative measures depend on the status of the child and range from volume expansion, tube thoracostomy for any pneumothorax, and consideration of hyperbaric O_2.

       g. This potentially life-threatening condition may require thoracotomy for children unresponsive to conservative therapy.

VII. Non–life-threatening chest injury

  A. Simple pneumothorax

    1. History and physical examination

      a. History of blunt or penetrating chest trauma

      b. Hyper-resonance on percussion

      c. Decreased breath sounds

    2. Diagnostic tests

      a. Chest radiograph reveals a radiolucent shadow between the rib margin and the lung parenchyma.

      b. Exclude rib fractures on chest radiograph.

    3. Management

      a. Apply face mask with 100% O_2 for the spontaneously breathing patient. A small simple pneumothorax (<20% diameter of the hemithorax) will resolve after breathing pure O_2 for several hours.

      b. Chest tube drainage to underwater seal is mandatory for a clinically significant pneumothorax before the patient is transported out of the emergency room or before induction of general anesthesia for repair of other injuries (see Section II and Figs. 21-2 and 21-3).

  B. Simple hemothorax

    1. History and physical examination

      a. History of blunt or penetrating chest trauma

      b. Dullness on percussion

      c. Decreased breath sounds

    2. Diagnostic tests: The decubitus view of the chest radiograph documents a radiopaque fluid layer between the rib margin and lung parenchyma.

    3. Management: Chest tube drainage (see Section II and Figs. 21-2 and 21-3).

  C. Rib fractures

    1. History and physical examination

      a. Palpable crepitus

      b. Rib deformity

      c. Asymmetrical chest wall movement

      d. Pain leads to splinting of thorax with impaired ventilation.

      e. Fracture of first and second ribs carries a risk for significant intrathoracic injury, including laceration of the great vessels and hemothorax.

    2. The middle ribs (5 to 9) are most commonly injured.

    3. Diagnostic tests: Chest radiography confirms the presence of rib fractures and excludes other chest injuries.

4. Management
   a. Supplemental O_2
   b. Pulmonary toilet
   c. Avoid atelectasis and pneumonia by providing analgesia and encouraging deep breathing.
   d. Analgesia is achieved with opioids (see Chapter 20) or regional nerve blocks (e.g., intercostal nerve blocks).
D. Chest wall contusion
   1. History and physical examination: Obvious evidence of blunt external trauma (soft tissue injury, abrasions, lacerations)
   2. Diagnostic tests: Use chest radiography to exclude other intrathoracic injuries.
   3. Management
      a. Local wound care
      b. Deep breathing exercises to avoid atelectasis and pneumonia

VIII. Resuscitative thoracotomy
Often, conventional resuscitative tactics fail for acute cardiopulmonary arrest after thoracic trauma, and thoracotomy for open chest cardiac massage must be considered. This drastic procedure has limited usefulness.
A. Goals
   1. Control of hemorrhage
   2. Effective cardiac compression
   3. Cross-clamping the pulmonary hilum in case of air embolism or bronchopleural fistula
   4. Cardiac tamponade
B. Indications
   1. All exsanguinating penetrating chest injuries with cardiopulmonary resuscitation started in the field and signs of life and cardiac electrical activity in the emergency department (ED)
   2. Blunt injury; patient arrives with vital signs and acutely deteriorates
   3. Contraindications
      a. Penetrating injury and no signs of life in the field
      b. Blunt trauma patients with pulseless electrical activity diagnosed in the ED

Chapter 22

Abdominal Trauma
Steven Stylianos, MD,
Anne C. Fischer, MD, PhD,
and Charles N. Paidas, MD, MBA

I. Overview
   A. Abdominal injury
      1. Blunt injuries cause 90% of abdominal trauma.
      2. Abdominal injury usually occurs with other multiple injuries involving the head, skeleton, and chest.
      3. Injury to the abdomen accounts for 10% of injuries.
II. Blunt injury
   A. Pathophysiology
      1. Injury results from energy transfer from compressive and/or crushing forces or from rapid deceleration.
      2. The liver and spleen are most commonly injured (solid organs): Spleen > liver > kidney > intestine > pancreas
      3. Hollow visceral (bowel) injuries are often insidious in presentation.
      4. Regardless of mechanism, examination and suspicion of abdominal injury begins at the level of the nipples. Thus, a presumed chest injury, at nipple level, may in fact represent intra-abdominal pathology.
      5. The bowel and pancreas are vulnerable to forces from rapid deceleration with seat belt injuries.
      6. Injuries to the kidney result in a spectrum of diagnoses, which vary from a simple contusion of the kidney or perinephric hematoma to vascular disruption (rare).
      7. Lower urinary tract injuries or urethral stenoses occur with pelvic fractures.
   B. Evaluation (look, listen, palpate)
      1. Any child with polytrauma and signs of hemorrhagic shock necessitates a high index of suspicion for abdominal trauma.
      2. Abdominal injury must be ruled out in any child with central nervous system (CNS) injury and an unreliable abdominal examination.
      3. Acute gastric distention occurs frequently; insertion of an orogastric tube is mandatory to examine thoroughly.

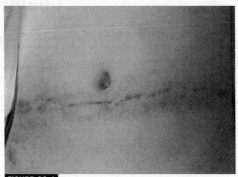

FIGURE 22-1

Lap belt sign. This injury occurs from a combination of deceleration and flexion distributed across the lap portion of the seat belt. The lap belt abrasion is an indication of extreme force and deserves a high index of suspicion for a constellation of injuries that include the abdominal wall; intra-abdominal, retroperitoneal traction, and avulsion-type injuries; and injuries to the lumbar spine.

4. Look
   a. External signs of soft tissue injury on the anterior abdominal wall (bruises, abrasions, lacerations, seat belt sign) (**Fig. 22-1**)
   b. Lateral flank bruising, hematoma
   c. Scaphoid or distended abdomen with or without masses
   d. Perineum: Blood at the urethral meatus
5. Listen
   a. Presence or absence of bowel sounds
   b. Bowel sounds are often present despite intra-abdominal injury.
6. Palpate
   a. Superficial and deep palpation—abdominal tenderness
   b. Guarding (voluntary) versus peritoneal irritation (involuntary response)
   c. Location: Anterior anatomic quadrants (hepatic, splenic), flanks (kidneys), suprapubic or epigastric region
   d. Rock the pelvis to check stability.
   e. Perineum, anorectal region, as well as urethral meatus, for injury
C. Diagnosis
   1. Radiography
      a. Anteroposterior and lateral cervical spine, chest, and pelvis for injured child

TABLE 22-1

PROPOSED GUIDELINES FOR RESOURCE UTILIZATION IN CHILDREN WITH ISOLATED SPLEEN OR LIVER INJURY

Parameter	CT Grade			
	I	II	III	IV
ICU days	None	None	None	1 day
Hospital stay	2 days	3 days	4 days	5 days
Predischarge imaging	None	None	None	None
Postdischarge imaging	None	None	None	None
Activity restriction*	3 weeks	4 weeks	5 weeks	6 weeks

Modified from APSA Trauma Committee. Evidence-based guidelines for resource utilization in children with isolated spleen or liver injury. J Pediatr Surg 2000;35:164-169; and Compliance with evidence-based guidelines in children with isolated spleen or liver injury. A prospective study. J Pediatr Surg 2002;37:453-456.

CT, Computed tomography; *ICU,* intensive care unit.

*Return to **full-contact competitive sports** (e.g., football, wrestling, hockey, lacrosse, mountain climbing) should be at the discretion of the individual pediatric trauma surgeon. The proposed guidelines for return to unrestricted activity include normal age-appropriate activities.

    b. Cross-table lateral film for free air

    c. Document the following:

        (1) Elevated diaphragm suggestive of subdiaphragmatic fluid

        (2) Gastric dilation or ileus suggestive of aerophagia or intraperitoneal blood

        (3) Extraluminal intraperitoneal air or fluid suggestive of perforation

        (4) Obliteration of retroperitoneal fat lines suggestive of retroperitoneal hematoma

        (5) Rib or spine fractures

        (6) Chance fractures: Lumbar spine fractures consistent with lap belt injury, presenting with abdominal ecchymosis and abdominal pain

  2. Computed tomography (CT)

    a. CT scanning is the standard of care for blunt abdominal trauma.

    b. Ideal for identifying organ-specific injury and important for nonoperative management of solid organ injury (spleen, liver, kidney) (**Table 22-1**)

    c. CT may miss intestinal and diaphragmatic injuries.

    d. Intravenous (IV) water-soluble contrast can demonstrate renal function.

    e. Oral contrast is not recommended for initial evaluation.

    f. Effective for evaluation of the retroperitoneum (pancreas)

    g. Free intraperitoneal fluid in the absence of solid organ injury is suggestive of hollow viscous injury.

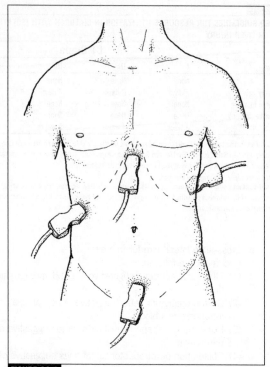

FIGURE 22-2

The FAST examination in trauma looks for hemoperitoneum using four positions to scan the abdomen. These include the subxiphoid position for pericardial fluid, right upper quadrant for hepatorenal fossa, left lateral position for splenorenal fossa, and suprapubic pelvic position for detecting fluid around the bladder.

3. Focused assessment sonography in trauma (FAST) (**Fig. 22-2**)
   a. Effective for detecting intraperitoneal and pericardial fluid or blood: Pericardium, hepatorenal fossa, splenorenal fossa, and pelvis.
   b. Evidence-based role for FAST yet to be defined.
   c. However, the presence of intraperitoneal fluid is not the criteria for operative management in children.
   d. FAST is not organ-specific.
4. Intravenous pyelography (IVP) and retrograde urethrocystography (RUG)
   a. Any blood at the urethral meatus **requires** RUG to exclude lower urinary tract injury **before** Foley catheter placement.

b. RUG is used for extensive pelvic fractures.

c. Hematuria (gross or microscopic) needs assessment by contrast CT scanning or IVP.

5. Diagnostic peritoneal lavage (DPL)

a. DPL provides rapid assessment of intra-abdominal blood or bowel perforation in an unconscious patient.

b. Positive study if blood is directly aspirated, or more than 50,000 to 100,000 red blood cells/mL, more than 500 white blood cells/mL, or vegetative material is present.

c. Indications (rare)

(1) Polytrauma patient requiring immediate operation (head or skeletal injury)

(2) Hemodynamically unstable patient

(3) Unavailability of CT

(4) Normal CT study in a child with presumed hollow viscous injury

D. Management

1. Primary survey: Initial assessment

a. Airway, breathing, and circulation (ABCs)

(1) Secure airway.

(2) Administer supplemental oxygen or mechanical ventilation.

(3) Two large-bore IVs in the upper extremities and/or large-bore central venous access (jugular or subclavian veins)

(4) During a trauma resuscitation, if the expertise required for central access is unavailable, intraosseous access is the route of choice for any age child (see Chapter 5).

b. Send blood for type and crossmatching, complete blood count (CBC), amylase, and electrolyte levels.

c. Place orogastric tube for decompression after the airway has been secured; inspect gastric contents for blood.

d. Monitor urinary output (Foley catheter); send urine for urinalysis.

e. Evaluate adequacy of resuscitation.

f. Warm blankets and warm IV fluids if body temperature is lower than 36° C

2. Secondary survey: Thorough head-to-toe system review

a. Further diagnostic studies (contrast CT or IVP) may be indicated after stabilization.

b. Patients with CNS injury and suspected abdominal injury need sequential noncontrast head and IV contrast abdominal CT scans.

c. Nonoperative management protocols for splenic, hepatic, or renal injury may be indicated (Table 22-1).

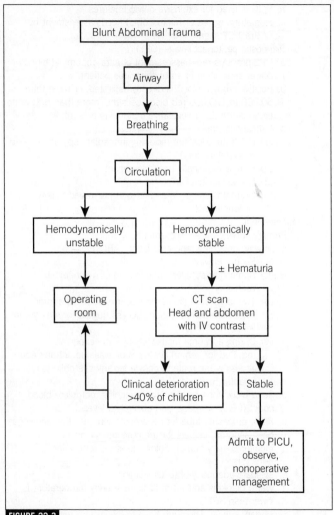

FIGURE 22-3
Operative intervention algorithm for abdominal injury. *CT,* Computed tomography; *IV,* intravenous; *PICU,* pediatric intensive care unit.

      d. Operative intervention is indicated if the patient becomes hemodynamically unstable (**Fig. 22-3**).

III. Penetrating trauma

These are generally gunshot and stab wounds.

  A. Pathophysiology

    1. Almost all intra-abdominal organs are at risk for injury.

    2. Associated with a high incidence of hollow visceral injury

    3. May manifest hemorrhagic shock

  B. Evaluation (look, listen, palpate)

With a history of penetrating injury, intra-abdominal injury should be assumed until proven otherwise.

    1. Thoroughly inspect for entrance and exit wound sites.

    2. Inspect for penetration through the fascia (particularly with stab wounds).

    3. Presence or absence of bowel sounds may not reflect the magnitude of injury.

    4. Evidence of peritoneal signs may suggest intra-abdominal blood and intestinal perforation.

  C. Diagnosis

    1. Radiographs should be obtained, with skin markings of all wounds.

    2. If possible, specify entrance and exit sites with different opaque shapes.

    3. Optimally, patient hemodynamic stability will allow for minimal studies to be obtained

      a. Chest radiograph

      b. Supine abdominal, pelvic radiograph with single-shot IVP (single-injection excretory urogram) to identify number and location of functioning renal units

  D. Management

    1. Primary survey: Initial assessment

      a. ABCs

      b. Send blood for type and crossmatching, CBC, amylase and electrolyte levels

      c. Immediately place orogastric tube for gastric decompression after the airway has been secured; inspect gastric contents for blood.

      d. Place Foley, assess for hematuria, and monitor for output.

      e. Minimal diagnostic imaging studies (as described earlier)

        (1) If unstable: Chest radiography and pelvis–one-shot IVP

        (2) If stable and stab wound to back and flank: Triple-contrast CT (IV, oral, rectal) for retroperitoneal injuries

    2. Secondary survey: Definitive

      a. Celiotomy: Abdominal surgery

      b. Selective nonoperative therapy in stab wounds that do not penetrate the fascia

Chapter 23

General Surgical Emergencies

Eric L. Lazar, MD, MS, FACS, FAAP,
Robert A. Cowles, MD,
and Charles Stolar, MD

I. Overview

Although children are often unable to articulate their symptoms fully, the progression of most pediatric surgical emergencies is so typical that asking parents the right questions, together with appropriate laboratory and diagnostic imaging studies, is usually more than sufficient to determine diagnosis. Once diagnosed, transfer to an inpatient setting and coordination of care with a pediatric surgeon are needed. The clinical presentation, diagnostic evaluation, and surgical treatment of common abdominal and thoracic pediatric surgical emergencies are presented here.

II. Abdomen

A. Malrotation and midgut volvulus

1. Definition

a. Malrotation describes a congenital anomaly.

(1) The midgut fails to fully rotate around its vascular axis during fetal development, leading to a narrow mesenteric base without normal retroperitoneal bowel attachments in the abdominal cavity.

(2) The small intestine then tends to twist around its vascular supply, resulting in midgut volvulus.

b. Midgut volvulus is a surgical emergency.

(1) Time is of the essence.

(2) Midgut volvulus leads to mesenteric vascular compromise, intestinal ischemia, and eventual necrosis, acidosis, and shock.

2. Presentation

a. Although usually presenting in the neonatal period or within the first year of life, malrotation can occur at any age as a midgut volvulus.

b. It presents as an obstruction with bilious emesis and usually abdominal distention.

3. Diagnosis

a. Plain abdominal radiographs may not be helpful.

    b. An upper gastrointestinal (GI) series is the gold standard; the normal pattern shows the following:
       (1) Passage of contrast from stomach to duodenum in left to right movement across the midline
       (2) Followed by contrast passing through the duodenal C loop (right to left crossing the midline)
       (3) Progression toward the greater curvature of the stomach
       (4) Finally, downward jejunal transit
       (5) Failure of the duodenum to cross the midline with the jejunum in the right abdomen defines simple malrotation.
       (6) If complicated by volvulus, distal duodenum is also often obstructed.
  4. Treatment
    a. Nasogastric tube insertion
    b. Aggressive intravenous (IV) fluid resuscitation
    c. An emergency celiotomy and Ladd procedure are performed.
       (1) Untwist volvulus in counterclockwise direction.
       (2) Take down congenital adhesions (Ladd bands) from malrotation.
       (3) Widen mesenteric base.
       (4) Perform appendectomy.
B. Bleeding, inflamed, or perforated Meckel diverticulum
  1. Definition: Meckel diverticulum is a remnant of the embryonic vitelline duct, the most common congenital anomaly of the GI system.
    a. Rule of *two:*
       (1) Incidence = 2%; located in distal ileum, 2 feet from the ileocecal valve
       (2) Approximately 2 inches in length
       (3) Symptomatic by 2 years of age
       (4) Two types of ectopic mucosa
    b. Overall, 30% to 50% will have ectopic mucosal (gastric > pancreatic) tissue.
  2. Presentation: Most Meckel diverticula are asymptomatic and may present with painless rectal bleeding secondary to peptic ulceration of downstream ileal mucosa, inflammation or perforation, or as a lead point for intussusception.
    a. Bleeding
       (1) Painless, at times intermittent, lower GI hemorrhage
       (2) Maroon-colored stools
    b. Inflammation or perforation
       (1) Acute abdominal pain with tender abdomen, guarding, and sometimes abdominal distention

    (2) Presentation similar to acute appendicitis
  c. Intussusception: Clinical picture of small bowel obstruction with crampy abdominal pain, vomiting, and abdominal distention
3. Diagnosis: The choice of diagnostic study depends on presentation.
  a. Lower GI bleeding thought to be caused by Meckel diverticulum
    (1) Technetium-99m pertechnetate isotope scan (Meckel scan)
    (2) Requires the presence of ectopic gastric mucosa in the diverticulum but active bleeding is not necessary
    (3) Good for active bleeding because the pathophysiology is related to the secretory action of ectopic gastric mucosa
  b. Acute abdominal pain or distention
    (1) Plain abdominal radiograph with decubitus views to evaluate for small bowel obstruction or for free air (uncommon)
    (2) Abdominal pain: Pelvic computed tomography (CT) scan can show inflammation, abscess, or phlegmon associated with an inflamed or perforated Meckel diverticulum or an ileoileal intussusception.
    (3) When preoperative studies are not helpful, these inflammatory complications can be diagnosed at exploratory celiotomy or laparoscopy.
4. Treatment
  a. Excision of asymptomatic Meckel diverticulum is controversial.
  b. When symptomatic (bleeding, inflammation, perforation, or intussusception), excision is necessary.
  c. Traditionally, a limited small bowel resection, including the intestine adjacent to the offending Meckel diverticulum, has been the procedure of choice.
    (1) Simple Meckel diverticulectomy, without formal small bowel resection and anastomosis, has been reported with increased frequency and is likely a reasonable alternative.
    (2) Both options are amenable to the laparoscopic approach.
  d. When a Meckel diverticulum serves as the lead point for intussusception, a simple diverticulectomy is sufficient.
C. Toxic megacolon
  1. Definition
    a. Toxic megacolon is not a primary condition but is secondary to another disease.

   b. Combination of a markedly dilated colon (usually transverse colon), abdominal distention, and a toxic or septic appearance should suggest the diagnosis.
 2. Presentation: Usually associated with *Clostridium difficile* colitis or ulcerative colitis
   a. Diagnosis and management of diarrhea
   b. Abdominal pain, abdominal distention
   c. Prior history of ulcerative colitis or antibiotic use
 3. Diagnosis can be difficult to make.
   a. History, physical examination, abdominal radiographs (obstruction series)
   b. Search for underlying cause—infectious, inflammatory, and metabolic
   c. Obtain IV access, assess clinical status, especially acid-base and electrolyte status.
   d. If transverse colon is dilated and child is critically ill, begin empirical antibiotic coverage (broad-spectrum oral metronidazole for possible *C. difficile* infection).
   e. Gentle enema, GI irrigation
   f. If condition does not improve or if clinical condition deteriorates, emergency operation should be considered.
   g. Subtotal colectomy with ileostomy may be necessary. In this case, a subsequent *pull-through* procedure may be possible weeks to months later.
 D. Acute cholecystitis
 1. Definition
   a. Acute inflammation of the gallbladder
   b. Typically related to gallstone disease with cystic duct obstruction and resultant inflammation of the gallbladder or, more rarely, may be *acalculous*
 2. Presentation
   a. Colicky, epigastric and right upper quadrant pain that does not improve with time
   b. At times, nausea, vomiting, or jaundice can be present.
 3. Diagnosis
   a. Complications of gallstone disease do occur, although are relatively rare in children; this represents a greater possibility of an alternative diagnosis.
   b. A history of known gallstones, hemolysis or hemolytic conditions, and obesity may be a clue; seek a previous history of symptoms of biliary colic.
   c. On physical examination, right upper quadrant pain is the hallmark of the disease; Murphy's sign (arrest of inspiration on palpation of the right upper quadrant) may be present.
   d. Imaging studies
     (1) Abdominal ultrasound

(a) Good at diagnosing pericholecystic fluid, gallstones, and gallbladder wall thickening

(b) Findings consistent with acute cholecystitis.

(2) Abdominal ultrasound is not definitive, but suspicion remains for acute cholecystitis.

(a) The patient may be further evaluated with a radionuclide scintigraphy scan.

(b) If the gallbladder fails to fill with tracer, this usually makes the diagnosis.

4. Laboratory studies

a. White blood cell count can be elevated or normal.

b. Elevated liver function

(1) This can signify the presence of stones in the common bile duct or may be related to inflammation adjacent to the liver.

(2) In these cases, the possibility of choledocholithiasis (common bile duct stones) must be considered.

c. Elevated amylase and lipase levels may suggest an alternative diagnosis of biliary pancreatitis; in this case, urgent operation may be contraindicated.

5. Treatment

a. IV fluids, IV antibiotics, and cholecystectomy (usually laparoscopic) in stable patients

b. Patients with hemodynamic instability should be admitted to an intensive care unit (ICU) for aggressive resuscitation and correction of physiologic derangements with enhanced monitoring.

c. With physiologic improvement of the unstable patient, a cholecystectomy may be performed as soon as possible.

(1) In moribund patients, a direct, percutaneous, image-guided cholecystostomy tube may be placed.

(2) This approach allows for expeditious treatment of ongoing sepsis without the morbidity of transporting the patient to the operating room for cholecystectomy.

E. Appendicitis

1. Definition

a. Inflammation of the appendix

b. Pathophysiology related to obstruction of the lumen of the appendix by a fecalith, lymphoid hyperplasia or, rarely, a tumor

2. Presentation

a. Begins with vague, periumbilical abdominal pain

(1) Over the next 12 to 48 hours, the character of the pain changes and localizes to the right lower quadrant.

(2) Anorexia is common.

(3) Nausea and vomiting usually begin *after* the onset of pain.

    (a) Physical examination with focal right lower quadrant tenderness or localized peritoneal signs

    (b) If perforation occurs, abdominal pain becomes more diffuse and severe.

b. In the ICU setting

    (1) Diagnosis of appendicitis is difficult to make.

    (2) A new onset of abdominal tenderness to palpation with involuntary guarding (in nonparalyzed, non–deeply sedated patients) may raise suspicion.

3. Diagnosis

  a. Clinical assessment: History and physical exam with focus on abdominal exam

  b. Leukocytosis is consistent with possible appendicitis.

    (1) Leukopenia, particularly neutropenia, raises the possibility of neutropenic colitis or typhlitis.

    (2) In this case, antibiotics and supportive care, not appendectomy, are the treatments of choice.

  c. Abdominal CT scan with IV and either oral or rectal contrast, if unable to perform a reliable physical examination or history is unclear

    (1) Usually required to make diagnosis in ICU setting

    (2) Usually allows a clear diagnosis

4. Treatment depends upon the results of the diagnostic evaluation:

  a. Acute appendicitis—Appendectomy (laparoscopic versus open)

  b. Phlegmon without systemic sepsis—Appendectomy or IV antibiotics with interval appendectomy 6 weeks later

  c. Walled-off abscess—Appendectomy with drainage of abscess or image-guided percutaneous drainage of the abscess, IV antibiotics, and interval appendectomy 6 weeks later

F. Necrotizing enterocolitis

1. Background

  a. Intestinal necrosis caused by mesenteric ischemia in newborns

  b. Premature newborns at highest risk

  c. Most common and most serious GI condition in premature infants

  d. Significant mortality despite advances in neonatal care

  e. Multifactorial pathophysiology

  f. Location

    (1) Terminal ileum most frequent, followed by colon

    (2) Pan-necrosis seen in 19%; of those; 100% mortality

2. Presentation: Abdominal distention is most common.
   a. Premature neonate who has begun feeding
   b. Abdominal distention with tenderness
   c. Sepsis syndrome
3. Diagnosis depends mainly on results of abdominal films.
   a. Begin with abdominal radiographs (supine, prone, and left lateral decubitus views) and assess the following:
      (1) Bowel gas pattern
      (2) Free air
      (3) Pneumatosis (diagnostic)
      (4) Portal venous gas
   b. Complete blood count (CBC): Thrombocytopenia and leukopenia or leukocytosis common
4. Treatment: Combination of medical and surgical treatment
   a. Pediatric surgical consultation
   b. Serial abdominal films (all views), especially to assess for perforation
   c. Serial CBC, including platelet count
   d. If unstable, follow blood gas, acid-base balance, and electrolytes.
   e. Nothing by mouth, nasogastric decompression, total parenteral nutrition, broad-spectrum IV antibiotics (ampicillin or vancomycin, gentamicin, metronidazole)
   f. If free intra-abdominal air is present, surgical therapy is indicated.
      (1) Exploration, bowel resection, enterostomy for treatable disease
      (2) In pan-necrosis, may elect to close without resection
   g. In a very low birth weight or unstable premature neonate, bedside intra-abdominal drainage can be performed in an attempt to avoid a major exploratory celiotomy.
   h. Other relative indications for surgery
      (1) Fixed intestinal loop
      (2) Abdominal wall erythema
      (3) Signs of abdominal compartment syndrome with respiratory or hemodynamic failure, portal venous gas, persistent metabolic acidosis, persistent thrombocytopenia
   i. Mortality remains high.
G. Enterocolitis in Hirschsprung Disease (HD)
   1. Background
      a. Intestinal infection seen in children with HD
      b. Can be initial presentation or can occur later when diagnosis of HD has already been made
   2. Presentation: Spectrum of mild to fulminant enterocolitis
      a. Diarrhea: Usually present and described as foul-smelling

    b. Abdominal distention
    c. Vomiting
    d. Fever
    e. *Explosive* rectal examination
  3. Diagnosis
    a. Requires high index of suspicion
    b. Any child with HD and who is ill may have some form of enterocolitis.
    c. History and physical examination look for above findings
    d. Abdominal radiographs to assess for distended bowel, thickened bowel wall, *intestinal cut-off sign*, pneumatosis, free intraperitoneal air
  4. Treatment: Should be aggressive and expeditious
    a. Children with enterocolitis can deteriorate quickly so treatment should be started as soon as possible.
    b. Pediatric surgical consultation
    c. Saline washouts of distal colon with rectal tube
    d. IV antibiotics, supportive care, nasogastric tube if necessary
    e. Oral metronidazole in mild cases
    f. If fulminant enterocolitis is unresponsive to therapy, an ileostomy may be necessary for intestinal decompression and diversion of the fecal stream.

H. Pyloric stenosis
  1. Definition
    a. Hypertrophy of the gastric outlet, resulting in obstruction
    b. Most common condition requiring surgery in the neonatal period
  2. Presentation
    a. Usually presents at 2 to 6 weeks of age
    b. Male preponderance of 4:1
    c. Hallmark symptom is progressive, nonbilious projectile vomiting after feeding.
    d. If diagnosis is delayed, infants many present with dehydration, weight loss, characteristic electrolyte abnormalities (hypokalemia, hypochloremia, metabolic alkalosis).
  3. Diagnosis
    a. Typical electrolyte abnormalities
    b. Abdominal ultrasound shows elongated, thickened pylorus, with fluid-filled stomach.
  4. Treatment
    a. In the dehydrated or unstable infant, volume repletion with electrolyte correction should occur before pyloromyotomy is attempted.
    b. Definitive treatment is laparoscopic or open pyloromyotomy.

III. Thorax
   A. Caustic ingestion
      1. Background
         a. Mortality is related to edema and airway obstruction from pharyngeal or laryngeal burns, perforation of upper GI tract, and complications from treatment of strictures (e.g., perforation from stricture dilation).
         b. Types of caustic materials
            (1) Strong alkalis (e.g., sodium or potassium hydroxide found in drain cleaners and lye) are viscous liquids or solids and create the worst injuries by causing deep, penetrating liquefaction necrosis.
            (2) Acids (e.g., paint thinners, metal cleaners, toilet cleaners) cause less penetrating injury by coagulation necrosis.
            (3) Bleach (sodium hypochlorite) and other detergents are the most commonly ingested caustic agents, usually causing mild esophageal and gastric irritation.
         c. Pathophysiology
            (1) Hemorrhage, inflammation, submucosal thrombosis, with possible ischemia or necrosis that occurs acutely and may lead to perforation and mediastinitis
            (2) Scar formation begins after 2 weeks with fibroblast proliferation leading to strictures, adhesions, and fistulas.
         d. Most commonly seen in children younger than 3 years (boys more than girls).
         e. Caustic ingestion by an adolescent is often intentional and should raise concerns of suicide attempt.
      2. Presentation
         a. Caustic solids (e.g., lye)
            (1) Create oropharyngeal burns and may cause excessive drooling
            (2) If the upper airway is involved, presentation includes hoarseness, stridor, wheezing, and/or dyspnea.
         b. Caustic liquids
            (1) Create more esophageal and gastric burns; may present with dysphagia, chest and abdominal pain, or aspiration
            (2) Esophageal and gastric perforation lead to mediastinitis and peritonitis, respectively, and may present as shock.
      3. Diagnosis
         a. Identify the ingested agent if possible; regional poison centers can supply product information.
         b. Endoscopic evaluation of esophagus and stomach delineates extent of disease and grades injury.
         c. Radiographic studies
            (1) CT scan of neck, chest, and abdomen should be obtained if perforation is suspected.

(2) Pneumomediastinum or extravasated oral contrast identifies perforation.

(3) Contrast esophagogram demonstrates perforation and ulcerations acutely and is often obtained several weeks after injury to evaluate for strictures.

4. Treatment
   a. Acute injury
      (1) Initial airway management, ventilation, and circulatory support are critical before any diagnostic procedures are performed.
      (2) Tracheal intubation or tracheostomy may be required for significant laryngeal edema and injury.
      (3) Forced vomiting is contraindicated and increases risk of aspiration.
      (4) Prophylactic antibiotics (including antifungals) and antacids may be used; prophylactic use of corticosteroids is more controversial.
      (5) Nutrition
         (a) Enteral nutrition is preferred, given via nasoenteric feeding tube or gastrostomy.
         (b) Some advocate a long-term nasogastric tube to stent the esophagus while providing enteral access; however, gastrostomy is more secure.
         (c) Total parenteral nutrition is given if enteral feeding is not possible.
      (6) Mild injuries
         (a) Require no further treatment.
         (b) If patient tolerates oral feeds, may be discharged home
      (7) Moderate injuries
         (a) Requires close observation, support, and follow-up
         (b) Prophylactic esophageal dilations may be needed.
      (8) Perforation or extensive necrosis requires immediate surgical intervention.
   b. Strictures
      (1) Dilations
         (a) Bougie or balloon dilations are performed several weeks after injury.
         (b) Strictures often recur and require repeated dilations.
         (c) Dilations may cause an esophageal tear, which can be treated nonoperatively if there are no signs of mediastinitis and the patient remains clinically stable.
      (2) Surgical
         (a) Focal segments can be resected with end-to-end anastomosis.

        (b) Diffuse disease or unsalvageable esophagus: Candidate for esophageal bypass or replacement with colonic or jejunal interposition, or gastric transposition procedure.

B. Foreign body

  1. Airway

    a. Background

      (1) Common in children.

      (2) Acute asphyxiation should be rapidly treated with back blows (in infants) or abdominal thrusts or Heimlich maneuver (in older children; see Chapter 5).

      (3) This section will cover retained foreign bodies.

      (4) Peanuts are the most common objects aspirated; other foods, toys, pins, and small objects are frequently aspirated.

      (5) Peak incidence: 1 to 2 years of age

      (6) Anatomy: Typically lodges in the right mainstem bronchus

    b. Presentation

      (1) History of choking episode is suggestive.

        (a) Coughing, wheezing, stridor, dyspnea, and fever are common.

        (b) Decreased breath sounds or wheezing on the affected side

      (2) May present as pneumonia from retained foreign body.

    c. Diagnosis: Must have high index of suspicion based on age, signs, and symptoms because most aspirations are not witnessed events.

      (1) Radiographs

        (a) Anteroposterior (AP) and lateral radiographs of neck and chest with both inspiratory and expiratory films

        (b) May see hyperinflation (ball valve mechanism of foreign body in bronchus), atelectasis (complete obstruction of a bronchus), or consolidation from pneumonia

        (c) Only 10% of aspirated foreign bodies are radiopaque.

      (2) Rigid bronchoscopy is the preferred method for diagnosis and treatment; flexible fiberoptic bronchoscope is helpful to visualize distal airways not accessible by the rigid bronchoscope.

    d. Treatment: Bronchoscopy should be performed in the operating room under general anesthesia.

      (1) Rigid bronchoscopy

        (a) Allows direct visualization with simultaneous ventilation through the bronchoscope

(b) Forceps or flexible grasping instruments can be used to extract the foreign body.

(2) Postoperative: Aggressive chest physiotherapy

2. Esophagus

a. Background

(1) Coins are the most frequently ingested foreign body by children; alkaline disc batteries, toys, pins, rings, bones are also frequently ingested, lodge in the esophagus.

(2) Batteries can cause caustic burns; bones and other sharp objects can cause esophageal tears and mediastinitis.

(3) Anatomy

(a) Usually lodge in upper esophageal sphincter at cricopharyngeus muscle, midesophagus where aortic arch crosses, and lower esophageal sphincter

(b) Also may lodge in areas of previous stricture or stenosis (i.e., previous tracheoesophageal fistula repair)

b. Presentation

(1) May be asymptomatic (one third)

(2) Common symptoms: Dysphagia, odynophagia, poor oral intake, drooling, fever, and irritability

(3) Wheezing, stridor, and coughing may be present if foreign body causes external compression of airway.

c. Diagnosis

(1) Radiographs

(a) AP and lateral radiographs of neck, chest, and abdomen

(b) Single AP view may miss superimposed foreign body in tracheobronchial tree.

(2) Rigid esophagoscopy

(a) Preferred method of diagnosis and treatment

(b) Flexible fiberoptic esophagoscopy may be used but lacks advantage of direct visualization and protection of sleeve of rigid esophagoscope when extracting objects.

(3) Contrast esophagogram with water-soluble contrast helps assess injury if immediate endoscopy not available.

d. Treatment

(1) All lodged esophageal foreign bodies must be removed; however, objects that are small, smooth, and inert may be pushed into the stomach and expected to pass through the GI tract.

(2) Treatment of choice: Rigid (or flexible) esophagoscopy under general anesthesia, which allows direct visualization and extraction of foreign body

C. Mediastinal masses
   1. Definition
      a. Classified as anterior (sometimes called anterosuperior), middle, or posterior mediastinal masses, depending on their relative location on a lateral chest radiograph
      b. Posteroanterior and lateral radiographs are initially obtained.
   2. Diagnosis
      a. CT scan of chest with IV contrast defines tumor involvement and possible airway compromise.
   3. Anterior masses: Compartment bound by sternum, anteriorly, and heart, pericardium, and great vessels, posteriorly.
      a. *Four Ts:* Terrible lymphoma, teratoma, thymoma, thyroid
      b. Lymphoma
         (1) Most common
         (2) Systemic disease treated by chemotherapy and/or radiation, and not by surgical resection, so adequate tissue biopsy required for diagnosis and planning chemotherapy
      c. Large anterior mediastinal masses can compress trachea and distal airways; are life-threatening
         (1) Sedation, general anesthesia, paralysis, and tracheal intubation cause loss of muscle tone and may compromise airway with real risk of distal airway collapse and total obstruction.
         (2) Other lymphoma sites (e.g., cervical or supraclavicular lymph nodes) should be sought for tissue biopsy.
         (3) If not available for biopsy and sedation/general anesthesia is not indicated, then may empirically treat with corticosteroids to first alleviate tracheal compression.
   4. Middle masses: Contain the heart, great vessels, trachea, esophagus
      a. Masses in children younger than 2 years
         (1) Usually remnants of embryologic foregut (esophageal duplication cysts, bronchogenic cysts)
         (2) Usually asymptomatic
      b. Diagnosis: Chest CT scan with contrast
      c. Treatment: Surgical excision
   5. Posterior masses: Compartment posterior to anterior surface of thoracic spine, including paravertebral sulci
      a. Usually a neurogenic tumor, including neuroblastoma or ganglioneuroma
      b. Diagnosis: Magnetic resonance imaging to evaluate involvement of neural foramina
      c. Treatment: Most are malignant and require surgical excision.

Chapter 24

Orthopedic Trauma

Joshua E. Hyman, MD, FAAP,
and Michael C. Ain, MD

I. Overview

Skeletal trauma accounts for 10% to 15% of emergency room visits related to trauma among children and teenagers. Pediatricians, trauma surgeons, and emergency room physicians must collaborate closely to care for this patient population effectively.

II. Pediatric anatomy

  A. Ligament properties

    1. Stronger than bones in children

    2. Therefore, dislocations and sprains are relatively uncommon in children, whereas growth plate disruption and bone avulsion are more common.

  B. Bone properties

   Increased bone vascularity, thicker periosteum, and more rapid callus formation lead to unique properties in pediatric fractures. Unique fracture patterns include the following:

    1. Plastic deformation: Bend in the bone without a fracture

    2. Greenstick fracture: Fracture of one cortex under tension while the contralateral cortex remains intact

    3. Torus (buckle) fracture: Fracture with buckling of one cortex in compression while the contralateral cortex is undamaged

    4. Spiral fracture:

      a. Created by low-energy rotational force

      b. Thick intact periosteum often prevents displacement

      c. Commonly associated with child abuse

    5. Growth plate fractures: Fractures at open growth plates

    6. **Figure 24-1** shows the Salter classification of growth plate injuries, which is useful when communicating with the orthopedic consultant.

III. Evaluation

  A. Secondary survey

   Once airway, breathing, and circulation have been addressed, a meticulous secondary survey evaluating for musculoskeletal injury should be performed.

    1. Skeletal

      a. The cervical spine remains immobilized until injury is ruled out. The spine is palpated for tenderness and swelling.

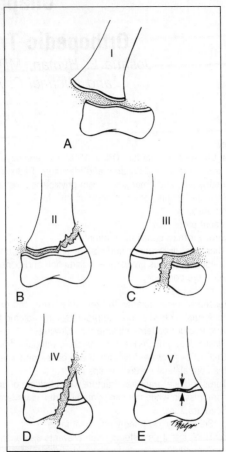

FIGURE 24-1

Salter classification of growth plate injuries. **A,** Type I: Fracture along but not across plate. **B,** Type II: Fracture along plate with metaphyseal extension. **C,** Type III: Fracture into joint. **D,** Type IV: Fracture across plate and joint. **E,** Type V: Crush injury to plate without obvious fracture.

    b. Pelvic stability is assessed by lateral compression.
        (1) Careful evaluation of every extremity includes
            inspection and palpation for gross deformity, abrasions,
            ecchymosis, and tenderness.
        (2) In the absence of obvious fractures, passive flexion and
            extension are performed on all extremities.
2. Neurologic
    a. Documentation of the neurologic examination before and
       after manipulation is essential.
    b. A rapid neurologic examination is focused on motor
       strength, including active flexion and extension of each
       major joint.
    c. Sensation should be tested on the dorsal and volar surfaces
       of each limb segment.
3. Vascular
    a. Fractures and dislocations around the elbow and knee are
       susceptible to vascular injury.
    b. Poor peripheral pulses and slow capillary refill suggest
       vascular injury and require an immediate orthopedic
       consult.
    c. Evaluate for compartment syndrome in all extremities even
       if no gross deformity exists (see Section VII).
4. Splinting
    a. Splint fractured limbs to reduce ongoing hemorrhages and
       decrease pain.
    b. Initial splints should be radiolucent or easily removable so
       they do not sacrifice the quality of screening radiographs.
B. Imaging studies
    1. An initial radiographic trauma series should be performed,
       including the following:
        a. Cervical spine series (anteroposterior [AP], lateral, and
           odontoid views)
        b. AP and lateral radiographs of the chest and pelvis
        c. **Figure 24-2** shows the algorithm for excluding cervical
           spine injury in children.
    2. Extremity radiographs
        a. These should be taken whenever there is any suspicion of
           injury.
        b. Always include the joint above and below the injury.
        c. If ossification is not complete, contralateral radiographs
           may be useful (especially true for pediatric elbow
           fractures).
    3. Specialized studies
        a. Computed tomography (CT), bone scans, magnetic
           resonance imaging (MRI) scans, or angiographs are
           obtained after consultation with an orthopedic surgeon.

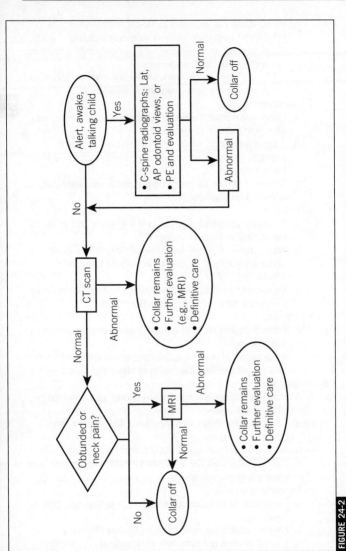

FIGURE 24-2

Algorithm for excluding cervical spine injury (cervical spine clearance) in children. *AP,* Anteroposterior; *CT,* computed tomography; *Lat,* lateral; *MRI,* magnetic resonance imaging; *PE,* physical examination.

b. An orthopedic surgeon should be called early to help coordinate proper imaging and management.

C. Child abuse
   1. Abuse is responsible for a high percentage of pediatric injuries; thus, a high index of suspicion is necessary.
   2. Fractures
      a. Second most common presentation of physical abuse after skin findings.
      b. Warnings that warrant a complete skeletal survey:
         (1) Spiral fractures
         (2) Metaphyseal corner fractures
         (3) Multiple fractures at different stages of healing
         (4) Fracture patterns inconsistent with patient history
         (5) Unwitnessed fractures
         (6) Suspicious skin lesions
   3. No fracture is pathognomonic for child abuse.

IV. Pain management
   A. Pediatric patients who have suffered orthopedic injury or who have diseased joints and bones all have substantial pain.
      1. Great care and sensitivity are required of all physicians who assess and treat these patients.
      2. The pain is related to the disease process and medical interventions. A full discussion of pain and sedation can be found in Chapter 20.
   B. Nonsteroidal agents such as ibuprofen and ketorolac might interfere with bone healing and are not recommended for bone injury–associated pain.
   C. In contrast, a combination of a narcotic and acetaminophen is an appropriate analgesic.

V. Compartment syndrome
   A. Mechanism
      1. Caused by swelling of muscle within an inelastic fascial compartment
      2. Muscle swelling can be caused by trauma or ischemia.
      3. Increase in compartment pressure leads to collapse of vessels and ischemic necrosis of tissues.
   B. Physical findings
      1. Compartment is firm.
      2. Pain is out of proportion to the expected findings.
      3. The most sensitive finding in the physical examination is exquisite pain with passive stretch of the involved muscles.
      4. Paresthesia, pallor, lack of pulse, and paralysis are late findings; diagnosis and management is not dependent on them.

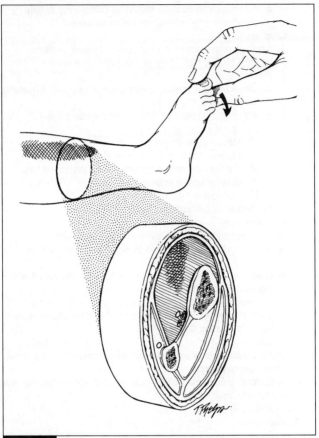

FIGURE 24-3

Physical examination for compartment syndrome. In the anterior compartment of the leg, plantar flexion of the toes stretches the toe extensors *(shaded),* causing pain, yet does not cause movement of any long bone fractures that may be present.

C. Diagnosis
   1. By physical examination (**Fig. 24-3**)
   2. Unconscious or unreliable patients
      a. Measurement of compartment pressure, preferably with a commercial device or manometer, is required (**Fig. 24-4**).

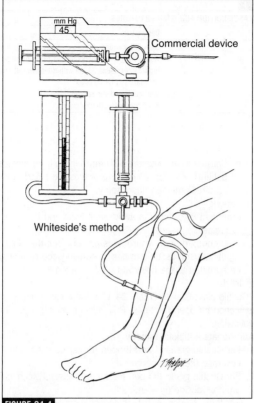

FIGURE 24-4

Whiteside's method for measurement of compartment pressure. The sterile needle, inserted into the compartment, is attached to fluid-filled tubing, three-way stopcock, and manometer. A 30-mL air-filled syringe is attached to the stopcock, which is open to the syringe and the tubing. Air is injected from the syringe until a small air bubble in the tubing is displaced toward the needle and the corresponding manometer pressure is recorded. Commercial devices measure compartment pressure automatically.

TABLE 24-1	
GUSTILO CLASSIFICATION FOR OPEN FRACTURES	
Type	Description
I	Low-energy wound <1 cm
II	Wound >1 cm with moderate soft tissue damage
III	High-energy wound >1 cm with extensive soft tissue damage
IIIA	Adequate soft tissue cover
IIIB	Inadequate soft tissue cover
IIIC	Associated with arterial injury

   b. Compartment pressure >30 mm Hg (in a normotensive
      patient) or within 30 mm Hg of diastolic blood pressure
      requires emergent fasciotomy.
   D. Treatment
      1. Emergent fasciotomy to avoid neurologic and ischemic
         sequelae
      2. If no compartment syndrome is present, but the child has
         significant soft tissue damage or swelling, the patient should
         be admitted to the hospital for observation.
VI. Open fracture
   The Gustilo classification (**Table 24-1**) is the most commonly used
   classification for open fractures. Principles in management include
   the following:
   A. Appropriate antibiotic therapy
      1. For Gustilo grades I and II open fractures: Antistaphylococcal
         coverage (cephalosporin)
      2. For Gustilo grade III open fractures: Antistaphylococcal and
         aminoglycoside (gentamicin)
      3. For farm injuries: Antistaphylococcal coverage, aminoglycoside
         (gentamicin), and penicillin
      4. Give tetanus prophylaxis, if indicated.
      5. Early operative débridement and irrigation are indicated in
         most cases.
   B. Fracture stabilization
      1. Temporary: Splints in emergency room
      2. Early: Often, external fixation
      3. Definitive: May convert to internal fixation after wound has
         healed and risk of infection has cleared
VII. Amputation and reimplantation
   Consider possibility of reimplantation in arm, hand, and finger
   amputations.
   A. Treatment
      1. Wrap amputated tissue in gauze and soak with sterile saline.
      2. Place tissue in plastic bag, seal, and place in ice water.

B. Call reimplantation center in advance of treating patient.
C. Reimplantation success
   1. Dependent on the interval from injury to revascularization
   2. Successful reimplantation likely with the following:
      a. Warm ischemia time <6 hours
      b. Cold ischemia time <12 hours

VIII. Spine and spinal cord trauma

A. Overview
   1. Once recognized, spine and spinal cord injuries are easy to manage; unrecognized, they may become catastrophic.
   2. Vertebral fractures may be present with or without spinal cord injury, and vice versa.
   3. Children may have spinal cord injury without radiographic abnormality.
      a. Therefore, even if radiographs are normal, the unresponsive child should be immobilized on a backboard and placed in a cervical spine (C-spine) collar until trauma evaluation is completed.
B. Pediatric anatomy
   1. Facet angle differences and greater ligamentous laxity lead to an increase in translational motion.
   2. Therefore, up to 4 mm of subluxation, known as pseudosubluxation, is considered normal (e.g., C2 on C3).
C. Evaluation
   1. Primary survey
      a. Airway, breathing
         (1) Observe breathing patterns.
         (2) An injury at level C3, C4, or C5 may affect the phrenic nerve and lead to loss of diaphragmatic breathing.
      b. Circulation
         (1) Spinal shock will lead to bradycardia with hypotension.
         (2) Vasodilation will cause the skin to be warm.
   2. Secondary survey
      a. A visual inspection of the back and abdomen should be performed for all trauma patients.
      b. Abdominal abrasions from lap belt injuries should raise suspicion for flexion injuries to the spine (see later).
   3. Neurologic examination: A complete neurologic evaluation, including sensorimotor function and level of consciousness, should be performed.
      a. Cranial nerve injuries
         (1) Vagus nerve: Stridor or alteration in phonation
         (2) Spinal accessory nerve: Trapezius muscle weakness
         (3) Hypoglossal nerve: Deviation of tongue

  b. Rectal tone
    (1) With a cord injury, the presence of rectal tone (sacral sparring) is a good prognostic sign and implies partial or complete recovery in 30% to 50% of patients.
    (2) In the absence of rectal tone, there is only a 2% to 3% chance of partial or complete recovery.
  c. Genitourinary system: Males may have priapism after spinal cord injury.
4. Radiographic evaluation
  a. Indications for complete **cervical spine imaging** include the following:
    (1) Acute neurologic deficit
    (2) Altered mental status resulting from injury
    (3) Intoxication
    (4) High-risk mechanism (e.g., diving, unrestrained passenger)
  b. A combination of plain radiographs of the neck, CT scan, and MRI are used, depending on the injury mechanism, age, physical examination, mental status, and presence of multisystem injury.
  c. While maintaining continuous C-spine immobilization during the entire injury evaluation, plain radiographs of the neck (taken as part of the initial trauma series) can be used as initial screening.
  d. Because of the magnitude of radiation, indiscriminate use of CT scanning of the neck is not warranted in children.
  e. MRI is reserved for suspicion of ligamentous injury within the first 48 hours of the event.
  f. Indications for thoracolumbar spine series
    (1) Back pain
    (2) Spine tenderness
    (3) Unreliable patient history following severe trauma
D. Common pediatric spine injuries
  1. C1 and C2 fractures
    a. Most common fractures of the spine in children
    b. Cervical spine injury may be associated with intimal tears of the carotid or vertebral arteries, so the following are warranted:
      (1) Screening CT arteriogram (CT-A) is suggested
      (2) Absolute indications for CT-A include vertebral fracture with subluxation and focal neurologic deficits of the upper and lower extremities.
    c. Odontoid fracture (C2) is treated with external immobilization using a halo vest.
  2. Atlantoaxial (C1-C2) instability, dislocation
    a. Excessive rotational mobility of C1 on C2 can lead to spinal cord injury.

      b. Instability can be caused by rupture of ligaments, increased ligamentous laxity (Down syndrome), or fracture of the odontoid.

      c. Flexion-extension studies

        (1) Will show greater than 5 mm of excursion from the anterior cortex of the dens to the anterior ring of C1 (predens space)

        (2) Perform only in awake cooperative patients who can terminate the movement at the onset of pain

      d. Treat with skeletal traction and/or posterior fusion.

   3. Jefferson burst fracture (C1)

      a. Bilateral fractures of the anterior and posterior arches of C1 resulting from axial load (e.g., diving, head-on collision against dashboard)

      b. Radiographs: Odontoid view shows displaced lateral aspects of the atlas (C1) relative to the axis (C2).

      c. Treat with external immobilization using a halo vest.

   4. Hangman fracture

      a. Extension injury leads to fracture of posterior neuronal arch C2.

      b. Treat with external immobilization using a halo vest.

   5. Chance fracture

      a. Hyperflexion injury (lap belt injury), usually at levels T10-L4

      b. Children are more susceptible than adults.

      c. Rule out cauda equine syndrome (urinary retention, decreased anal tone, saddle anesthesia, loss of ankle reflexes, and leg pain or weakness) from disc herniation.

      d. Most are stable injuries and will heal with closed management.

      e. Small bowel and pancreatic injuries may be associated with the Chance fracture.

E. Incomplete spinal cord syndromes

   1. Anterior cord syndrome

      a. Bilateral loss of motor, pain, and temperature function below injury; preservation of proprioception and touch

      b. Flexion, axial compression, blast effect, or thrombosis cause damage to the anterior spinal artery, leading to ischemic injury to the anterior cord.

   2. Central cord syndrome

      a. Caused by hyperextension injury

      b. Affects variable amounts of spinothalamic (pain, temperature), corticospinal (motor), and posterior columns (proprioception, touch, vibratory sense)

      c. Motor weakness in arms worse than legs

   3. Posterior cord syndrome

      a. Caused by hyperextension injury

      b. Loss of proprioception, touch, and vibratory sense

        4. Brown-Séquard syndrome
          a. Cord hemisection caused by penetrating injuries
          b. Ipsilateral loss of motor, proprioception touch, and vibratory sense
          c. Contralateral loss of pain, temperature sensation

   F. Therapy for spinal cord injury
        1. There is lack of evidence to support the use of high-dose steroids as a requirement for the management of nonpenetrating spinal cord injury.
        2. If the decision is made to use steroid therapy for nonpenetrating injury, the drug protocol must begin within 8 hours of injury (administer methylprednisolone, 30 mg/kg IV loading dose over 15 min, followed by methylprednisolone 5.4 mg/kg/hr for 23 hr if therapy is initiated less than 3 hr after injury; if therapy is initiated 3 to 8 hr after injury, infusion should continue for 48 hr). Methylprednisolone is not indicated for nonpenetrating injuries more than 8 hours after injury, nor for penetrating spinal cord injuries.
        3. Spinal cord perfusion
          a. Depends on mean arterial pressure (MAP)
          b. Maintain MAP at the 75th to 90th percentile for age with phenylephrine, 0.1 to 10 mcg/kg/min, after fluid resuscitation is completed.

IX. Femur fractures
   A. Femoral shaft fractures
        1. Represent 1.6% of all fractures in the pediatric population
        2. Most common fractures requiring hospitalization
   B. Fractures in adolescents
        1. Caused by high-energy trauma (90% are motor vehicle accidents [MVAs])
   C. Fractures in younger children
        1. Femur fractures are caused by low-energy injuries.
        2. Abuse is responsible for 80% of femur fractures in children not yet walking and 30% in toddlers.
        3. The remainder are caused by low-energy injuries, such as falls.
   D. Fracture management
        1. Directed by the following:
          a. Age of the child
          b. Amount of energy causing the fracture
          c. Presence of additional injuries
        2. **Table 24-2** provides guidelines for age-based treatment.

X. Tibia fractures
   A. Causes
        1. Tibia fractures represent the third most common pediatric fracture after femur and forearm fractures.

TABLE 24-2	
FEMUR FRACTURE MANAGEMENT	
Age (yr)	**Isolated Injury**
Neonate	Splinting for 2-3 wk until united
1-5	If <1.5 cm of shortening, then immediate spica cast in emergency room under moderate to deep sedation
	If >1.5 cm shortening, then external fixation, intramedullary flexible nailing, or skeletal traction in the operating room
6-10	External fixation, flexible nailing, plating, or skeletal traction
10-14	Flexible nailing for stable fractures
>14	Reamed, locked intramedullary nailing using trochanteric entry point if growth center is open

24

      2. Causes include the following:
        a. 50%, pedestrian (versus motor vehicle) accident
        b. 22%, indirect rotational forces
        c. 17%, falls
        d. 11%, MVA
   B. Evaluation
   There should be a high index of suspicion for compartment syndrome.
   C. Proximal tibia metaphyseal fractures
      1. These fractures constitute 11% of pediatric tibia fractures and have a peak incidence at 3 to 6 years of age.
      2. Nondisplaced fractures are treated with a long leg cast in 10 degrees of flexion at the knee.
      3. Displaced fractures
        a. Reduced under general anesthesia
        b. Long leg cast is applied in full extension with varus molding to prevent valgus collapse and malunion.
      4. If interposed tissue prevents closed reduction, an open reduction should be performed.
   D. Diaphyseal fractures of the tibia
      1. Of all tibia fractures, 39% occur in the diaphysis.
      2. Most of these fractures can be managed nonoperatively with closed reduction under conscious sedation, followed by immobilization.
      3. Immobilization is performed with a long leg cast and the knee flexed to provide rotational control and prevent weight bearing.
      4. Indications for operative correction (<5% cases) include the following:
        a. Open fractures
        b. Complex fractures that cannot be reduced
        c. Compartment syndrome
        d. Neurovascular injury
        e. Multiple long bone fractures

E. Distal metaphyseal tibia fractures
   1. Fractures of the distal third of the tibia
      a. Comprise approximately 50% of pediatric tibial fractures
      b. Peak incidence between 2 and 8 years of age
   2. For minimally displaced fractures, treatment includes reduction under conscious sedation, followed by long leg casting.
   3. Surgical intervention is reserved for open fractures or complex fractures for which stable reduction is not possible by closed means.
F. Toddler fracture
   1. A spiral fracture of the tibia without involvement of the fibula is caused by a low-energy torsional force.
   2. Most of these fractures occur in children younger than $2\frac{1}{2}$ years.
   3. Management consists of the following:
      a. Long leg cast for 2 to 3 weeks, followed by 2 to 3 weeks in a short leg cast
      b. Manipulation is usually not necessary.
   4. This is a low-energy injury.
      a. The suspicion for compartment syndrome is less than for other tibia fractures.
      b. Therefore, it is usually not necessary to admit the patient for observation.
XI. Ankle fractures (Figure 24-1)
   A. Overview
      1. Ankle injuries are common.
         a. Peak incidence is from 8 to 15 years.
         b. After age 16, adult fracture patterns are seen.
      2. 58% of ankle injuries occur during athletic participation.
      3. If proximal fibula tenderness presents, rule out a high fibula fracture.
   B. Isolated lateral malleolus injuries
      1. In children, ligaments are relatively stronger than bones.
         a. Therefore, bones and growth plates tend to fracture before ligaments tear.
         b. For this reason, ankle sprains are less common in children than adults.
         c. More common is a Salter-Harris I fracture of the distal fibula (Figure 24-1)
         d. Because both have negative radiographic findings, the only way to distinguish them is by careful physical examination.
         e. Examination may reveal the following differences:
            (1) Ankle sprain: Swelling and tenderness directly over the talofibular ligament
            (2) Distal fibula physis fracture: Tenderness over the lateral malleolus growth plate

2. Treatment of a sprained ankle includes an Ace bandage, ice, elevation, and weight-bearing as tolerated.
3. Treatment for an isolated Salter-Harris I of the distal fibula is a short leg cast with weight bearing as tolerated for 3 to 6 weeks.

C. Isolated distal tibia growth plate (physeal) fractures

1. Fractures of the distal tibia growth plate pose a diagnostic challenge.
   a. Can have a poor prognosis secondary to physeal growth arrest
   b. Delayed diagnosis may lead to premature physeal closure, with a leg length discrepancy.
2. Closed reduction and casting
   a. Treatment of choice for Salter-Harris I and II fractures (Figure 24-1)
   b. A long leg cast for 3 weeks, followed by a short leg cast for 3 weeks, is standard.
3. For Salter-Harris III and IV fractures, anatomic reduction is required; a CT scan is often essential for diagnosis.
   a. If there is <2 mm of displacement following closed reduction, then treatment is a long leg cast for 4 weeks, followed by a short leg cast for 3 weeks.
   b. If >2 mm of displacement remains, then reduction under general anesthesia is followed by percutaneous pinning or open reduction and internal fixation.

XII. Clavicle

A. Overview

1. The clavicle is one of the most commonly fractured bones in children.
2. These tend to occur in the region of the middle of the clavicle.

B. Treatment

1. Sling
   a. Most can be managed with a sling for 2 to 3 weeks.
   b. The purpose of the sling is for comfort, not to reduce the ends of the fractured bones.
2. Operative intervention is reserved for the following:
   a. Rare open fractures
   b. Severe tenting of the skin
   c. Neurovascular compromise
   d. Symptomatic nonunion

XIII. Elbow

A. Overview

1. Common (~9% of all fractures in children)
   a. Often difficult to diagnose because the fracture line can be difficult to view on plain radiographs

TABLE 24-3

ELBOW INJURY FREQUENCY

Fracture Type	Elbow Injuries (%)	Peak Age (yr)	Requires Operative Procedure
Supracondylar fractures	41	7	Majority
Radial head subluxation	28	3	Rarely
Lateral condylar physeal fracture	11	6	Majority
Medial epicondylar apophyseal fracture	8	11	Minority
Radial head and neck fractures	5	10	Minority
Elbow dislocations	5	13	Rarely
Medial condylar physeal fractures	1	10	Rarely

b. Anterior and posterior fat pad signs (i.e., lucencies anterior and posterior to the elbow joint on lateral radiographs) suggest distention of the joint capsule and play an important role in the diagnosis of fracture when combined with the clinical examination.

2. **Table 24-3** shows the frequencies of different elbow fractures, peak incidence, and need for surgery.

B. Radial head subluxation

1. More commonly known as *nursemaid*'s *elbow*, these injuries are most common in children from 2 to 5 years of age.

2. The injury is caused by longitudinal traction applied to an extended arm, leading to subluxation of the radial head and interposition of the annular ligament into the radiocapitellar joint.

3. A child with radial head subluxation tends to hold the elbow flexed and the forearm pronated; pain will be localized to the lateral aspect of the elbow.

4. There are no abnormal radiographic findings with this injury.

5. Reduction is performed by manually supinating the forearm, with the elbow in 60 to 90 degrees of flexion.

a. While holding the arm supinated, the elbow is then maximally flexed.

b. During this maneuver, the physician's thumb applies pressure over the radial head.

c. A palpable click is often heard with reduction of the radial head.

6. Immobilization is not necessary, and the child may immediately resume use of the arm.

7. Follow-up is only needed if the child does not resume normal use of the arm in the following weeks.

C. Supracondylar fractures
  1. This is an **acute emergency because of potential for vascular injury** and resulting compartment syndrome–Volkmann contracture.
  2. Closed reduction often relieves impingement on the artery and should not be delayed when there are diminished pulses.
  3. Neurologic deficits occur in 7% to 15% of supracondylar fractures; most nerve injuries are neuropraxias and do not require treatment.
  4. Only a completely nondisplaced fracture is amenable to nonoperative treatment in a long arm cast, with the elbow at 90 degrees for 2 to 3 weeks.
  5. Displaced fractures are treated surgically with closed reduction and percutaneous pinning, followed by casting.
D. Lateral condyle fractures
  1. An increased risk of malunion and nonunion occurs with these fractures; in these cases, cubitus valgus and tardy ulnar nerve palsy may result.
  2. Swelling and tenderness are usually limited to the lateral side of the elbow.
  3. If the lateral condyle and capitellum have not ossified, then radiographic findings can be subtle.
  4. To obtain good treatment results, the articular surface must be perfectly reduced.
    a. Only a completely nondisplaced fracture should be treated nonoperatively.
    b. More often, the fracture is displaced and should be treated by open reduction and percutaneous pinning in the operating room.
E. Medial epicondyle fractures
  1. 50% of medial epicondyle fractures are associated with elbow dislocations.
  2. Ulnar nerve dysfunction is found in 10% to 16% of these fractures.
  3. Minimally or nondisplaced medial epicondyle fractures
    a. Splinted in a posterior molded splint, with the elbow flexed to 90 degrees
    b. After 3 to 4 days, the splint is discontinued and active range of motion is begun.
    c. A sling can be worn for comfort.
F. Radial head and neck fractures
  1. In children, fractures of the proximal end of the radius typically involve the radial neck and physis.
  2. Patients typically present with lateral swelling and pain exacerbated by supination and pronation.

    3. A portion of the radial neck is extraarticular; therefore, an effusion and fat pad signs are sometimes absent.
    4. A radiograph with the beam directed 40 degrees in the proximal direction, known as the Greenspan view, is helpful to visualize the fracture.
    5. Nonoperative treatment is indicated for minimally displaced fractures with less than 30 degrees of angulation.
    6. If there is more than 30 degrees of angulation, closed reduction with or without percutaneous pinning should be done in the operating room.
  G. Elbow dislocations
    1. Elbow dislocations are rare and occur in older children as the result of a fall on a hyperextended elbow. Most dislocations are posterolateral.
    2. A careful neurovascular examination must be performed because injury to the brachial artery, median nerve and, less commonly, the ulnar nerve, can occur.
    3. Reduction should be performed in a timely matter under conscious sedation.
    4. If the elbow is stable after reduction, immobilize for 1 week and then begin range-of-motion (ROM) exercises.
    5. If unstable, immobilize in a position of stability for 3 weeks and then begin ROM exercises, making sure to avoid full extension until 6 weeks.
    6. The need for surgery is rare and is reserved for the following:
      a. Open dislocations
      b. Median nerve entrapment
      c. Brachial artery injuries
      d. Treatment of an associated fracture
XIV. Forearm and wrist
  A. Overview
    1. Pediatric forearm fractures are very common, comprising 45% of all pediatric fractures.
    2. Rare compartment syndrome should be carefully ruled out in forearm fractures.
  B. Management
    1. Most forearm and wrist fractures are treated nonoperatively with closed reduction under conscious sedation, followed by casting.
    2. The reduction maneuver and accepted angulation are defined on a case-by-case basis depending on the following:
      a. Age of the patient
      b. Location of the fracture
      c. Type of deformity

3. Immobilization
   a. Consists of a long arm cast for 6 to 8 weeks with the possibility of conversion to a short arm cast after 4 weeks, depending on the type of fracture and healing response
   b. One exception is the torus fracture, which may be immobilized in a short arm cast for 2 to 3 weeks.
4. Operative treatment is indicated for the following:
   a. Fractures in which acceptable angulation cannot be obtained through closed reduction
   b. Comminuted fractures with segmental bone loss
   c. Open fractures

24

Chapter 25

Ocular Emergencies and Trauma

Michael X. Repka, MD

I. Overview

Although an ophthalmologist should be consulted for almost all eye injuries, the first person to see the patient or talk to the parents can be of enormous value. The results of the initial assessment of most eye injuries often determine the degree of damage to ocular structure and function. In addition, care during this evaluation can prevent further injury and visual loss.

II. Field treatment

A. Never try to pry the eyelids of a child apart to see the eye.

1. If a view cannot be obtained, a shield, a disposable drinking cup, or similar device should be applied over the eye. Avoid placing a gauze bandage directly over the eye or applying pressure on the eye, and immediately transport the patient to an appropriate facility.

2. The shield should rest on the facial bones beyond the orbital rim, with no pressure placed on the eyeball or the orbital contents.

3. Inadvertent pressure on the globe by the examiner's fingers may make a perforating injury worse.

B. Other appropriate emergency field treatment for an eye that has been splashed with a chemical:

1. Prompt irrigation with saline or water (if saline not available) for at least 30 minutes is essential.

III. History

A. Establish time, mechanism of injury, and what was done to the child after the injury.

B. In cases of possible foreign body, obtain some of the material.

C. Determine the following:

1. Preexisting eye disorders

2. Allergies

3. Tetanus immunization history

4. Time of the last meal

TABLE 25-1

CLINICAL ASSESSMENT OF THE OCULAR MOTOR SYSTEM

Cranial Nerve	Primary Movement	Muscle Innervated
III—Oculomotor	Adduction	Medial rectus
	Depression	Inferior rectus
	Elevation	Superior rectus
	Elevation in adduction	Inferior oblique
IV—Trochlear	Depression in adduction	Superior oblique
VI—Abducens	Abduction	Lateral rectus

IV. Visual acuity
   A. Every child should have an assessment of vision.
      1. This is done monocularly, testing the visual acuity of each eye in the responsive patient.
      2. For unresponsive patients, determination of pupillary reactivity to direct and indirect stimulation is useful in evaluating the state of the afferent visual pathway.
   B. Techniques to test visual acuity
      1. A near card that includes picture optotypes (symbols)
      2. Allowing preverbal children to reach for (and follow) a small toy with one or the other eye covered
V. Ocular motor system
   A. Tested by voluntary eye movement
      1. As the child follows a toy in all directions of gaze
      2. See **Table 25-1.**
   B. Unresponsive patient
      1. Testing is performed by head rotation (doll's eye maneuver; see Chapter 15).
      2. This induces ocular movements in the opposite direction.
      3. In the unresponsive injured child, the doll's eye maneuver can be performed only after cervical spine injury has been excluded.
VI. Physical examination
   A. Perform the following:
      1. Inspect the orbital bones, eyelids, and ocular adnexa.
      2. Palpate the orbital rim around each eye for fracture and crepitus.
      3. Evaluate the infraorbital nerve by comparing sensation to light touch on the upper lip and cheeks.
      4. Inspect the skin and conjunctival surfaces of the eyelids for laceration or foreign body.
      5. Observe the position of the globes and note presence of enophthalmos or exophthalmos.
      6. Examine the pupils with a flashlight and note size, shape, and response to light.
      7. Note corneal opacities and defects.

VII. Corneal abrasion

This is the most common ocular emergency. The pathophysiology involves injury and removal of a portion of the corneal epithelium, but the eyeball remains intact. Patients complain of pain and photophobia. Vision is variably reduced and depends on the extent of the abrasion.

A. Diagnosis

1. Instill fluorescein eye drops, which adhere to areas of exposed basement membrane.
2. Illumination with a cobalt blue light source causes the fluorescein to fluoresce bright green.

B. Treatment

1. Administer oral analgesics (e.g., acetaminophen, ibuprofen, codeine, or oxycodone) (see Chapter 20).
2. Protect the cornea with an antibiotic ointment.
   a. The antibiotic should have gram-positive coverage and not be toxic to the epithelium (erythromycin or bacitracin ointment).
   b. The use of a pressure patch is optional, although most children find it uncomfortable.
   c. Monitoring of the cornea should continue until the fluorescein staining is gone.
3. Never prescribe topical anesthetics (e.g., proparacaine); prolonged use can lead to a corneal perforation or ulceration.

VIII. Corneal foreign body

This is a common cause of acute ocular pain, especially with eyelid movement. Apply a topical anesthetic such as proparacaine HCL 0.5% or tetracaine 1% and examine the eye with magnification. Rapid but temporary relief of pain strongly suggests corneal trauma or corneal foreign body.

A. Examination

1. Lower lid: Apply downward pressure on the lower lid while the patient looks upward.
2. Upper lid: Single eversion
   a. Place the wood end of a cotton-tipped swab on the upper eyelid 7 to 10 mm above the lid margin.
   b. Grasp the lashes and lid margin firmly and flip the lid up and over the swab.

B. Treatment

1. Remove the foreign body with a moistened cotton-tipped applicator.
2. In a cooperative patient, the foreign body can be flushed out with the tip of a hypodermic needle.
3. Apply an antibiotic ointment, possibly a patch, and schedule an examination for the following day.

IX. Eyelid injuries
   A. Contusions
      1. These injuries are usually associated with marked eyelid swelling from blood.
      2. Most such ecchymoses resolve with little sequelae.
      3. However, these injuries may be associated with orbital bone fractures or orbital bleeding and can be identified by physical examination and by a reduction in ocular motility or vision.
   B. Lacerations
      1. Always check for an occult globe perforation and assess visual acuity and pupillary function.
      2. Reduced vision may mean deep orbital or globe damage or retrobulbar hemorrhage.
      3. In the latter case, an ophthalmologist may perform a lateral canthotomy to relieve the pressure elevation.
      4. If the globe is intact, check for orbital damage (see later).
      5. A moistened dressing may be applied over an intact eye protected with a shield.
      6. Primary closure, tetanus toxoid, and antibiotics should be instituted.

X. Orbital trauma
   Orbital trauma may be blunt or penetrating. Acuity is determined and the integrity of the globe ensured in all cases.
   A. Blunt
      1. Palpation of the orbital rim for step-offs will suggest a fracture of the orbital rim and crepitus will suggest a fracture of the medial or nasal orbital bones.
      2. Proptosis usually suggests retrobulbar hemorrhage.
      3. The pressure may be sufficient to occlude the central retinal artery.
      4. *Retinal necrosis from ischemia will be irreversible within 1 hour*.
      5. If acuity is reduced, determine the intraocular pressure; if elevated, an emergency lateral canthotomy can save vision.
   B. Penetrating
      1. The history of the type of trauma is crucial for suspecting this diagnosis.
      2. If the injury could have included orbital penetration, neuroimaging is needed to locate retained material.
      3. If a foreign body is present, leave it in place, stabilize it, and obtain imaging of the location prior to removal.

XI. Chemical injuries
   A. Causes
      1. Chemical burns occur in the home and on the job.
      2. They are both accidental and intentional.

25

3. Alkali burns are more devastating than acid burns.
4. Both require urgent treatment.

B. Management
1. Acute therapy begins at the site of the injury with copious irrigation with saline or water.
2. Continue for at least 30 minutes, holding the lids open.
3. Intravenous tubing is a useful way to administer the irrigation.
4. Evert the lids (see Section VIII) to remove any retained solid chemicals.
5. The irrigation can be discontinued when the pH of the surface is 7.0.

XII. Perforating globe injuries
All injuries to the ocular region should be suspected to have ocular perforation until proven otherwise. The presence of normal visual acuity will argue against perforation. Never apply pressure to the lids. Place a shield over the eye until an ophthalmologic examination can be performed.

XIII. Orbital cellulitis
A. Diagnosis
1. Infectious inflammation in the orbital region occurs in two basic types: Preseptal and orbital cellulitis. Delay in therapy can lead to permanent visual loss and even death.
2. Computed tomography scanning or magnetic resonance imaging of the orbit and paranasal sinuses can be used for diagnosis.
3. Preseptal cellulitis
a. An inflammation of ocular structures anterior to the orbital septum
b. Acuity, ocular motility, and white blood cell count are usually normal.
c. There is no proptosis.
d. There may be fever.
e. Associated with skin trauma, dacryocystitis, and upper respiratory disease
4. Orbital cellulitis
a. Inflammation of the orbit associated with proptosis, reduced acuity and mobility, and constitutional symptoms
b. Associated with sinusitis

B. Management
1. Initial parenteral antibiotics: Cefotaxime or ceftriaxone, plus clindamycin
2. Drainage of infected sinuses

XIV. Glaucoma
A. Overview
1. Glaucoma is associated with increased intraocular pressure.
2. Most glaucoma is not emergent.

3. However, angle closure glaucoma must be treated rapidly or the patient will suffer irreparable vision loss from optic nerve damage.
   a. Quite rare in childhood
   b. The central retina vessels are occluded by the intraocular pressure and the inner retina becomes ischemic.
   c. This entity is associated with severe ocular pain, a red eye, cloudy cornea, loss of vision, nausea, and vomiting.
   d. The latter gastrointestinal symptoms may obscure the correct diagnosis, especially in the pediatric patient.
   e. The diagnosis can be made with palpation of a hard eye through the eyelids or tonometry.

B. Management
   1. Timolol 0.5%, one drop every 12 hours
   2. Pilocarpine 4%, one drop every 2 hours; four doses, then every 6 hours
   3. Parenteral carbonic anhydrase inhibitor (e.g., acetazolamide, 15 mg/kg) or osmotic agent (e.g., 20% mannitol, 5 mL/kg) Note that all carbonic anhydrase inhibitors have reduced function in the setting of ciliary body ischemia.
   4. Oral acetazolamide, 30 mg/kg/day in four divided doses
   5. Topical carbonic anhydrase inhibitors, one drop every 8 hours (e.g., brinzolamide)

25

Chapter 26
Soft Tissue Injuries
Karen Michiko Kling, MD, FACS

I. Definition
  A. Tissues involved
    1. Soft tissue injuries (STIs) involve integumentary, subcutaneous (SC), or muscular elements and their nerves, vessels, and tendons.
    2. Although often associated, they are independent of skeletal, intra-abdominal, intrathoracic, and intracranial compartments.
    3. In children, these injuries usually heal promptly and without significant scarring because of the plasticity of tissues and good preinjury condition.
    4. However, some injuries with tissue loss or neurovascular components require complex reconstruction and prolonged rehabilitation and can have lasting morbidity.
II. Priority
  A. Airway, breathing, circulation (ABCs)
    1. Control of hemorrhage from STIs is an important part of supporting circulation (the C in ABCs).
    2. This is accomplished via manual compression with tourniquet use and is limited to rare situations, such as limb amputations.
    3. Fracture reduction also minimizes blood loss.
    4. The primary survey is then completed, and fractures or injuries penetrating body cavities are identified and addressed.
  B. Secondary survey
    1. This includes rolling the patient.
    2. It readily identifies the extent of most STIs, including underlying fractures.
    3. Electrical burns, however, are underestimated by outward appearance.
  C. Contamination
  This must be assessed and treated by irrigation, débridement, antibiotics, and tetanus prophylaxis.
    1. Classification of wounds
      a. Clean—tetanus unlikely
        (1) Free of debris or devitalized tissue
        (2) <6 hours old
        (3) Well vascularized
        (4) <1 cm deep, and linear

      b. Dirty—tetanus-prone
        (1) Grossly soiled by environmental (e.g., rust, particulate matter, soil) or bodily (gastrointestinal) contaminants
        (2) Made by a dirty object
        (3) >6 hours old
        (4) Crushed or significantly distorted wounds
        (5) Wounds with a devascularized component
  2. Tetanus prophylaxis (see Chapter 30)
  3. Antibiotic coverage is rarely required if superficial wounds are irrigated immediately and sufficiently; however, antibiotics are indicated for the following:

26

    a. Open fractures or exposed bone
    b. Facial, periorbital, hand, or foot wounds
      (1) 24 hours of cephalosporin, aminoglycoside
      (2) Potential for spread along potential spaces, tendon sheaths, and functional and cosmetic consequences of infection
    c. Erythematous wounds
    d. Immunocompromised patients (diabetes, transplantation, cancer)
    e. Animal bites
    f. Foreign bodies (e.g., catheters, hardware)
    g. Cardiac anomaly
  4. Irrigation and débridement
    a. Required promptly to remove particulate matter
    b. Irrigation within the first 6 hours decreases bacterial count, preventing subsequent infection.
    c. Devitalized tissue must be excised.
D. Pain control
  1. Required for safe, adequate, and humane examination and repair of STIs
  2. May require local anesthetics or regional nerve block, systemic analgesics, sedation, or even general anesthesia.
  3. The vasoconstrictive effects of epinephrine added to local anesthetics improve hemostasis and prolong the anesthetic effect.
  4. Epinephrine, however, should *not* be used in areas with end arteries in which blood supply can be compromised (e.g., ears, nose, digits, penis).
  5. See Chapter 20 for a list of local anesthetics and techniques for peripheral nerve blockade.
E. Foreign body removal from wounds with potential neurovascular or tendinous involvement
  1. Can cause bleeding or tissue damage during extraction
  2. Sometimes requires the following:
    a. Anesthesia

       b. Dissection of the important anatomy

       c. Direct visualization

    3. Intraoperative fluoroscopy significantly diminishes the risk of iatrogenic injury; thus, surgical consultation is advisable.

    4. Local wound exploration is recommended only if adequate pain control, equipment, and competent personnel are available.

III. Specific injuries

Precise description of a wound is essential for appropriate medicolegal adjudication with respect to child abuse.

  A. Contusion (bruise)

    1. Tissue edema and blood pooling from broken vessels leading to discoloration, but without loss of skin integrity or circumscribed hematoma formation; caused by blunt force

    2. Can be deep within muscle and rarely with enough edema for compartment syndrome (CS)

    3. Treatment

       a. Identify and address associated hematoma, fracture, or CS.

       b. **R**est, **i**ce, **c**ompression, and **e**levation (RICE)

       c. Pain control

       d. Self-limited, but immobilization can increase comfort

  B. Hematoma

This is a blood collection in SC tissues, muscles, or joints caused by blunt force.

    1. Identify and address associated fractures, CS

    2. Accumulation in a closed space may warrant evacuation to avoid or treat elevated compartment pressures.

    3. RICE: Immobilization improves comfort and resolution.

    4. Pain control

    5. Usually self-limited

       a. Seeding of the hematoma may lead to abscess formation (rare) and require drainage.

       b. An encysted hematoma (persistent mass with fluid center) can be managed expectantly unless infected.

  C. Abrasion

An abrasion is denuded epithelial (superficial) or dermal (deep) tissue caused by tangential force and friction applied to the skin.

    1. Superficial: Cleanse with soap and water or saline.

    2. Deep: Cleanse with scrub brush or gauze to remove debris. Particles may become incorporated and leave a *tattoo*.

    3. Pain control

    4. Topical antibiotic ointment and Vaseline-impregnated gauze to minimize wound adherence

  D. Laceration

This is an interruption in the skin caused by cutting or shearing, which can lead to a linear, stellate, superficial, or deep defect.

    1. Identify, treat fractures and vascular, nerve, tendon injuries

2. Pain control with systemic or regional techniques
3. Decontaminate and prepare wound for repair
   a. Hair can be shaved to facilitate closure. **Never** shave eyebrows because they may not regrow.
   b. 500 to 1000 mL sterile saline irrigation delivered by pulse using a syringe
   c. Débride all devitalized tissue (**Fig. 26-1**)

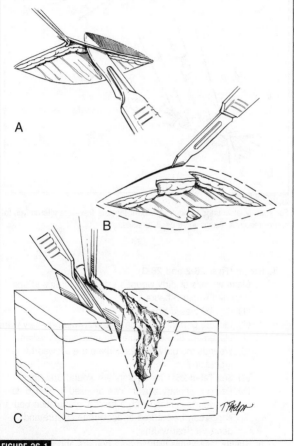

FIGURE 26-1

A, Undermining the superficial skin of the wound edges decreases tension on the repair. **B, C,** Débridement of irregular wound edges or devitalized tissue is necessary.

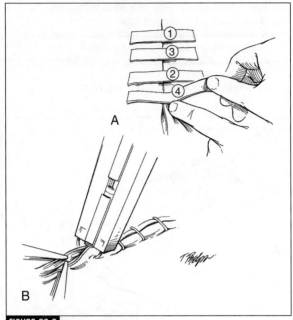

FIGURE 26-2

For superficial wounds without significant tension, there are alternatives to suture repair. **A,** Adhesive strips. **B,** Staples.

4. Repair (**Figs. 26-2** and **26-3**)
   a. **Clean wounds** or dirty wounds extensively irrigated and débrided within 6 hours
      (1) Can be closed primarily
      (2) Closure of minimally contaminated wounds may warrant placement of a drain to avoid fluid accumulation.
      (3) Wounds too dirty to approximate are allowed to granulate.
      (4) See **Table 26-1** for appropriate wound dressings.
      (5) Delayed primary closure can be used if, after 5 days, the wound is clean with a healthy granulation bed; the edges can be sutured to accelerate closure and decrease scar width.
   b. **Simple lacerations** with smooth borders and without distortion are repaired by coapting tissue edges with glue, adhesive strips, staples, or monofilament suture on a cutting needle.

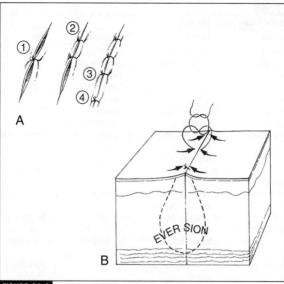

FIGURE 26-3

A, Sutures are placed with the needle perpendicular to the entry point on one side. Then, by supination of the forearm, the needle is rotated within its circumference to exit the other side, opposite the first entry point. **B,** This technique everts the repair. Sutures can be placed, splitting the difference in the wound's length to ensure proper alignment.

   (1) Glue and adhesive strips are useful in small superficial wounds without tension (Fig. 26-2, *A*).
   (2) Staples are useful in noncosmetic areas (Fig. 26-2, *B*).
   (3) Evert wound edges and allow for swelling so sutures do not cause tissue necrosis (see Fig. 26-3).
   (4) Interrupted sutures are most often used to allow drainage of potential fluid (see Fig. 26-3).
   (5) Mattress sutures help distribute tension.
   (6) Heavier suture (3-0) is recommended for thicker tissue; finer suture (6-0 or 7-0) is recommended for cosmetic repair (**Table 26-2**).
   c. Facial lacerations
   (1) Should be repaired with 6-0 or smaller suture, with special attention paid to approximating the vermillion border of the lip
   (2) Significant lesions should be repaired in the operating room with anesthesia for proper exposure.

TABLE 26-1

WOUND DRESSING ALTERNATIVES

Dressing Type	Advantages	Disadvantages	Uses
Gauze packing (wet → dry saline gauze)	Débrides exudates, readily available	Change twice daily; débridement of healthy granulation tissue, skin maceration	Dirty wounds
Polyurethane film (Tegaderm)	Skin barrier, keeps wound moist	No drainage or débridement	Clean skin tears
Polyurethane foam	Conformable, keeps wound moist, permeable	Little débridement	Moderate defects
Hydrocolloid gel (Duoderm)	Autolytic débridement of eschar		Dry eschar
Hydrocolloid (Duoderm)	Impermeable barrier with some padding	No drainage	Clean pressure sores
Calcium alginates (Aquacell, Kaltostat)	Nonantigenic, fewer dressing changes, hemostatic, bioabsorbable	Residual from alginates can be confused with purulent discharge	Clean wounds with moderate drainage
Starch copolymers	Absorb many times their weight		Moist wounds
Vacuum-assisted devices	Actively remove excess exudate, change 2-3 times/wk, accelerate contraction, promote granulation	May cause irritation of normal perimeter skin if improperly applied	Large or deep wounds that need accelerated contraction

Courtesy of Kimberly Haus McIltrot, Pediatric Nurse Practitioner, Johns Hopkins Children's Center, Baltimore.
For challenging wounds, consult your wound enterostomal health care provider.

TABLE 26-2

SUTURE GUIDELINES

Location of Injury	Type of Suture		Duration (days)
	Monofilament*	Absorbable†	
Scalp	4-0	3-0	5-7
Face, ear	6-0	5-0	3-5
Eyebrow	6-0	5-0	3-5
Eyelid	7-0		3-5
Hand	4-0 or 5-0	4-0	5-7
Sole	3-0 or 4-0	3-0	7-10
Across joint	4-0	3-0	10-14
Extremity	3-0 or 4-0	3-0	7-10
Trunk	3-0 or 4-0	3-0	5-7

*Nylon, polypropylene (Prolene).
†Polyglycolic.

(3) In general, intraoral buccal mucosa components do not require suturing.

d. **Scalp lacerations** with significant bleeding
   (1) Should be closed with continuous suture, encompassing all layers of the scalp to ensure hemostasis
   (2) Saline injection directly into the scalp wound produces effective hemostasis.

e. **Deep lacerations** with significant interruption of SC tissue and fat require a layer of deep, interrupted, absorbable suture (3-0 or 4-0)
   (1) Brings tissue together
   (2) Minimizes dead space
   (3) Takes tension off the superficial closure

f. **Complex** or stellate disruptions of tissue with distortion of the anatomy, possible crush component, or loss of tissue
   (1) Require careful débridement and assessment for remaining vascularized tissue
   (2) Relaxation of surrounding skin and SC tissues and reapproximation with multiple layers of deep absorbable sutures may be required to restore form.
   (3) Irregular borders should be trimmed.
   (4) Then a superficial layer is used to approximate the skin.
   (5) If significant tissue loss precludes simple primary closure, consultation with a reconstructive surgeon is warranted to decide among plasty, tissue advancement, or delayed closure with soft tissue transfer.

g. **Animal and human bites** often include puncture, laceration, crush, and tissue loss.
   (1) Rabies treatment may be warranted (see Chapter 27).
   (2) Antibiotics are required for *Pasteurella* (animal) and *Eikenella corrodens* (human) (see Chapter 27).
   (3) Interrupted sutures should be used to allow drainage.
   (4) Have a low threshold to leave the wound open.
   (5) An injury from a *fist into teeth* should be considered an open joint.

h. **Avulsions** in which the proximal component (blood supply) is intact are likely to heal—large devascularized flaps will necrose.

i. **Perineal wounds** (large) and anorectal lacerations may require fecal diversion and drainage; thus, surgical consultation is mandatory.

5. Dry gauze can be applied.
   a. Occlusive dressings should be avoided.
   b. If the wound is in an area of frequent motion or stress, immobilization is advisable for 3 to 5 days.

6. Most sutures should be removed at 7 days, but facial sutures should be removed at 3 days (see Table 26-2).
   a. Even after the epidermal layer has healed, scars mature for several months and should be kept out of the sun for 6 months to avoid irreversible pigmentation.
   b. Evaluation for scar revision should generally wait until the scar is mature.

E. Types of fractures
1. Closed fracture
   a. Fracture without skin disruption over the fracture site
   b. May be associated with neurovascular injuries from entrapment, stretch, or laceration by bone fragments
   c. Treatment
      (1) Control bleeding and pain via reduction, immobilization.
      (2) Conduct neurovascular examination for palpable pulse and capillary refill.
         (a) Reduction of the fracture often relieves stretch or entrapment injuries.
         (b) Persistent abnormal vascular examination warrants a duplex scan or angiography.
      (3) Evaluation for CS
      (4) Orthopedic reduction and fixation
2. Open fracture
   a. Fracture with overlying STI in which there is loss of skin integrity
   b. Treatment
      (1) Pressure, reduction, immobilization to control bleeding
      (2) Coverage with sterile dressing that also controls bleeding
      (3) Definitive intraoperative irrigation and débridement within 6 hours, including the following:
         (a) Removal of any foreign materials (may require radiography)
         (b) Fixation of the fracture (see Chapter 24)
         (c) Repair of the STI
      (4) Antibiotics

IV. Special situations requiring surgical consultation
   NOTE: Nerve, tendon, and vascular injuries, amputations, injections, and complex or cosmetic lacerations should be referred for surgical evaluation.
   A. CS
   1. See Chapter 24.
   2. Caused by edema, hematoma, reperfusion injury, or injection injury
   3. The pressure leads to severe pain, tightness, weakness, and vascular compromise.

4. If not treated within 6 hours of onset, muscle necrosis and nerve injury lead to future dysfunction.
5. Can be seen in conjunction with orthopedic injuries that lead to edema or vascular compromise
6. Treatment
   a. Recognize it! Measure compartment pressure.
   b. Relieve pressure via fasciotomy or evacuation.
   c. Monitor for myoglobinuria and renal damage.
      (1) Hydration
      (2) Forced diuresis ± mannitol
      (3) Alkalinization of urine
   d. Delayed primary closure or skin grafting after edema subsides
   e. Physical therapy
B. Nerve injury
   1. Neurapraxia
      a. Nerve bruising but no interruption
      b. Recovers spontaneously over days, weeks
   2. Axonotmesis
      a. Axon but not myelin sheath interruption
      b. Regenerates 1 to 3 mm/day
   3. Neurotmesis
      a. Interruption of both axons and myelin
      b. Requires reapproximation for regeneration (primary or delayed)
C. Tendon injury
   1. Should be reapproximated
   2. A partial tendon tear can convert to complete disruption days after the injury.
   3. Sudden onset of pain, not associated with infection or vascular compromise, requires reevaluation for tendon disruption.
D. Vascular injury
   1. Includes dissections and partial or complete transections
   2. Recognize a vascular problem! Use the five Ps:
      a. Pain
      b. Pallor
      c. Pulselessness
      d. Paresthesia
      e. Poikilothermia
   3. Obtain surgical consultation.
   4. Angiography may be required for diagnosis or treatment (e.g., long intramural dissection), or vascular injury may be obvious (e.g., arterial bleeding).
   5. Treatment
      a. Primary repair
      b. Interposition grafting

   c. Ligation and bypass
   d. Ligation alone
   e. Possible anticoagulation
E. Amputations
   1. Amputated elements can be reimplanted if vascular supply can be established, and functional recovery can occur if nerve regrowth is successful.
   2. The amputated part should be cleaned of gross contamination, sealed in a plastic bag (to avoid direct contact with ice), with most of the air evacuated, and this bag placed in iced slush.
F. High-pressure injection injury
   1. This causes significant tissue injury because of ischemia and chemical contamination.
   2. Tissue necrosis and CS may occur.
   3. Treatment
      a. Immediate and wide débridement
      b. Antibiotics
      c. Elevation and splinting
   4. Despite these measures, these injuries often require amputation or result in stiff, dysfunctional digits.
G. Crush injury
   This may lead to rhabdomyolysis and myoglobinuria (see Chapter 30).

Chapter 27

Human and Animal Bites and Stings

G. Patricia Cantwell, MD, FCCM, and Allen R. Walker, MD, MBA

I. Overview

Bites and stings are common injuries in childhood. Sources include humans, cats, dogs, insects, and wild or marine animals. Early management reduces serious, occasionally life-threatening complications.

Controversy exists regarding, for example, antimicrobial prophylaxis and wound closure techniques. The material presented here represents a conservative approach.

II. Human bites

A. Sources and classification

1. An *occlusional bite* is a wound from human teeth actually biting an anatomic structure.
2. A *fight bite* is an injury and laceration from a clenched fist striking an opponent's teeth and is particularly problematic. The configuration of the resultant laceration may change dramatically when the fist is unclenched.

B. Colonization

1. Human bites are typically colonized with multiple aerobic and anaerobic bacteria (e.g., *Eikenella corrodens*).
2. Other infectious risks include hepatitis B (HB), hepatitis C, tuberculosis, syphilis, and actinomycosis.
3. The potential for transmission of human immunodeficiency virus (HIV) is currently undefined.

C. Deep injury

1. Deep injury may be present, particularly with clenched fist injuries.
2. Deep injury (particularly) of the hand increases risks of tenosynovitis and/or osteomyelitis.

D. Essential early care

1. Copiously irrigate bite wounds with large volumes of normal saline under pressure.
   a. Use a needle or intravenous (IV) catheter.
   b. If bitten by a person infected with or at high risk for HIV, wound irrigation should be accomplished with a virucidal agent, such as 1% povidone-iodine or chlorhexidine.
2. Remove any foreign material or devitalized tissue.

3. Whenever a fracture or foreign body is suspected, obtain radiographs, particularly for hand injuries.
4. Give tetanus toxoid booster (given as DT or Td), if indicated (see Chapter 30).
5. Give hepatitis B immune globulin and hepatitis B vaccine (HBV) if the patient is unvaccinated (or had a poor antibody response to HBV) and the biter is HB surface antigen (HBsAg)–positive or from a high-risk group.
6. Give HBV to the patient with unknown or low HBsAg titer if the biter is HBsAg-negative or untested (but thought to be low risk); testing of the biter is recommended, if possible.

E. Indications for antibiotic prophylaxis
   1. Err on the side of prophylactic antibiotics for any human bite, but especially for the following:
      a. Any bite on the hand, especially clenched fist injuries
      b. Any deep or occlusional bite or bite involving devitalized or crushed tissue
      c. Bites older than 12 hours when first seen

F. Antibiotic prophylaxis
   1. The goal is to offer antibiotics with activity against *Eikenella*, anaerobes, and *Staphylococcus aureus*.
   2. Preferred choice: Amoxicillin/clavulanic acid (45 mg/kg/day) orally (PO) divided every 12 hours
   3. Alternative choices require two antibiotics.
      a. Trimethoprim-sulfamethoxazole, 5 mg/kg trimethoprim/dose PO/IV twice daily *plus* metronidazole 10 mg/kg/dose PO/IV three times daily; doxycycline may be substituted for trimethoprim-sulfamethoxazole in children older than 8 years.
      b. Cefuroxime 10-15 mg/kg (max 500 mg) IV/intramuscularly (IM) twice daily *plus* clindamycin, 10 mg/kg/dose PO/IV three times daily; penicillin VK may be substituted for cefuroxime.
   4. IV antibiotics for established infections based on the clinical examination or wound culture (particularly if the hand, face, bone, or joint are involved)

G. HIV testing or antiretroviral therapy
   1. At present, there is no indication for HIV testing or antiretroviral therapy if the biter's HIV status is unknown.
   2. If the biter is known to be HIV-positive or considered at high risk, rapid HIV testing and postexposure prophylaxis with antiretroviral drugs is recommended.
   3. Treatment should be individualized based on the HIV status of the biter and recommendations of experts in infectious disease and special immunology.

III. Mammalian nonhuman bites
  A. Dogs and cats
    1. Dogs and cats account for millions of bites annually.
      a. Most are insignificant.
      b. Most bites that come to medical attention involve the face or upper extremity.
      c. Cat bites are more likely to present as puncture wounds; dog bites are more often tearing injuries, with devitalized tissue.
    2. Likely pathogens
      a. *S. aureus*
      b. *Streptococcus*
      c. *Pasteurella* spp.
        (1) *P. multocida* is the most virulent.
        (2) Although considered more common in cats than in dogs, it has been a significant pathogen in dog bites.
      d. *Clostridium tetani*
      e. Anaerobes
    3. Rabies
      a. High index of suspicion if dog or cat attack was unprovoked or if rabies known to be present in the species or area
      b. If the dog or cat can be observed for 10 days, there is no need to administer rabies immune globulin (RIG) and human diploid cell vaccine (HDCV) emergently unless the animal exhibits rabid signs.
      c. If the animal escapes, consultation with local health authorities is recommended.
      d. Consult the Centers for Disease Prevention and Control website (http://www.cdc.gov/rabies) for updated information.
  B. Other animals
    1. Raccoons, skunks, bats, foxes, and other wild animals are considered rabid unless the geographic area is known to be free from rabies in these species.
    2. Postexposure prophylaxis is required for the child bitten by a wild animal.
      a. The patient should receive active immunization with the rabies vaccine and passive immunization with RIG.
      b. RIG is infiltrated first at the wound site and the rest of the dose given IM.
      c. The rabies vaccine (HDCV or purified chick embryo cell vaccine) is given IM in the deltoid (but at a site separate from the RIG injection site) on days 0, 3, 7, 14, and 28.

27

C. Wound care
  1. Meticulous local care is essential.
     a. Cleanse wound with hand soap that has bactericidal and virucidal properties.
     b. Thoroughly irrigate with a syringe containing saline, tap, or drinking water under pressure; 1% povidone-iodine irrigation solution is preferred for its virucidal properties.
     c. Remove dirt and foreign objects with a clean cloth or sterile gauze after irrigation and cleansing—simple irrigation without swabbing of wound edges may not remove rabies virus.
  2. Bites causing tissue contusion receive ice and cold pack application during the initial 24 hours.
  3. Closure of wounds for cosmetic purposes may be appropriate, generally after consultation with a plastic surgeon.
  4. Leave wounds open, if they:
     a. Are punctures rather than lacerations
     b. Are not potentially disfiguring
     c. Involve a limb, particularly hand or foot
     d. Are clearly infected at the time of presentation
  5. Delayed repair may be indicated for the following:
     a. Bites to arms or legs older than 6 to 12 hours
     b. Bites to the face older than 12 to 24 hours; however, many surgeons now advocate primary closure for dog bites to the face, even when several days old, because dog bites have lower infection rates than human or cat bites.
  6. Recommend antimicrobial prophylaxis for the following:
     a. Most cat bites, puncture wounds
     b. Hand or foot bites
     c. Any injuries that require extensive débridement
D. Standard recommendations for prophylaxis
  1. Amoxicillin, clavulanic acid (45 mg/kg/day divided every 12 hours)
  2. Alternative choices: Require two antibiotics
     a. Trimethoprim-sulfamethoxazole (5 mg/kg trimethoprim/dose) twice daily *plus* metronidazole (10 mg/kg/dose) three times daily; doxycycline may be substituted for trimethoprim-sulfamethoxazole in children older than 8 years.
     b. Cefuroxime (10-15 mg/kg/dose, max 500 mg) twice daily *plus* clindamycin (10 mg/kg/dose) three times daily; penicillin VK may be substituted for cefuroxime.
IV. Insect stings
A. Causes of significant insect stings
  1. Hymenoptera
  2. Bees

      3. Yellow jackets

      4. Wasps

      5. Hornets

      6. Nonwinged fire ants

B. Reactions to stings

    1. Local reaction

      a. Normal:

        (1) Diameter of swelling <2 inches

        (2) Duration <24 hours

      b. Large local reaction

        (1) Diameter of swelling >2 inches

        (2) Duration, 1 to 7 days

    2. Toxic reactions to multiple stings: Introduction of large volumes of insect venom simultaneously may lead to central nervous system symptoms (e.g., headache, syncope, seizures) or gastrointestinal symptoms (e.g., nausea, vomiting, diarrhea).

    3. Delayed reaction (serum sickness)

      a. Very rare

      b. Symptoms: Urticarial rash, fever, joint pains, adenopathy, fatigue occurring 7 to 10 days after sting

    4. Isolated skin reactions: Urticaria, morbilliform rash, erythema, pruritus

C. Life-threatening anaphylaxis

    1. Presentation

      a. Immediate generalized reaction

      b. Cutaneous presentation: Erythema, pruritus, angioedema, morbilliform rash

      c. Respiratory presentation: Hoarseness, dysphagia, dyspnea, tightness in throat and chest, wheezing, tachypnea

      d. Cardiovascular presentation: Syncope, palpitations, hypotension, tachycardia, bradycardia

      e. Cardiorespiratory arrest

    2. Risks factors for anaphylaxis

      a. Prior episode of anaphylaxis (but 50% of cases occur with no prior history)

      b. Children > adults

      c. Males > females

D. Treatment of anaphylaxis

    1. Administer 100% oxygen (O_2) and secure the airway.

    2. Administer epinephrine subcutaneously (1 : 1000): 0.01 mg (mL)/kg given every 20 to 30 minutes, maximum adult dose 0.5 mg (0.5 mL).

    3. Correct hypotension with volume expansion.

    4. Administer an antihistamine such as diphenhydramine 1 mg/kg IV or IM, maximum dose 50 mg.

     5. Epinephrine aerosol may be helpful in acute upper airway obstruction.

     6. If symptoms last longer than 20 minutes, give methylprednisolone 2 mg/kg IV, followed by prednisone 2 mg/kg/day for 1 to 2 days; max dose 80 mg, given once.

  E. First aid management of stings

     1. Emergency epinephrine self-treatment for anaphylaxis

       a. Dose: <30 kg, 0.15 mg

       b. Dose: >30 kg, 0.3 mg

     2. Remove the stinger with a horizontal scraping motion.

       a. Avoid squeezing the sac

       b. This could force more venom into the victim.

     3. Apply ice or cool compresses.

     4. Give acetaminophen for pain and antihistamines for pruritus.

V. Tick bites

  A. Tick paralysis

     1. Presentation

       a. Afebrile muscle weakness

       b. Acute, ascending, flaccid paralysis preceded by 12 to 24 hours of general malaise and anorexia

       c. Rapid progression of paralysis

       d. Rapid resolution on removal of the tick

     2. Treatment

       a. Tick removal is best accomplished by grasping the tick as close to the skin as possible with tweezers and pulling straight up.

       b. Avoid squeezing the body and injecting blood into the patient.

       c. There is no evidence that prophylactic antibiotics given at the time of the tick bite are effective in preventing illness.

  B. Lyme disease

     1. Presentation

       a. Erythema migrans (red macule at site of tick bite 1 to 2 weeks after bite).

       b. Without treatment, the macule expands greatly in diameter, sometimes with central clearing (target lesion).

     2. Commonly associated symptoms: Fatigue, fever, headache, arthralgia

     3. Disseminated Lyme disease

       a. Meningitis

       b. Carditis (heart block): See Chapter 7.

       c. Facial nerve or (other cranial nerve) palsy

     4. Treatment choices: Amoxicillin or cefuroxime, or doxycycline

  C. Rocky Mountain spotted fever

     1. Presentation

a. Early constitutional symptoms: Fever, arthralgia, myalgia, abdominal pain
b. Rash: Maculopapular rash, usually on day 3 of illness, which becomes petechial in character
    (1) Begins on ankles and wrists, spreads to the palms and soles and centrally to involve the entire body.
    (2) Rash is absent in rare cases.
c. Other findings: Neurologic (confusion, seizures, coma, focal deficits), ophthalmologic (conjunctivitis, retinal abnormalities), bleeding, cough

  2. Treatment
    a. For children >45 kg, doxycycline 100 mg PO or IV every 12 hours
    b. For children <45 kg, doxycycline 2 mg/kg/dose every 12 hours

VI. Snake bites
  A. Causes
    1. Most U.S. snake bites are caused by pit vipers (rattlesnakes, water moccasins, copperheads).
    2. Very few bites are caused by coral snakes.
    3. Venomous snakes are located in every state except Maine, Hawaii, and Alaska.
    4. See **Figure 27-1.**
  B. Risk to children
    1. Compared with adults, children are at increased risk of death and significant injury.
    2. Children generally require more antivenom per kilogram because the dose is based on the venom load, not the child's weight.
  C. Symptoms
    1. May be mild, moderate, or severe
    2. May be local or systemic
    3. Venom can cause tissue necrosis at the site of the bite, hypotension, frank shock, hemorrhage and clotting dysfunction, renal failure, and respiratory distress.
      a. Pit vipers (crotalid): Cytotoxic, hemotoxic, cardiotoxic
      b. Coral snakes (elapid): Neurotoxic, cardiotoxic
  D. First aid measures
    1. Rapid transport to the emergency department should be the first priority; few deaths occur in the first 6 hours (17%).
    2. Calm the victim.
    3. Immobilize the limb, ideally with a crepe pressure bandage and splint or any available substitute.
      a. If possible, the entire extremity proximal and distal to the bite and over the bite itself is bandaged.

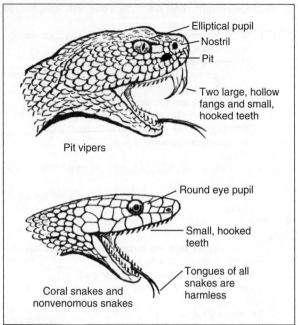

Physical differences between pit vipers, coral snakes, and nonvenomous snakes include pupil shape, presence of a nostril, and hollow fangs in the pit viper. *(Courtesy of Florida Game and Fresh Water Fish Commission, Tallahassee, Fla.)*

       b. Apply just tightly enough (approximately 20 mm Hg) to occlude lymphatic and superficial venous flow while sparing arterial and deep venous perfusion.

       c. If patient presents with bandage in place, sudden removal may lead to systemic absorption of venom.

    4. Ineffective or dangerous measures include the following:

       a. Cruciate cuts at the site of the bite

       b. Suction at the bite (mouth suction is ill advised)

       c. Tourniquets

       d. Electrotherapy

       e. Cryotherapy

E. Early treatment

    1. Emergent attention to airway, breathing, and circulation

    2. IV antivenom within 4 hours of a significant envenomation is crucial; there are two types of crotaline antivenom.

- a. Crotalidae Polyvalent Immune Fab (Ovine) antivenom (CroFab, Protherics, Brentwood, Tenn.) is preferred because of diminished risk of allergic reaction.
  - (1) Fab fragments from sheep immunized with venom from four types of rattlesnakes
  - (2) Effective against all North American rattlesnakes, copperheads, and water moccasins
  - (3) Dose by venom load (signs and symptoms), not by child's age or weight.
  - (4) Starting dose of CroFab is four to six reconstituted vials within 6 hours of bite.
    - (a) Repeat every hour until symptoms are controlled.
    - (b) Then give two vials every 6 hours three times.
  - (5) No recommended skin test
- b. Antivenom (Crotalidae) Polyvalent (pit vipers) is no longer distributed by the manufacturer and should not be used.
- c. Elapid antivenom (coral snake) is also no longer available; consult Poison Control Center (1-800-222-1222) for management guidelines.
  3. Antivenom skin testing no longer recommended—often unreliable results and delays antivenom administration
  4. Cardiorespiratory monitoring is mandatory during antivenom administration; epinephrine and other resuscitation drugs should be immediately available.
  5. Administer tetanus toxoid, if indicated.
  6. Administer broad-spectrum antibiotic coverage in the face of significant local tissue damage.
- VII. Spider bites
  - A. Dangerous venomous spiders in the United States
    1. *Latrodectus* spp., most notably *Latrodectus mactans* (black widow)—venom more potent than that of pit vipers
    2. *Loxosceles* spp., especially *Loxosceles reclusa* (brown recluse)
  - B. *Latrodectus mactans* (black widow)
    1. Geographic distribution—throughout the United States
    2. Symptoms
      - a. Local pain at the bite site
      - b. Muscular pain, cramping
      - c. Hypertension, tachycardia
      - d. Sudden irritability
      - e. Generalized muscle pain in back, abdomen, and chest
      - f. Nausea, vomiting, headache
      - g. Periorbital swelling
      - h. Cholinergic effects: Local or generalized diaphoresis, salivation, lacrimation, bronchorrhea
    3. First aid
      - a. Administer local wound care.

27

        b. Apply ice.

        c. Immobilize and elevate the bite site, if possible.

    4. Treatment

        a. O_2, IV access, cardiac monitoring

        b. Antivenom indications

           (1) Severe pain or muscle cramping

           (2) Dyspnea

           (3) Nausea and vomiting

        c. Consult poison control center for dosing.

        d. Cardiorespiratory monitoring and epinephrine should be available in the rare event of allergic reaction to antivenom (containing horse serum).

        e. Supportive medication to alleviate muscle pain and cramping

           (1) Morphine

           (2) Diazepam

           (3) Calcium gluconate 10%

           (4) Methocarbamol (muscle relaxant)

           (5) Apply cardiorespiratory monitoring and be prepared to assist ventilation.

C. *Loxosceles reclusa* (brown recluse)

    1. Geographic distribution in the United States

        a. Primarily the southern half of the Midwestern states (from Illinois in the north to Louisiana in the south)

        b. From Tennessee to Texas and Oklahoma

    2. Symptoms

        a. Red macule within minutes of the bite

        b. Red papule progressing to bruiselike macular lesion occurring within hours

        c. Hemorrhagic blister, 48 to 72 hours after the bite

        d. Black necrotic eschar and ulcer within 7 to 14 days

        e. Systemic reactions are rare but can be life-threatening.

        f. Progressive hemolysis can result in hemolytic anemia, thrombocytopenia, disseminated intravascular coagulation, and myoglobinuria.

        g. Milder systemic symptoms include fever, chills, nausea, vomiting, weakness, joint and muscle pain, headache, and fleeting rashes.

    3. Treatment

        a. Local wound care

        b. Ice compresses

        c. Immobilization and elevation

        d. Non-narcotic analgesics, antipruritics; avoid salicylates because of the potential for bleeding.

        e. Antibiotic for secondary infection, usually *Staphylococcus* or *Streptococcus*

f. Tetanus prophylaxis

g. Systemic steroids may be considered for severe hemolysis, although there is no proven benefit.

h. Dapsone inhibits leukocyte chemotaxis.
  (1) May be administered to prevent necrosis in the wound
  (2) Patients must be proven not to have glucose-6-phosphate dehydrogenase deficiency prior to dapsone administration.

i. Hyperbaric O_2 therapy has been used to treat soft tissue necrosis.

j. Early excision of the bite wound is ineffective.

k. Delayed surgery for débridement

VIII. Scorpion bites

A. Southwestern desert scorpion: *Centruroides exilicauda* (*C. sculpturatus*)
  1. Main species of medical importance in the United States
  2. Found mainly in Arizona, Texas, and California

B. Local symptoms
  1. Pain
  2. Paresthesias
  3. Edema
  4. Skin inflammation

C. Systemic symptoms
  1. Hyperexcitability
  2. Convulsions, ataxia
  3. Hypertension or hypotension
  4. Tachycardia
  5. Vomiting
  6. Dysphagia
  7. Lacrimal, nasal, salivary secretions

D. Treatment
  1. Primarily supportive care
  2. Antivenom (hyperimmune goat serum) if locale permits; use *only* for life-threatening symptoms with severe envenomation.
  3. Local wound care
  4. Propranolol for tachyarrhythmias and severe hypertension
  5. Anticonvulsants, generally phenobarbital

IX. Marine envenomations

Marine envenomations are increasing in frequency. It is important to consider the dermatologic manifestations of marine envenomations in the differential diagnosis of insect bites, varicella, viral exanthems, or urticaria from other causes. High fevers can sometimes occur. Minor lacerations or abrasions in an aquatic environment can be catastrophic in the immunocompromised host. The following outline provides a general approach to the most commonly encountered marine species with problematic envenomations.

A. Invertebrate
   1. Coelenterate envenomations include the following:
      a. Portuguese man-of-war
      b. Fire coral
      c. Sea wasp
      d. Sea nettles
      e. Sea anemones
      f. Jellyfish
      g. Sea lice
   2. Symptoms
      a. Mild
         (1) Local reaction: Burning, pruritus, paresthesias, throbbing radiation of pain, red-brown-purple discoloration (tentacle prints), local edema, erythema, wheal, blisters
         (2) Secondary reaction: Local necrosis, desquamation, infection
         (3) Resolution
            (a) Lesions usually resolve within 1 to 2 weeks.
            (b) Hyperpigmentation, 1 to 2 months
            (c) Permanent scarring possible
            (d) Keloids, fat atrophy
            (e) Vascular spasm
      b. Moderate to severe
         (1) Anaphylaxis possible
         (2) Nausea, vomiting, diarrhea
         (3) Abdominal rigidity, diffuse myalgia, muscle cramps, spasm
         (4) Conjunctivitis, chemosis, corneal abrasions
         (5) Loss of consciousness
   3. Treatment
      a. Remove swimwear because the stinging apparatus (nematocyst) can be trapped in clothing (e.g., sea lice)
      b. Inactivate the nematocyst with 5% acetic acid (vinegar).
      c. Remove the nematocyst with shaving or horizontal scraping.
      d. Topical therapy includes diphenhydramine cream, hydrocortisone cream, and lidocaine.
      e. Tetanus prophylaxis
      f. Do not use tap water, hot water, tourniquets, prophylactic antibiotics, or irrigation of eyes with vinegar.
      g. Showering with fresh water can exacerbate the symptoms.
   4. Sea urchins, sponges, and starfish
      a. Symptoms
         (1) Puncture results in immediate pain and burning.

        (2) Multiple punctures may result in paresthesias, nausea, vomiting, and muscular paralysis.

        (3) Granulomatous lesions can occur with retained spines.

        (4) Rare anaphylaxis

        (5) Sponges and sea cucumbers are generally associated with pruritic dermatitis and burning, edema, and possible vesiculation.

  b. Treatment

        (1) Sea cucumbers, sponges: Detoxify skin with application of 5% acetic acid, papain, or 40% to 70% isopropyl alcohol.

        (2) Sponge and bristleworm spicules may be removed with adhesive tape.

        (3) Immerse sea urchin or starfish wound in hot water (113° F).

          (a) Gently remove spines.

          (b) **Do not** break up the spines.

          (c) Consider soft tissue radiography.

        (4) Meticulous wound care

        (5) Diphenhydramine PO for severe pruritus

        (6) Topical therapy: Corticosteroid cream, calamine lotion

        (7) Prophylactic antibiotics for deep wounds (must cover *Staphylococcus*, *Streptococcus*, and especially *Vibrio* spp. (e.g., ciprofloxacin, imipenem, cilastatin, third-generation cephalosporins, trimethoprim-sulfamethoxazole)

B. Vertebrate (lion fish, scorpion fish, stonefish, catfish, stingray)

  1. Symptoms

    a. Immediate intense pain

    b. Edema

    c. Systemic symptoms may include weakness, nausea, vomiting, diarrhea, vertigo, and tachycardia.

  2. Treatment

    a. Immediately irrigate with water to remove venom.

    b. Place affected area in hot water (113° F) to inactivate venom proteins.

    c. If heat is unavailable, apply ice packs for up to 30 minutes.

    d. Inject 1% lidocaine directly into and around the site of envenomation to ease pain.

    e. Obtain radiograph of wound for evidence of spines or stingers (radiopaque).

    f. Explore the wound and remove all traces of broken barb.

    g. Meticulous wound care

    h. Analgesia

    i. Allow the wound to remain open to granulate.

27

      j. Penetrating wounds to abdomen or chest must be referred for surgical evaluation.

      k. Tetanus prophylaxis

      l. Antibiotic therapy if the wound is more than 6 hours old

X. Prevention

Common sense precautions must be taken when exploring the environment. It is imperative to respect the habitats of animals. Most species are not aggressive unless their territories are invaded or they are otherwise threatened.

Chapter 28

Hypothermia and Hyperthermia

George Ofori-Amanfo, MD,
G. Patricia Cantwell, MD, FCCM,
and Charles L. Schleien, MD, MBA

I. Temperature regulation
   Temperature homeostasis is maintained by a fine balance between heat production and heat loss in the presence of normal mechanisms of heat conservation. Normothermia is defined as a rectal temperature of 36° to 37.5° C.
   A. Heat-generating mechanisms: Response to cold
      1. Thyroid hormone: Increases metabolic rate and heat production by stimulating Na^+,K^+-ATPase
      2. Sympathetic stimulation
         a. Cold temperature stimulates β receptors in brown fat, resulting in an increased metabolic rate.
         b. Norepinephrine and epinephrine uncouple oxidative phosphorylation, leading to heat generation.
      3. Shivering: Most potent mechanism for increasing heat production
         a. Cold temperature activates the primary motor center in the posterior hypothalamus to cause shivering.
         b. Alpha (α) and gamma (γ) motor neurons are activated, causing contraction of skeletal muscles and then heat production.
   B. Heat conservation mechanisms
      1. Skin vasoconstriction through posterior hypothalamic sympathetic stimulation
      2. Piloerection
   C. Heat loss mechanisms: Response to heat and fever
      1. Vasodilation of skin vessels caused by inhibition of the sympathetic centers of the posterior hypothalamus
      2. Full vasodilation → eightfold increase in heat transfer rate to the skin → heat loss by the following mechanisms:
         a. Radiation
            (1) Heat loss via infrared heat waves from the body to the environment

           (2) 60% of all heat loss in a nude person at room temperature occurs via radiation.

    b. Conduction: Transfer of heat from the body to adjacent objects with which it is in direct contact

    c. Convection: Transfer of heat to moving air that is temporarily in contact with the body surface

    d. Evaporation

        (1) Heat loss through the conversion of liquid into vapor

        (2) When water evaporates from the body surface, 0.58 kcal of heat is lost per gram of water that evaporates.

D. Special considerations in the newborn

Newborn infants are prone to hypothermia.

  1. Thermoregulatory system is underdeveloped, increasing risk of heat loss.

  2. Relative to body weight, the body surface of a newborn infant is approximately threefold greater than that of an adult.

    a. The relatively large head forms approximately 20% of the total body surface area.

    b. Therefore, for a given ambient temperature, heat loss in a newborn is fourfold higher than in an older child or adult.

  3. Minimal subcutaneous tissue results in suboptimal insulation against heat loss.

  4. Absence of shivering results in the impaired ability to generate heat.

  5. Thermogenesis

    a. Dependent on the metabolism of brown fat, which is highly vascular, rich in mitochondria, and located near the major vessels of the neck, chest, and abdomen

    b. Hypothermia stimulates the release of norepinephrine, which causes nonshivering thermogenesis via oxidation of brown fat.

II. Hypothermia overview

  A. Definition

    1. Core temperature below 35° C (95° F)—associated with impairment of muscular and cerebral functions

    2. Core temperature reflects the average temperature in the brain, heart, lungs, and viscera.

    3. Severity levels

      a. Mild: 32° to 35° C

      b. Moderate: 28° to 31.9° C

      c. Severe: <28° C

  B. Causes

    See **Table 28-1**.

  C. Signs, symptoms, and laboratory abnormalities

    See **Table 28-2**.

TABLE 28-1

CAUSES OF HYPOTHERMIA

Environmental Causes	Neurologic Disease	Acute Illness, Organ Dysfunction	Skin Diseases	Endocrine or Metabolic Failure
Drug intake (alcohol, opioids, barbiturates, antidepressants, alpha blockers)	Any CNS disease (tumor, infection, trauma)	Sepsis Shock Pancreatitis	Burns Exfoliative dermatitis	Hypothyroidism Hypoadrenalism Hypopituitarism
Cold exposure (infancy, older adults, immersion, resuscitation [cold IV fluids], emergency delivery)	Spinal cord transection Peripheral neuropathy	Diabetic ketoacidosis Uremia Water intoxication	Epidermolysis bullosa	Hypoglycemia Malnutrition

CNS, Central nervous system; *IV*, intravenous.

28

D. Treatment
   1. Initial steps
      a. Ensure adequate airway, breathing, and circulation.
      b. Move patient to a warm environment.
      c. Remove wet or constricting clothing.
      d. Begin monitoring and assess degree of hypothermia.
   2. External warming
      a. Mild hypothermia
         (1) Warm blankets can rewarm at a rate of 0.5° to 1° C/hour.
         (2) Forced heated air convection devices (e.g., Bair Hugger, Eden Prairie, Minn.) can rewarm at a rate of 1° to 2.5° C/hour.
         (3) Never apply a heating lamp directly onto skin (burn risk); heating lamp may be applied to patient who is covered with a blanket.
      b. Moderate hypothermia
         (1) Same measures as with mild hypothermia
         (2) Administer warmed intravenous (IV) fluid through a blood warmer at 40° to 42° C.
   3. Invasive warming techniques: Reserved for severe hypothermia
      a. Delivery of humidified oxygen (O_2) warmed from 40° to 42° C via mechanical ventilation
      b. Peritoneal lavage with K^+-free dialysate (or normal saline [NS]) warmed from 40° to 42° C
      c. Closed thoracic lavage with K^+-free dialysate (or NS) warmed from 40° to 42° C if patient is also unstable hemodynamically

```
TABLE 28-2
```

ASSESSMENT OF THE HYPOTHERMIC PATIENT

	Degree of Hypothermia	
Site	Mild (32°-35° C)	Moderate to Severe (<32° C)
PHYSICAL EXAMINATION		
Skin	Cold, pale	Sclerema, edema
CNS	Impaired judgment	Obtunded, comatose, weak, flaccid
	Amnesia	Dilated nonreactive pupils (<25° C)
	Lack of coordination	Diminished deep tendon reflexes
	Slurred speech	
	Decreased appetite	
Respiration	Tachypnea	Slow, shallow respirations
		Impaired airway protective reflexes
		Aspiration and pneumonia
		Respiratory arrest
Cardiac	Tachycardia	Bradycardia, hypotension
Gastrointestinal	Decreased bowel sounds	Ileus
PHYSIOLOGIC MONITORING		
CNS	6%-7% ↓ in CBF for each 1° C lowering of brain temperature	↓ Cerebral metabolic rate
		↑ Cerebral ischemic tolerance
ECG	Sinus tachycardia	Sinus bradycardia
		First-, second-, or third-degree heart block
		Prolongation of QRS and QT intervals
		ST elevation or depression
		T wave inversion
		J wave (Osborne wave)
		Atrial fibrillation
		Ventricular ectopic beats
		Ventricular fibrillation
Hemodynamics	↑ Cardiac output	↓ Cardiac output
	↑ SVR	↓ Mean arterial pressure
	Mean arterial pressure—may be unchanged	
Urine output	Polyuria	Oliguria
LABORATORY TESTING		
Hematologic	↑ Hct, ↓ WBC count	↑ PT, ↑ PTT, platelet dysfunction
Metabolic	↓ Na$^+$ level	↓ pH
	↑ K$^+$ level	↑ BUN level
	↑ Glucose level	↑ Amylase level
Radiography	Ileus	Ileus
		Pulmonary edema

BUN, Blood urea nitrogen; *CBF*, cerebral blood flow; *CNS*, central nervous system; *ECG*, electrocardiogram; *Hct*, hematocrit; *PT*, prothrombin time; *PTT*, partial thromboplastin time; *ST*, skin temperature; *SVR*, systemic vascular resistance; *WBC*, white blood cell.

    d. Extracorporeal membrane oxygenation (ECMO) or cardiopulmonary bypass (CPB) in severely hypothermic patients with nonperfusing rhythms

    e. Proceed as rapidly as possible to ECMO or CPB in the presence of nonperfusing rhythm induced by severe hypothermia.

    f. Use ECMO or CPB to rewarm to >32° C and return of stable perfusing rhythm.

4. Cardiopulmonary resuscitation (CPR) during severe hypothermia

    a. If possible, the electrocardiogram (ECG) should be monitored in the field to determine the presence of cardiac activity because patients will appear comatose with barely palpable pulses.

    b. If the patient has no pulse but has an organized cardiac rhythm on the ECG, CPR should **not** be initiated because of the risk of precipitating ventricular fibrillation (V Fib).

    c. There is controversy over the advisability of starting CPR in the profoundly hypothermic patient in whom electrocardiographic confirmation of asystole or V Fib is not possible.

       (1) Initiation of and continued CPR are recommended until the patient has remained unresponsive to CPR efforts, despite being rewarmed to >34° C.

5. Ventricular fibrillation

    a. In severe hypothermia, V Fib is extremely refractory to cardioversion until rewarming has been successfully achieved.

    b. Unless extracorporeal circulatory support can be rapidly established, prolonged CPR may be necessary until sufficient rewarming (>32° C) has occurred to allow defibrillation.

    c. Do not administer resuscitative medications until temperature is higher than 30° C.

    d. Currently available antiarrhythmic agents

       (1) Have not been shown to be efficacious in hypothermia-induced V Fib

       (2) However, there has been some success with the use of IV magnesium sulfate ($MgSO_4$) (100 mg/kg).

       (3) Amiodarone should be used with extreme caution because it may worsen QT prolongation induced by hypothermia.

6. Invasive access

    a. Peripheral venous lines

       (1) Preferred over central venous lines in the right atrium because of risk of inducing arrhythmias during placement

28

TABLE 28-3

MONITORING DURING REWARMING

Parameter	Expected Change
BP; preferably invasive measurement	↑ BP; recirculation of cold blood may lead to severe ↓ BP.
ECG	Sinus rhythm or ventricular tachycardia associated with after-drop; prolonged QT may persist for hours or even days.
Urine output (with Foley catheter in place)	↑ Urine output
Serum K^+ level	↑ Serum K^+ level
P_{CO_2}	↑ P_{CO_2} with ↑ temperature
Serum glucose level	↑ or ↓
Central venous pressure	↓ Caused by vasodilation

BP, Blood pressure; *ECG,* electrocardiogram; *P_{CO_2},* partial pressure of carbon dioxide.

(2) If peripheral venous access is unobtainable, consider femoral venous line or careful placement of a central venous line terminating in the superior vena cava rather than the right atrium (RA). Also, do not advance the guidewire into the RA during line placement.
    b. Pulmonary artery catheterization is contraindicated.
    c. Nasogastric tube insertion may be needed for management of ileus, but avoid until core temperature is higher than 30° C.
7. Monitoring (**Table 28-3**)
    a. ECG
    b. Core (rectal or esophageal) temperature with low-temperature thermometer
    c. Invasive blood pressure (BP) monitoring
    d. Arterial blood gases
    e. Urine output
III. Frostnip
    A. Definition
        1. Superficial and reversible ice crystal formation
        2. Associated with intense vasoconstriction
    B. Symptoms and signs
        1. Cold, white areas on the face, ears, or extremities.
        2. Severe discomfort at the affected site
        3. Symptoms reversible with rewarming; usually does not result in tissue loss
        4. Blistering and peeling may occur over the next 24 to 72 hours following exposure.
    C. Treatment
        1. Goal is early and rapid warming in the field and rapid transfer to a warm environment.
        2. Remove wet clothing.

3. Consider skin-to-skin rewarming (place hand in axilla).
4. Immersion into warm water, 40° to 42° C, for 30 to 40 minutes
5. Topical treatment with soothing agents (e.g., aloe)
6. Analgesia (e.g., ibuprofen)

IV. Frostbite

A. Definition

Frostbite is localized, cold-induced injury caused by tissue freezing.

B. Pathophysiology

1. Frostbite occurs at temperatures lower than 0° C (32° F).
2. Following hypothermia
   a. Local vasoconstriction
   b. Decreased perfusion of warm blood to the affected site
   c. Ice crystals form in the extracellular fluid compartment and compress the surrounding tissues.
   d. Red blood cell sludging and microthrombus formation
   e. Increased vascular permeability resulting in edema formation and decreased circulation
   f. Microvascular aggregates form in nerves, blood vessels, and skeletal tissue 1 to 2 hours after these tissues thaw.
   g. Most commonly affected tissues: Ear lobes, fingers, and feet
   h. Relatively resistant tissues: Fascia, connective tissue, bone, and tendon

C. Risk factors

1. Results from exposure to cold; influenced by the following:
   a. Air temperature
   b. Duration of exposure
   c. Relative humidity (conductive losses)
   d. Wind conditions (convective losses)
2. Constrictive clothing and drugs that interfere with peripheral circulation may increase predisposition to frostbite.
3. Other exacerbating factors include hypoxia (high altitude) and inactive dependent extremities.

D. Clinical course

1. Begins with an initial tingling and aching sensation at the affected site that progresses to a cold anesthetic area
2. Blanching at the affected area: With progression, the tissue changes consistency from doughy to rock hard.
3. Throbbing pain persists for up to 2 to 4 days after tissue thawing.
4. Edema occurs shortly after thawing and blister formation occurs within 24 to 48 hours.
5. Eschar formation develops over 2 to 3 weeks.
6. Demarcation occurs over the subsequent days to months, and spontaneous amputation may occur.

E. Degrees of injury

Frostbite is graded by degrees similar to burn injuries.

28

1. First degree
   a. Numbness and erythema, followed by hyperemia and edema
   b. White or yellowish plaque in the area of injury
   c. After rewarming, the tissue becomes mottled, cyanotic, and painful; intense pruritus or burning occurs.
   d. Desquamation of superficial tissue develops 5 to 10 days after the injury.
2. Second degree
   a. Superficial skin vesiculation with clear or milky fluid within blisters, surrounded by erythema and edema
   b. After rewarming, the skin becomes deep red and feels hot and dry to the touch.
   c. Swelling occurs within 2 to 3 hours after rewarming.
   d. Blebs form after 6 to 12 hours.
3. Third degree
   a. Violaceous bullae, necrosis of the skin and cutaneous tissues
   b. Edema occurs within 6 days after rewarming.
   c. Early anesthesia is followed by deep aching or throbbing in 1 to 2 weeks.
4. Fourth degree
   a. Complete necrosis of the skin as well as loss of tissue, including bone
   b. After rewarming, the area becomes deep red, cyanotic, and mottled with anesthesia of the involved area.
      (1) The proximal area swells after 6 to 12 hours.
      (2) The injured area does not become edematous; rather, dry gangrene and mummification occur.
      (3) When this degree of frostbite affects the digits, development of the growth plate is impaired, resulting in deformities.
F. Treatment
   1. General principles
      a. Remove from cold environment and rewarm.
      b. Correct systemic hypothermia to at least 34° C (93° F) prior to frostbite treatment.
      c. Protect against vascular spasms, hyperviscosity, and thrombosis.
      d. Prevent inflammation and infection.
      e. Identify and treat associated traumatic or medical conditions.
      f. Avoid rubbing, pressure, and mechanical trauma.
         (1) Splint affected extremity with bulky dressing.
         (2) Insert sterile cotton pledgets between digits.
      g. Avoid reexposure to the cold.
         (1) Warming and refreezing are associated with more permanent tissue damage.

        (2) Therefore, rewarming methods should be delayed until cold reexposure is unlikely and definitive rewarming measures are available.

    h. Vasodilators and sympathetic blockade have been used to aid faster rewarming.

  2. Rewarming

    a. Rapid rewarming is accomplished by placing the affected extremities in a water bath from 40° to 42° C.

      (1) Rewarming is continued until a hyperemic flush reaches the tips of the extremities.

      (2) This process may take from 30 to 40 minutes.

      (3) It is often associated with itching and pain requiring narcotic analgesia.

    b. Obtain a digital angiogram.

      (1) If rewarming fails to improve perfusion

      (2) If angiogram shows significant perfusion defects, administer tissue plasminogen activator (tPA) and heparin intra-arterially (i.e., directly through the angiography sheath).

    c. Do not use dry heat to rewarm because it can cause burns.

  3. Post-thaw therapy

    a. Administer tetanus immunization, if indicated.

    b. Administer cefazolin to prevent infection.

    c. Administer ibuprofen (10 mg/kg) for arachidonic acid cascade inhibition and fibrinolysis.

    d. Appropriate wound care must be instituted.

    e. Patients are followed until wounds are stable.

V. Trench foot (immersion foot)

  A. Definition

    1. Localized cold injury caused by prolonged exposure of the feet to cold, wet conditions.

    2. This can occur even at temperatures as high as 60° F if the feet are constantly wet, in poorly ventilated boots.

  B. Clinical course

    1. The affected foot becomes cold and numb.

    2. The skin is pale, mottled, and edematous.

    3. The affected tissue generally becomes necrotic and sloughs off.

    4. In severe cases, the toes, heel, or entire foot can be affected.

    5. If circulation is impaired for more than 6 hours, permanent damage can occur.

    6. This may be associated with autonomic disturbance leading to excessive sweating, pain, and hypersensitivity to temperature changes.

    7. Impaired circulation for more than 24 hours may result in loss of the affected foot.

28

C. Treatment
   1. Management includes careful washing and drying the affected foot.
   2. Because the foot is not frozen, only gentle warming is required; ibuprofen or other pain medication may be administered.
VI. Hyperthermia
   A. Definition
      1. Hyperthermia is an extreme body temperature elevation (>41° C) beyond the hypothalamic set point.
      2. It is caused by inadequate heat loss or excessive heat gain and is to be distinguished from fever, in which cytokine activation has raised the set point to a higher level.
      3. The classification of hyperthermia syndromes includes environmental (heat stroke), drug or toxin-induced, and genetic or unknown causes.
   B. Heat stroke
      1. Overview
         a. Heat stroke is a life-threatening emergency characterized by a core temperature exceeding 41° C and central nervous system (CNS) dysfunction resulting in delirium, convulsions, and/or coma.
         b. Heat exhaustion and heat stroke are two extremes of a continuum of disorders.
         c. The boundary between heat exhaustion and heat stroke is arbitrarily defined as 41° C and the presence of altered mental status.
         d. Despite appropriate therapy and adequate lowering of the body temperature, heat stroke is often fatal.
         e. Survivors may sustain permanent neurologic damage.
      2. Causes
         a. Classic heat stroke: Environmental overheating and the body's inability to dissipate heat through sweating
         b. Exertional heat stroke: Hyperthermia occurs when metabolic heat production exceeds the body's normal ability to dissipate the heat.
         c. Environmental overheating can, however, worsen exertional heat stroke (**Table 28-4**).
      3. Pathophysiology of heat stroke: General considerations
         a. Direct cytotoxicity
         b. Adverse host inflammatory and coagulation responses resulting in alterations in microcirculation and damage to vascular endothelium
         c. Physiologic derangements include cardiovascular collapse, hypoxia, stupor, and increased metabolic demands, which may progress to multiorgan dysfunction syndrome.

TABLE 28-4

CLASSIC VERSUS EXERTIONAL HEAT STROKE

Parameter	Heat Stroke	
	Classic	Exertional
Age group	Older adults	Younger age
Activity	Sedentary	Strenuous exercise
Acid-base status	Respiratory alkalosis	Respiratory alkalosis
		Lactic acidosis
Hyperkalemia	Unusual	Often present
Hypocalcemia	Uncommon	Frequent
Hyperuricemia	Rare	Severe
Rhabdomyolysis	Unusual	Frequent, severe
Acute renal failure	<5% of patients	25% to 30% of patients
Coagulopathy	Mild	Severe
Mechanism of disease	Poor dissipation of ambient heat	Excessive endogenous heat production >heat loss

28

    d. Intestinal ischemia may lead to gut hyperpermeability, resulting in endotoxemia.

    e. Increased infection risk because of immunosuppression

    f. The severity of the thermal injury depends on the **critical thermal maximum.**

       (1) This is defined as the level and duration of hyperthermia that will induce tissue injury.

       (2) The critical thermal maximum in humans is a body temperature of 41.6° to 42° C for 45 minutes to 8 hours.

4. Infant predisposition: The relatively larger body surface area of infants makes them more prone to heat stroke because of increased conduction of heat from the environment.

5. Protective mechanism

    a. Hyperthermia is associated with the induction of heat shock proteins that protect cells from damage by heat, hypoxia, ischemia, inflammatory cytokines, and endotoxin.

    b. There is profound attenuation of this adaptive response during an episode of heat stroke.

6. Evaluation

    a. Hyperthermia: Core temperature 40° to 47° C.

    b. CNS dysfunction is key to the diagnosis of heat stroke.

    c. Subtle to severe symptoms

       (1) Prodrome: Headache, dizziness, and confusion

       (2) Progression to prostration, coma, and shock

       (3) Seizures may occur, especially during cooling.

7. Laboratory findings (**Table 28-5**)

    a. Respiratory alkalosis in nonexertional heat stroke; mixed respiratory alkalosis and lactic acidosis in exertional heat stroke

---

TABLE 28-5

LABORATORY ABNORMALITIES IN HEAT STROKE

Laboratory Test	Abnormality
Complete blood cell count	↑ Hct, ↑ WBC, ↓ platelets
Coagulation profile	↑ PT, ↑ PTT, ↓ fibrinogen level
Chemistry	↑ BUN, ↑ creatinine, ↓ Ca^{2+}, ↓ PO$_4$; ↑ AST and ALT
Urinalysis	Proteinuria, myoglobinuria
ECG	Sinus tachycardia, nonspecific ST-T changes, prolonged QT interval
Arterial blood gas	↓ or ↑ pH, ↓ Pco$_2$

ALT, Alanine aminotransferase; *AST,* aspartate aminotransferase; *BUN,* blood urea nitrogen; *ECG,* electrocardiogram; *Hct,* hematocrit; *Pco$_2$,* partial pressure of carbon dioxide; *PT,* prothrombin time; *PTT,* partial thromboplastin time; *WBC,* white blood cell.

   b. Evidence of diffuse myocardial injury
      (1) Increased serum troponin level
      (2) Tachyarrhythmias
      (3) Nonspecific ST-T changes
      (4) QT prolongation (probably caused by hypokalemia or hypomagnesemia)
      (5) Bundle branch block
   c. Pulmonary edema may be seen on a chest radiograph, although usually the result of fluid overload during resuscitation
   d. Acute renal failure, which is seen in 30% of exertional heat stroke cases, is related to rhabdomyolysis, hypotension, and direct thermal injury to renal parenchyma.
8. General management
   a. Maintain adequate airway and breathing.
   b. Treat shock and maintain normal hemodynamic status.
   c. Lower core body temperature.
      (1) Cooling methods should be rapidly instituted.
         (a) The core temperature should be lowered at least 0.1° C/min to <39° C.
         (b) At this point, active cooling must be discontinued to avoid induced hypothermia.
      (2) External cooling methods include the following:
         (a) Application of cold packs to the skin
         (b) Spraying cool water onto the skin
         (c) Fanning
         (d) These modalities enhance heat loss by conduction, evaporation, and convection, respectively.
      (3) Invasive cooling methods such as iced gastric or peritoneal lavage may be used, but typically not required.
      (4) External iced water cooling poses the theoretical disadvantage of causing peripheral vasoconstriction, with shunting of blood away from the skin.

        (a) Results in a paradoxical rise in body temperature
        (b) May also cause shivering, which can induce an additional elevation in body temperature
    (5) Do **NOT** use antipyretics.
        (a) Use of antipyretics is generally potentially harmful in heat stroke.
        (b) Acetaminophen and aspirin lower body temperature by normalizing the elevated hypothalamic set point.
        (c) In heat stroke, the set point is usually normal.
    (6) Do **NOT** use alcohol baths; systemic absorption of alcohol may lead to poisoning and coma.
    (7) Dantrolene is ineffective in heat stroke.

9. Initial field management
    a. Document core body temperature (with rectal probe).
    b. If unconscious, patient should be positioned to maintain a patent airway.
    c. Move patient to cooler environment.
    d. Remove clothing.
    e. Initiate external cooling.
        (1) Cold packs on the neck, axillae, groin
        (2) Continuous fanning
        (3) Spray the skin with water at 25° to 30° C.
    f. Administer supplemental O_2.
    g. Administer IV crystalloid solution.
    h. Transfer to the emergency department.

10. In-hospital management
    a. Secure airway if patient is unconsciousness or impaired gas exchange is present.
    b. Confirm diagnosis with repeat core temperature assessment.
    c. Continue cooling measures described, plus cooling blanket.
    d. Administer lorazepam, 0.1 mg/kg, or fosphenytoin, 20 mg/kg, for seizures.
    e. Aggressive management of hypotension with fluids and vasopressors
    f. Monitor central venous pressure in refractory hypotension.
    g. Treat rhabdomyolysis with the following:
        (1) Crystalloids, diuretics (furosemide, 0.5 mg/kg, or mannitol, 250-500 mg/kg)
        (2) Alkalinization of the urine
            (a) $NaHCO_3$, 1- to 2-mEq/kg boluses
            (b) Followed by continuous infusion of $NaHCO_3$, 100 mEq/L in D5W or 100 mEq/L in D5 1/4NS (depending on the serum Na), at 1.5 to 2 times maintenance to achieve urine pH of 7 to 8

28

    h. Correct serum electrolyte abnormalities to prevent
       life-threatening arrhythmias.
    i. Treat metabolic acidosis (pH <7.2) with NaHCO$_3$ 1 to
       2 mEq/kg.
    j. Assess for multiorgan system failure and treat appropriately.
 11. Complications: The most serious complications of heat stroke
     are due to multiorgan dysfunction; these include the following:
    a. Encephalopathy
    b. Acute renal failure
    c. Rhabdomyolysis
    d. Acute respiratory distress syndrome
    e. Hepatocellular injury
    f. Myocardial injury
    g. Intestinal ischemia or infarction
    h. Disseminated intravascular coagulation
 12. Outcome
    a. Recovery of CNS function during cooling is a favorable
       prognostic sign.
    b. Residual neurologic deficit, especially cerebellar syndrome,
       may occur despite prompt treatment in about 20% of
       patients.
C. Malignant hyperthermia-like syndrome
  1. Definition
    a. Hyperthermia syndrome associated with diabetes and insulin
       use
    b. No prior history of exposure to anesthetics or succinylcholine
       (as in classic malignant hyperthermia)
    c. More common in obese African American males with
       acanthosis nigricans
    d. Usually progresses to rhabdomyolysis
    e. Cause unknown but the insulin preservative, *m*-cresol, has
       been implicated in some cases
  2. Management
    a. Dantrolene (a muscle relaxant), 2.5 mg/kg IV every 1 to 6
       hours, until temperature <39° C
    b. Cooling measures (see Section VI.B)
    c. Supportive care (see Section VI.B)
D. Neuroleptic malignant syndrome
  1. Definition: Hyperthermia syndrome associated with the use of
     antipsychotic drugs (e.g., haloperidol, chlorpromazine,
     fluphenazine, clozapine, olanzapine, risperidone) and
     antiemetic drugs (e.g., promethazine, metoclopramide)
  2. Classic signs: Muscle rigidity, mental status changes,
     hyperthermia, and autonomic instability (e.g., diaphoresis,
     tachycardia, hypertension)

3. Risk factors: Rapid dose escalation, concomitant use of lithium, comorbid diseases
4. Management
   a. Dantrolene, 2.5 mg/kg IV every 1 to 6 hours, until temperature <39° C
   b. Discontinue all potential triggering agents.
   c. Cooling measures (see Section VI.B)
   d. Supportive care (see Section VI.B)
   e. Control agitation with benzodiazepines.
E. Serotonin syndrome
   1. Definition: Hyperthermia syndrome characterized by signs of increased serotonin release
      a. Abnormal mental status: Agitation, delirium
      b. Hyperactive neuromuscular function: Hyperreflexia, clonus, hypertonicity, tremor
      c. Excess autonomic function: Tachycardia, hypertension, vomiting, diarrhea, diaphoresis, hyperthermia
   2. Management
      a. Discontinue all serotonergic drugs.
      b. Cyproheptadine, a histamine-1 receptor antagonist with nonspecific serotonergic (5-HT1A and 5-HT2A) antagonistic properties
         (1) Total daily dose is 0.25 mg/kg divided every 6 hours via nasogastric tube; no parenteral formulation available
         (2) Maximum daily dose: 12 mg for children 2 to 6 years old and 16 mg for children 7 to 14 years old
      c. Cooling measures (see Section VI.B)
      d. Treat hypotension with IV fluids and direct-acting vasoconstrictors, such as phenylephrine.
      e. Other supportive measures (see Section VI.B)

28

Chapter 29

Terrorism and Mass Casualty Events
Ronald Pauldine, MD

I. Overview

On September 11, 2001, our perceived immunity from the threat of biologic, chemical, or nuclear terrorism was shattered. Conventional warfare, unconventional weapons (weapons of mass destruction), acts of terrorism, and natural disasters have enormous importance in terms of threats to immediate public safety and long-term public health. In turn, planning for the response to such events is of great concern to federal, state, and local government agencies and the medical community at large.

It is essential for health care professionals to have a fundamental understanding of disaster response and become active participants in disaster preparedness. This chapter includes quickly accessible, useful, and accurate information to aid in the management of illnesses produced by biologic, chemical, and radiologic weapons and to help recognize that an attack has taken place.

II. Disaster preparation and management

A. General considerations

1. Advances in health care and financial considerations have resulted in the near-elimination of excess bed space in U.S. hospitals.

2. There is limited hospital management experience with regard to response to mass casualty incidents.

3. Coordination between medical personnel and emergency managers is limited.

4. In the early hours or days following a mass casualty incident, the local hospital must be prepared to operate without support from local, state, or federal agencies.

5. Institution and geographic specific concerns should be addressed through a hazard vulnerability analysis.

a. This analysis is required by The Joint Commission.

b. The assessment considers the types of incidents likely to occur as well as the preparedness at a particular institution.

c. Considerations include surge capacity and contingency plans.

6. All hospitals are required to have a disaster plan and written guidance in the form of a disaster manual.

7. An incident command system (ICS) has been recommended as a tool to assist hospital administrators in operating medical facilities in times of crisis.

B. Incident command systems
   1. The ICS coordinates and synchronizes all activities relating to a nuclear, biologic, chemical, or natural disaster mass casualty event.
   2. The ICS may exist at the local hospital or local, state, or federal government level.
   3. The hospital ICS is responsible for conducting internal operations and coordinating with other hospitals, first responders, and local, state, and federal organizations, with or without the presence of a public ICS.
   4. The head of the ICS is the incident commander.
      a. This person is directly responsible to the hospital or health care system chief executive.
      b. This individual should be clearly identified as the person in charge.
   5. The system should be designed to be flexible and modular, with components based on the nature, severity, and duration of the incident.
   6. The various components of the ICS should be tailored to meet the size and needs of the specific facility and community served.
   7. Possible core functional areas include the following:
      a. Staffing and human resources
      b. Security and intelligence
      c. Operations
      d. Logistics
      e. Finance
      f. Public affairs and media relations
      g. Communications
      h. Environmental affairs
      i. Liaisons
   8. The ICS staff conducts their work in an area designated as the emergency operations center.
      a. This area should ideally be located away from triage and patient care areas.
      b. The space should be adequate for the number of individuals employed and should possess redundant communication technology and media sources, such as radio and local and national television.

C. Personal protective equipment (PPE)
   1. When treating contaminated casualties, protection for health care workers and responding personnel is essential.

2. PPE is designated by levels of protection ranging from A to D; A is the equipment offering the greatest amount of protection.
3. Separate designations are made for the suit ensemble (suit, gloves, boots, boot covers) and mask.
4. The appropriate level of protection required for hospital personnel is controversial because it depends on the capacity and capability of each institution.
5. Increasing levels of protection with increased levels of complexity require greater training and cost.
6. The level of PPE required depends on the known or anticipated contaminant or agent.
7. Hospital personnel requiring PPE include the following:
   a. Those involved in decontamination
   b. Security personnel working at casualty collection and decontamination areas
   c. Initial reception and triage personnel
8. Hospitals may not have sufficient resources to purchase, store, and maintain appropriate PPE.

III. Unconventional weapons: General principles
   A. Definitions
      1. Unconventional weapons are classified as nuclear, biologic, or chemical.
         a. Nuclear warfare: The use of radioactive materials to cause damage and destruction, usually in the form of explosive devices
         b. Biologic warfare: The use of microorganisms or toxins derived from living organisms to produce death, disease, or toxicity in humans, animals, or plants
         c. Chemical warfare: The use of any chemical substance that because of its physiologic, psychological, or pharmacologic effects, can be used to kill, seriously injure, or incapacitate humans
      2. Contamination from unconventional weapons may come in the form of solid particles, liquids, or vapors.
         a. Exposed casualties require special precautions.
         b. Decontamination involves the removal and/or neutralization of such hazards.
      3. Terrorism is the use or threat of violence made for ideologic reasons.
      4. Dirty bombs: Nuclear dispersion devices
         a. Use conventional explosives to disperse radioactive material
         b. Not likely to result in high-dose radiation exposure
         c. May contaminate areas, including food and water sources, and necessitate resource allocation for cleanup

IV. Nuclear contamination
  A. Historical perspective and data
    1. Hiroshima, Japan, August 6, 1945
    2. Nagasaki, Japan, August 9, 1945
    3. Ground tests
  B. Components of nuclear explosion
    1. Flash effect is more intense than the sun; may cause temporary or permanent blindness
    2. Shock effect
      a. Results from rapid increase in air pressure at ground zero
      b. Produces air concussion that may lead to rupture of lungs or eardrums in nearby victims
    3. Thermal effect
      a. Caused by heat released during the explosion
      b. Heat begins at 100,000° F, the temperature at which sand changes to glass.
      c. Thermal burns may be prevalent many miles away.
    4. Electromagnetic pulse is an electrical disturbance.
      a. Created in the atmosphere
      b. May disable equipment, including vehicles, communication, and medical devices
    5. Blast wind is a high-pressure area at a blast site that produces winds in excess of 400 mph.
      a. Immediately followed by a low-pressure area pulling high winds back
      b. Serious injury may result from flying debris, collapsing structures, and victims thrown into stationary objects.
    6. Fallout
      a. Late effect secondary to radioactive particles blown into the atmosphere
      b. Particles return to earth and are widely disseminated, with potential to cause radiation sickness.
  C. Radiation exposure
    1. Measured in radiation absorbed dose (rad) or gray (Gy) (1 rad = 0.01 Gy)
    2. May be detected with specialized equipment, such as a Geiger counter
  D. Triage of victims
    1. Initial triage is based only on conventional injuries and may include multiple trauma, burns, and eye injuries.
    2. Secondary triage is based on the degree of exposure.
  E. Radiation sickness: Three stages
    1. Initial stage: Weakness, nausea, rapid-onset vomiting, short duration

29

TABLE 29-1

LYMPHOCYTE LEVELS AFTER RADIATION EXPOSURE

- Measure levels initially and after 24 hr for comparison.
- Decrease of 50% to values <1000/mm^3 is associated with significant exposure.
- Lymphocyte levels may be unreliable in the presence of other injuries.

Level (/mm^3)	Comments
>1500	Significant exposure is unlikely.
1000-1500	May require treatment for granulocytopenia and thrombocytopenia within 3 wk.
500-1000	Indicates severe radiation injury; anticipate hemorrhagic and infection complications within 2-3 wk.
<500	Possible fatal exposure; pancytopenia is inevitable.
Undetectable	Lethal exposure; survival beyond 2 wk is unlikely.

---

2. Latent stage
   a. Virtually no signs or symptoms
   b. May last only several hours with high-dose exposure and up to weeks with lower-dose exposure
3. Clinical stage: Syndrome associated with major organ systems injured
4. Relative radiosensitivity of organs: Hematopoietic system and gastrointestinal (GI) system > skin, cornea, and lens > growing cartilage and bone > mature cartilage and bone > muscle, brain, and spinal cord

F. Decontamination
   1. Remove clothing and wash with soap and water.
   2. Usually effective (95%)

G. Treatment
   1. Treat conventional injuries first.
   2. Risk stratification is based on:
      a. White blood cell count (**Table 29-1**)
      b. Symptom complex
         (1) Hematopoietic syndrome is manifested by patients receiving low to moderate levels of radiation resulting in pancytopenia.
         (2) GI syndrome
            (a) Results from higher levels of exposure
            (b) Manifested by severe vomiting, diarrhea, and hemorrhage
            (c) Likely to be accompanied by nonrecoverable bone marrow suppression
         (3) Neurovascular syndrome is associated with extreme exposure.
            (a) Thus, victims usually die of other causes.
            (b) Symptoms include mental confusion, convulsions, and coma.

      c. The presence of conventional injuries considerably decreases the lethal dose of radiation.

      d. Supportive care for survivors includes bone marrow–stimulating agents.

      e. Aggressive treatment of infection is indicated.

      f. Children and adolescents are at high risk for developing thyroid cancer after exposure to radioactive iodine.

        (1) The most likely sources of exposure include the following:

          (a) Nuclear reactors (following a containment mishap)

          (b) Contaminated vegetation, meat, and dairy products

        (2) Potassium iodide

          (a) Effectively competes for thyroid uptake with radioactive iodide, preventing organification and storage of iodine

          (b) Recommended after exposure to radioactive iodide

          (c) Should be continued for the duration of the exposure

        (3) Radioactive iodine release is likely following detonation of a nuclear bomb; however, other radioactive isotopes would also be present and contribute to radiation sickness (see earlier).

V. Bioterrorism

  A. Definition

    1. The intentional or threatened release of disease-producing living organisms or biologically active substances derived from living organisms for the purpose of causing the following:

      a. Death

      b. Illness

      c. Incapacity

      d. Economic damage, and/or

      e. Fear

    2. Considered weapons of mass destruction or mass casualties

  B. Biologic considerations

    1. Advantages of biologic agents

      a. Ease of manufacture

      b. Low cost

      c. Dispersed with simple delivery systems

      d. Kill or incapacitate in large numbers

      e. Incite panic and fear, paralyzing a nation

      f. Overwhelm medical services

      g. Can be targeted at the food supply and not directly at human beings (e.g., foot-and-mouth disease)

29

2. Detection of a biologic attack
   a. Usually associated with a delay in onset of illness
   b. The attack may occur without obvious signs that anything unusual is happening.
   c. These factors may make detection very difficult.
   d. Look for epidemic trends such as the following:
      (1) Large groups of people with similar unexplained signs and symptoms
      (2) Dead or sluggish animal life
      (3) Decaying plants
      (4) Unusual organisms for a geographic area
      (5) Increase in the mortality rate from a specific disease
      (6) Contaminated food or water sources
3. Prevention
   a. Immunizations
   b. Sanitation
   c. Personal hygiene
   d. Prophylactic therapy
   e. Vectors removed
4. Decontamination
   a. Soap and water
   b. Check all food and water sources.
C. Categories of biologic agents
   The Centers for Disease Control and Prevention has designated three categories of biologic agents based on their potential for use as terrorist weapons and potential for contagiousness, social disruption, injury, and death.
   1. Category A agents: Considered the most likely to be used in a biologic attack; have the following features:
      a. Can be easily disseminated or transmitted (not all agents are transmittable from person to person)
      b. Result in high mortality
      c. Have the potential to cause panic and extensive social disruption
      d. Place a burden on the health care system to be prepared for such an attack
      e. These agents include the following:
         (1) *Bacillus anthracis* (anthrax)
         (2) Variola (smallpox)
         (3) *Yersinia pestis* (plague)
         (4) *Francisella tularensis* (tularemia)
         (5) *Clostridium botulinum* (botulism)
         (6) Viral hemorrhagic fevers
   2. Category B agents have the following features:
      a. Moderate ease of dissemination
      b. Cause moderate morbidity and low mortality

      c. Require enhanced diagnostic capacity and disease surveillance

      d. These agents include the following:

         (1) *Coxiella burnetii* (Q fever)

         (2) *Brucella* spp. (brucellosis)

         (3) *Burkholderia mallei* (glanders)

         (4) Alphaviruses (Venezuelan, eastern and western equine encephalomyelitis)

         (5) Ricin toxin *(Ricinis communis* [Castor beans])

         (6) Epsilon toxin *(Clostridium perfringens)*

         (7) Enterotoxin B *(Staphylococcus aureus)*

         (8) Foodborne or water-borne agents

   3. Category C agents are pathogens that could be engineered and produced in the future because of the following:

      a. Availability

      b. Ease of production and dissemination

      c. Potential for high morbidity and mortality

      d. These agents include the following:

         (1) Nipah virus

         (2) Hantavirus

         (3) Tickborne hemorrhagic fever viruses

         (4) Tickborne encephalitis viruses

         (5) Yellow fever

         (6) Multidrug-resistant *Mycobacterium* tuberculosis

D. Clinical presentation

   1. Many biologic weapons present with flulike illness or have other syndromic associations (**Table 29-2**).

      a. Flulike symptoms include fever, malaise, myalgia, headache, cough, sore throat, and nasal congestion.

      b. Other syndromic associations include respiratory distress, widened mediastinum, hemorrhage, petechia, and arthralgias (**Tables 29-3** and **29-4**).

   2. Types of fever

      a. Remittent fever: Temperature increases and decreases without ever returning to normal

      b. Intermittent fever: Temperature that irregularly returns to normal

      c. Relapsing fever: Temperature that regularly returns to normal

   3. Differentiation from influenza

      a. Chest pain

      b. Hemoptysis

      c. GI symptoms

      d. Sore throat and nasal congestion are rare with biologic weapons.

29

TABLE 29-2

BIOLOGIC AGENTS: SYMPTOMS AND MANAGEMENT

Disease, Agent	Incubation (days)	Symptoms	Medical Management	Contagion Risk	Infection Precautions
Anthrax	1-6	FLI, widened mediastinum, pleural effusion, malaise, fever, RD	Doxycycline, ciprofloxacin	Low	Standard
Botulism	0.5-1.5	Diplopia, ptosis, slurred speech, progresses to complete paralysis	*Botulinum* antitoxin, mechanical ventilation	None	Standard
Cholera	0.2-5	Severe rice water diarrhea	Doxycycline	Very low	Standard
Ebola and other hemorrhagic fevers	3-14	FLI, diarrhea, rash, bleeding, shock	None (supportive care)	Moderate	Airborne
Hantavirus	7-35	FLI, dyspnea, RD, headache, GI symptoms	None (supportive care)	Very low	Standard
Plague	1-6	FLI, high fever, hemoptysis, RD	Gentamicin, ciprofloxacin, doxycycline	High	Droplet
Ricin	0.2-0.4	Fever, cough, RD, cough, arthralgias	None (supportive care)	Very low	Standard
Smallpox	3-19	FLI, vesicular rash starting on arms, backache	Preventive vaccine or none (supportive care)	Very high	Airborne and cohort patients
Tularemia	1-21	Hemoptysis, chest pain	Gentamicin, ciprofloxacin	Low	Standard

Airborne, Standard + isolation, negative-pressure room, HEPA filter; *droplet,* standard + HEPA filter mask; *FLI,* flu-like illness; *GI,* gastrointestinal; *RD,* respiratory distress; *standard,* gloves, hand washing, gown, mask, eye protection.

TABLE 29-3

BIOLOGIC AGENTS AND MAJOR SYNDROMES

Fever and Arthralgia	Fever and Respiratory Distress	Fever and Petechiae	Fever and Lymphadenopathy	Fever and Acute Neurologic Symptoms	Fever and Acute Gastrointestinal Symptoms
Blastomycosis	Anthrax	Dengue fever	Coccidiomycosis	Hemorrhagic fever	Aflatoxins
Brucellosis	Blastomycosis	Hemorrhagic fever	Hemorrhagic fever	Q fever	Anthrax
Coccidiomycosis	Coccidiomycosis	Lassa virus	Plague	Rocky Mountain spotted fever	Brucellosis
Dengue fever	Hantavirus	Rocky Mountain spotted fever	Psittacosis	Smallpox	Cholera
Hemorrhagic fever	Legionnaire's disease	Typhus	Tularemia	Typhoid fever	Dengue fever
	Leptospirosis	Yellow fever	Typhus	Typhus	Ebola
	Plague, Q fever, ricin, tularemia			Viral encephalitis	Leptospirosis, ricin, salmonellosis, shigellosis, tularemia
					Typhoid fever, viral encephalitis, yellow fever

29

TABLE 29-4

BIOLOGIC AGENTS AND MAJOR SYNDROMES

Hemorrhage and Coagulopathy	Hilar Adenopathy	Cutaneous Lesions or Ulcerations	Gastrointestinal Symptoms without Fever	Neurologic Symptoms without Fever	Acute Liver Failure
Dengue fever	Blastomycosis	Anthrax	Cholera	Botulism	Ebola
Ebola	Brucellosis	Blastomycosis	Mycotoxin	Saxitoxin	Dengue fever
Hemorrhagic fever	Coccidiomycosis	Coccidiomycosis	Ricin	Tetrodotoxin	Leptospirosis
Hantavirus	Tularemia	Plague	Saxitoxin		Q fever
Lassa virus		Smallpox	Tetrodotoxin		Ricin
Leptospirosis		Tularemia			Rift Valley fever
Ricin		Typhus			
Rift Valley fever					

4. Illness out of season
   a. Influenza-like outbreak in spring or summer
   b. Arthropod borne–like illness (e.g., Rocky Mountain spotted fever) in the winter
5. Illness out of context
   a. Sudden increase in flulike illness in healthy population
   b. Absence of positive cultures
   c. Sudden increase in mortality or need for intensive care unit admission
   d. Increase in complications such as pneumonia, hemorrhage, hepatitis, acute respiratory distress syndrome
   e. Disease cluster in one locale or hospital
   f. Illness in an area in which it is not expected to occur
E. Personal precautions
   Most biologic weapons are not easily transmitted from person to person; exceptions include smallpox and plague. One of the goals of biologic weapons is to induce fear and panic and to disable the medical community. Accepted isolation precautions include the following:
   1. Standard precautions
      a. Hand washing
      b. Mask, glove, gown
      c. Clean stethoscopes and other equipment between patients
   2. Airborne precautions
      a. Negative air pressure handling
      b. High-efficiency particulate air filter mask
      c. Mask on the patient

3. Droplet precautions
4. Contact precautions

F. Considerations for selected biologic agents

1. Anthrax

   a. Dissemination: Inhalation of spores; not transmitted person to person

   b. Incubation period: As short as 1 to 2 days or as long as 6 weeks

   c. Symptoms

      (1) Fever, cough, and weakness progressing to acute respiratory distress

      (2) Septicemia

      (3) Shock

      (4) Meningitis

   d. Mortality: Greater than 80%

   e. Treatment: Naturally occurring strains usually susceptible to the following:

      (1) Penicillin

      (2) Amoxicillin

      (3) Chloramphenicol

      (4) Tetracyclines

      (5) Ciprofloxacin

      (6) Other quinolones

      (7) Strains have been engineered with resistance to penicillin and doxycycline.

   f. Vaccine

      (1) Available but limited to military use

      (2) Should be administered postexposure if available

   g. Postexposure prophylaxis

      (1) Ciprofloxacin, 10 to 15 mg/kg PO bid (max dose 500 mg PO bid)

      (2) Treatment should be changed to amoxicillin, 80 mg/kg/day PO, divided q8hr for children <20 kg when susceptibility to penicillin is confirmed. For children >20 kg, dose is 500 mg PO q8hr.

      (3) Ciprofloxacin has potential to cause cartilage damage and arthropathy in children; however, weaponized anthrax has high likelihood of resistance to penicillin.

2. Smallpox

   a. Cause: Variola virus

   b. Dissemination

      (1) Respiratory droplet or aerosol

      (2) Contact with skin lesions of infected persons, their bedding, or clothing

   c. Epidemiology: Eradicated worldwide in 1977

   d. Incubation period: 7 to 17 days

    e. Clinical symptoms
      (1) Febrile prodrome followed by rash after 2 to 4 days
      (2) Rash marked by slow evolution from papules to
          vesicles to pustules, followed by scabs
      (3) Lesions all at the same stage in any one area
    f. Morbidity and mortality
      (1) Virus is highly transmissible
      (2) Mortality rate of 20% to 30% in unvaccinated
          patients
    g. Vaccine (prophylaxis)
      (1) Not currently recommended for children
      (2) Available and mandatory for deploying military
          personnel and available on an elective basis for health
          care providers likely to be exposed to patients following
          a biologic incident.
    h. Treatment
      (1) Postexposure vaccination
          (a) Can decrease the rate of severe or fatal smallpox if
             administered within the first 4 days
          (b) Should be considered regardless of age
      (2) The antiviral agent cidofovir may be useful in severe
          cases.

VI. Chemical agents
  A. Overview
    1. Like their biologic counterparts, are designed to cause death,
       incapacitation, economic damage, and terror
    2. Synthetic and not derived from living organisms
    3. Once released, they produce almost instantaneous
       effects.
    4. There are exceptions—for example, mustard agents take 1 to
       2 days to manifest their effects.
    5. First used by the Spartans against Athens, the modern age of
       these weapons was ushered in by Germany in World War I
       when chlorine gas was released to kill and panic Allied
       troops.
    6. Since World War I, many chemical agents have been
       developed; sarin is the most well known because of the
       following:
      a. Its use by Iraq on its own civilian population
      b. Its release in the Tokyo subway in 1995
    7. Chemical agents can be divided into lethal and nonlethal
       agents (**Table 29-5**).
  B. Advantages of chemical agents
    1. Low cost
    2. Limited technology required for production

TABLE 29-5

LETHAL VERSUS NONLETHAL CHEMICAL AGENTS

Lethal Agent (Example)	Nonlethal (Incapacitating) Agent
Nerve agents (VX, sarin)	Anticholinergics
Pulmonary agents (chlorine, phosgene, mustard)	Hallucinogens (LSD)
Cyanides	Fentanyl aerosol
Ammonia	Tear gas (lacrimators)
High-dose vesicants (mustard)	Vomiting agents
High-dose urticants (phosgene)	Low-dose vesicants and urticants

LSD, Lysergic acid diethylamide.

C. Increased risk in **children**

Children have increased risk from exposure to chemical (or biologic) agents because of their anatomic and physiologic differences from adults.

1. Infants and children are at greater risk for dehydration, with limited physiologic reserve.
2. Agents causing GI effects, such as diarrhea or vomiting, may lead to profound hypovolemia in children.
3. More rapid respiratory rates may result in greater uptake of aerosolized agents.
4. Some chemical agents have a high vapor density.
   a. This leads to higher concentrations closer to the ground, thus encroaching on a child's breathing space.
   b. Therefore, exposure may be greater for children with these agents.
5. Greater skin surface area relative to body mass
   a. This places children at greater risk for agents directly affecting the skin, such as vesicants, or agents absorbed through the skin, such as nerve agents.
   b. Lower levels of keratin in child's skin may further enhance cutaneous uptake.

D. Treatment of children
1. May be problematic because of lack of availability of appropriate pediatric medications and doses.
2. Most treatments for chemical agents have been developed for military personnel.
3. Testing of specific antidotes and delivery systems in children is lacking.

E. Classification of chemical agents into functional categories
1. Incapacitating agents
   a. Definition
      (1) Least harmful of the chemical agents
      (2) Used mainly for riot control

29

      b. Symptoms: Disorientation, nausea, and vomiting; dissipates quickly

      c. Example: Tear gas

  2. Vesicants (blister agents)

      a. Definition: Irritants affecting skin and mucous membranes

      b. Signs and symptoms

         (1) Airway damage occurs if inhaled.

         (2) Initial small blisters coalesce into larger areas of involvement.

         (3) Symptoms may be delayed 6 to 12 hours.

         (4) Bone marrow suppression can occur.

      c. Mechanism of action: Alkylation of DNA, RNA, and protein, leading to cell death

      d. Examples: Mustard gases and lewisite

      e. Treatment

         (1) Decontamination and burn care as indicated

         (2) Airway involvement may require tracheal intubation and aggressive pulmonary toilet.

         (3) Consider marrow-stimulating agents for supportive treatment.

  3. Pulmonary toxicants (choking agents)

      a. Definition: Cause irritation to the eyes and respiratory tract

      b. Examples: Phosgene and diphosgene chloride

      c. Mechanism of action: Reactions that produce hydrochloric acid and oxidative injury (e.g., phosgene)

      d. Symptoms: Range from minor pulmonary irritation and bronchospasm to severe pneumonitis

      e. Treatment

         (1) Supplemental oxygen (O_2)

         (2) Positive pressure ventilation

         (3) Bronchodilators

         (4) Steroids

  4. Cyanides (blood agents)

      a. Examples: Hydrogen cyanide and cyanogen chloride

      b. Mechanism of action: Uncoupling of oxidative phosphorylation and profound metabolic acidosis

      c. Treatment: Supportive treatment includes the following:

         (1) Supplemental O_2

         (2) Generation of methemoglobin via administration of amyl nitrite (inhaled) or sodium nitrite (9-10 mg/kg IV)

         (3) Increasing detoxification to thiocyanate by administration of sodium thiosulfate (1.65 mL/kg of 23% solution, up to 50 mL).

         (4) Chelation with hydroxocobalamin may also be useful.

  5. Nerve agents

      a. Definition: Odorless, tasteless, deadly neurotoxins

TABLE 29-6

EFFECTS OF NERVE AGENTS

ACh Receptor	End Organ	Response
Nicotinic	Skeletal muscle	Fasciculations
		Weakness
		Paralysis
	Ganglia	Tachycardia
		Initial hypertension, then hypotension
Muscarinic	Smooth muscle	Miosis
		Bronchoconstriction
		GI hyperactivity
	Glands	Increased secretion
	Heart	Bradycardia

ACh, Acetylcholine; *GI,* gastrointestinal.

   b. Spread: Absorbed through the skin or inhaled
   c. Examples: Tabun (GA), sarin (GB), soman (GD), VX
      (1) The G agents are volatile at room temperature.
      (2) VX is a persistent liquid and becomes volatile at high temperatures.
   d. Mechanism of action
      (1) Inhibition of acetylcholinesterase, leading to accumulation of acetylcholine and overstimulation of nicotinic and muscarinic receptors (**Table 29-6**).
      (2) The binding of nerve agents to acetylcholinesterase becomes irreversible over time through a process known as aging.
      (3) GD aging occurs very rapidly, with 50% irreversible binding in about 2 minutes.
      (4) Other agents age more slowly over periods of hours.
   e. Signs and symptoms
      (1) Cholinergic crisis
         (a) Bronchoconstriction
         (b) Apnea
         (c) Visual changes
         (d) Miosis
         (e) Urination
         (f) Diaphoresis
         (g) Defecation
         (h) Lacrimation
         (i) Emesis
         (j) Seizures
      (2) However, children may present atypically without miosis or the usual glandular muscarinic effects.
      (3) Following a significant exposure, children may present with only weakness and hypotonia.

29

  f. Treatment

   (1) Clinical management includes decontamination, triage, and administration of anticholinergics and antidotes.

   (2) Large doses of atropine may be necessary and should be administered until bronchospasm improves.

   (3) Oximes, including pralidoxime chloride (2-PAM), are specific antidotes for organophosphate poisoning.

    (a) Work by cleaving nerve agents from acetylcholinesterase; dramatically less effective after aging occurs.

    (b) Limited dosing data in children. Loading doses range from 15-20 mg/kg followed by continuous infusion of 50 mg/kg/hr for moderate to severe intoxication.

    (c) For adults, repeat doses may be given every hour.

    (d) However, the half-life of pralidoxime may be considerably longer in children.

    (e) Decreasing the dosage interval may be necessary.

   (4) Nerve agent–induced seizures are best treated with benzodiazepines; intramuscular midazolam may be the agent of choice.

   (5) Nonconvulsive status epilepticus should be considered in unconscious victims.

F. Strategies for decontamination

 1. Natural method

  a. Involves waiting it out because effects of contamination naturally decrease over time

  b. Too time-consuming and strongly influenced by weather

 2. Soap and water

  a. Requires large amounts of water

  b. Technique limited by availability of clean water and air temperature

  c. Must use passive water flow because pressurized water will drive contamination deeper

  d. Must avoid hot water because pores may open, contributing to deeper contamination

 3. Dry decontamination

  a. Useful when no water is available

  b. Technique isolates contaminants but will not neutralize them.

  c. Examples include Fuller's earth.

VII. Mass casualty

 A. Phases of care during mass casualty incidents

  1. **First phase: Ongoing arrival of patients**

   a. Magnitude of event is unknown.

   b. Communication at scene and possibly beyond is impaired.

  c. Conservation of key resources is the overriding concern.
  d. Patients may not arrive by emergency medical services.
   (1) May not be subject to triage or decontamination at the scene
   (2) Consider risk of secondary spread of biologic or chemical agents
  e. Transportation is difficult.
  f. Information may be unreliable.
  g. The nearest hospital will receive the greatest number of patients.
  h. Hospital security may require assistance from local police.
  i. Requests from the public and media for information will occupy more resources than expected.
 2. **Second phase: Represents definitive care**
  a. Achieved only after patients stop arriving at the hospital
  b. Involves retriage and reassignment of resources after prioritization is complete
B. Special considerations for children
 1. Children may arrive unaccompanied.
 2. Children may be more susceptible to unconventional weapons (see earlier) and may require a greater degree of monitoring postexposure.
 3. Children are at greater risk for hypothermia during decontamination.
 4. Consider designating a pediatric-only triage area.
  a. Permits staffing with pediatric specialists
  b. Concentrates resources
  c. Allows attention to be given to behavioral issues
 5. Psychological response and needs depend on age and developmental stage of the child.
  a. Anxiety, confusion, and fear are normal reactions.
  b. Risk of long-term emotional effects
C. Tactics to conserve resources during first phase of mass casualty event:
 1. Triage: Differs from usual method in that focus is on providing care to the maximum number of salvageable patients with the realization that the care may be suboptimal because of situational and environmental circumstances
 2. Minimal acceptable care: May be necessary to accept temporary suboptimal care and deliberately delay the definitive diagnosis and treatment of non–life-threatening injuries
 3. Goals for surgery: Strategy for the staged management of critically injured patients
  a. Restore patient stability without definitive anatomic reconstruction.

29

    (1) Short operating room time

    (2) Goals include the following:

     (a) Control of both bleeding and spillage of intestinal contents or urine

     (b) May involve temporary vascular shunts, abdominal packing, ligation of bowel, and temporary abdominal closure with artificial materials

  b. Definitive repair occurs later, during planned reoperation, after restoration of physiologic stability, including correction of hypothermia, coagulopathy, and acidosis.

VIII. Conclusions

 A. Disaster preparation requires coordination of multiple systems, provision of appropriate resources, and extensive planning on the part of health care organizations and government agencies.

 B. Health care providers must be familiar with the threat, response, and interventions indicated for possible incident scenarios.

 C. Practice and planning have vast potential to improve the response to mass casualty incidents and favorably affect outcome.

Chapter 30

Burns

Richard J. Redett, MD,
and Charles N. Paidas, MD, MBA

I. Overview

Burns are the third most common cause of injury-related death in children. Although major improvements in prehospital, intrahospital, and rehabilitative care have increased the numbers of survivors and the quality of their lives, permanent physical and psychological disability and suffering remain a heavy burden on survivors, families, health care delivery systems, and the taxpayer. In this chapter, we will discuss the epidemiology, pathophysiology, and Golden Hour management of pediatric burn patients. However, we must emphasize that prevention remains the best and most effective treatment method for these injuries.

II. Epidemiology in North America

A. Unintentional injury

1. Leading cause of death in children younger than 15 years

2. Burn deaths account for 12% to 14% of all accidental deaths in children to 10 years of age.

3. The incidence of accidental deaths caused by burns decreases to 4% in the 11- to 15-year age group.

B. Child abuse

1. Associated with up to 10% to 20% of burns in young children

2. *Stocking* distribution scald burn to the legs most common presentation

C. Scald injury

1. Most common burn in children younger than 5 years

2. Flame burns predominate in children older than 5 years

D. **Global death toll** from burns in children

1. Worldwide, the death rate from burns in children is 3.9 per 100,000 population. The highest rates are in infants.

2. The rate declines through childhood and then increases in the elderly. (World Health Organization, Global Burden of Disease, 2004).

E. **Overall survival** in massively burned children

1. Defined as more than 80% total body surface area (TBSA)

2. Survival has improved.

3. Many of these children recover and grow to be independent, with normal psychosocial adjustment and development.

F. **Young age:** Survival not worsened
G. Mortality
1. Increases with advancing age, TBSA burned, and presence of inhalation injury
2. Fire consumes oxygen (O_2) and may reduce O_2 concentration in an enclosed space to 10% to 11%.
3. Factors related to morbidity and mortality include the following:
   a. TBSA and depth of burn
   b. Hypoxemia
   c. Cellular anoxia (carbon monoxide [CO] poisoning).

III. Pathophysiology
All organ systems (as well as the psyche) are affected by a major burn; appropriate and timely interventions are based on understanding this fact.
A. Basic principles
1. The degree of tissue injury is proportional to the following:
   a. Length of exposure
   b. Temperature of the agent
   c. Inversely proportional to the age of the child (thinner skin)
2. The skin can tolerate temperatures up to 40° C for lengthy periods of time before tissue injury occurs.
3. In large burns, inflammatory mediators are released, causing a systemic inflammatory response leading to the following:
   a. Edema
   b. Fluid loss
   c. Circulatory stasis
   d. Protein and muscle breakdown
   e. Coagulopathies
   f. Impaired immunity
4. Significant metabolic responses include the following:
   a. Alterations of the hypothalamic-adrenal axis
   b. Insulin resistance
   c. Edema
   d. Severe catabolism
   e. Impaired gastrointestinal barrier function, resulting in translocation of bacteria
B. Burn wound zones
There are three concentric areas of vascular change in the soft tissue following a burn.
1. Zone of coagulation
   a. The center of the wound that represents the area of direct cellular injury secondary to the thermal effects of the burn

    b. The surface temperature of this area of the burn exceeds 45° C.
    c. This tissue is nonviable and there is no capacity for cellular repair or regeneration.
  2. Zone of stasis
    a. Extends peripherally from the zone of coagulation
    b. Characterized by regions of injured cells, vasoconstriction, and decreased perfusion
    c. Cellular viability depends on adequate fluid resuscitation and perfusion.
    d. Evaluation of tissue recovery or necrosis may require 2 to 3 days.
  3. Zone of hyperemia
    a. Lying further peripherally, this is the margin of the burn wound where cells have sustained minimal damage.
    b. With proper burn wound care, this area should recover in 7 to 10 days.
C. Scald injuries
  1. Skin thickness varies with age, gender, and body part.
  2. Infant skin may be less than half the thickness of adult skin.
  3. There is a logarithmic increase in tissue injury as the temperature rises above 40° C.
  4. Exposure to 70° C (158° F) results in full-thickness burns in less than 1 second.
  5. Exposure to 52° C (125° F) results in full-thickness burns in 2 minutes.
  6. Parents should be counseled to set hot water heaters at <48.9° C (120° F).
D. Fluid shifts
  1. Partial-thickness and full-thickness injuries result in the following:
    a. Increased capillary permeability
    b. Loss of intravascular oncotic pressure
    c. Edema formation
    d. Third spacing (sequestration) of large quantities of fluid
  2. Without the protection of the skin
    a. Fluid loss at the air-wound interface is high, 5 to 10 times greater than from undamaged skin.
    b. The larger surface area–to–weight ratio in children results in more fluid and body heat loss than adults.
E. Systemic manifestations
  1. Cardiovascular system
    a. Burn shock
      (1) Fluid losses, increased capillary permeability, decreased circulating blood volume, and release of

    toxins lead to a decreased cardiac output of
    approximately 20%.
    (2) The risk of burn shock increases significantly with
    burns >40% body surface area (BSA).
  b. With adequate fluid resuscitation, cardiac output returns
    to normal within 2 days.
2. Renal system
  a. Loss of fluid leads to renal artery vasoconstriction,
    reduced renal blood flow, and decreased glomerular
    filtration.
  b. Extensive tissue damage (e.g., electrical burns) may result
    in rhabdomyolysis, acute renal failure, and hyperkalemia.
3. Metabolism
  a. Hypermetabolism occurs with the metabolic rate
    increasing linearly to a maximum of 150% to 200%
    of normal in children older than 3 years with severe
    burns.
  b. The onset of hypermetabolism occurs within 24 to 36
    hours of the burn and lasts for up to 12 months.
  c. This leads to severe catabolism, with the following:
    (1) Decreased body weight
    (2) Negative nitrogen balance
    (3) Decreased energy stores
    (4) Anabolic hormones (e.g., human growth hormone,
      insulin growth factor) are decreased (in boys more
      than girls) for months after a severe burn.
F. Inhalation injuries
  1. Caused by products of incomplete combustion, toxic fumes,
    and/or direct thermal injury
  2. Most inhalation injuries occur in a closed space.
  3. Manifestations (radiographic and clinical) may not be
    apparent for 24 to 36 hours.
IV. Burn depth and extent
  See **Table 30-1.**
  A. Terminology
    Although still relevant, the more comprehensive terms of
    superficial, superficial-partial, deep-partial, and *full thickness*
    better describe the injury and method of treatment than first-,
    second-, and third-degree burns.
  B. Superficial (first degree)
    1. Injury involving only the epidermis
    2. Characterized by erythema, edema, pain, and absence of
      blisters (e.g., sunburn)
    3. Heal without scar formation, pigmentation changes, or
      contractures
  C. Partial thickness (second degree)

TABLE 30-1

CLASSIFICATION OF BURNS BASED ON DEPTH

	First Degree	Second Degree		Third Degree
Parameter	Superficial	Superficial-Partial Thickness	Deep-Partial Thickness	Full Thickness
Affected layers	Epidermis	Epidermis and superficial dermis	Epidermis and deep dermis	Epidermis, dermis, subcutaneous tissue
Causes	Sun, scald	Scald, flame	Prolonged scald, flame	Prolonged scald, flame, electrical, oil, chemical
Characteristics	Red	Red	Red or white	White or gray
	No blisters	Blisters	Blisters	No blisters
	Dry	Moist	Moist or dry	Dry
	Pain	Severe pain	Dull pressure	No sensation
	Brisk capillary refill	Delayed capillary refill	No capillary refill	No capillary refill

1. The injury extends from the epidermis into the dermis.
2. Partial-thickness injury can be superficial or deep.
   a. Superficial injury heals in 2 weeks and has minimal risk of scarring; structures such as nails, hair, and nerves are left intact and function without disruption.
   b. Deep-partial thickness burns require longer healing and have greater risk of scarring and disruption of nails and hair; itching and hypersensation are common.
3. Swelling, erythema, and pain: Hallmark is skin blisters.
D. Full thickness (third degree)
   1. The entire epidermis, dermis, and subcutaneous tissue are destroyed and require extensive healing times.
   2. Burned areas can be insensate, but itching and hypersensitivity in the affected area are common.
   3. Skin appears pale and leathery; scars and contractures are common.
E. Fourth degree
   1. Burn involves underlying muscle, tendon, or bone
F. Estimation of TBSA
   1. An age-specific chart based on the Lund and Browder diagram is used to estimate the TBSA (**Table 30-2** and **Fig. 30-1,** in that order).
   2. Assessment of the zone of stasis can make it difficult to determine the depth of the burn during the first 24 hours.
   3. Clinical evaluation by an experienced burn specialist is the most accurate means of determining burn depth and extent.

TABLE 30-2

BURN ESTIMATE (AGE VERSUS AREA)

| Area | Age (yr) | | | | | Degree of Burn | | |
	Birth-1	1-4	5-9	10-14	15	Second	Third	Total
Head	19	17	13	11	9			
Neck	2	2	2	2	2			
Anterior trunk	13	13	13	13	13			
Posterior trunk	13	13	13	13	13			
Right buttock	2½	2½	2½	2½	2½			
Left buttock	2½	2½	2½	2½	2½			
Genitalia	1	1	1	1	1			
Right upper arm	4	4	4	4	4			
Left upper arm	4	4	4	4	4			
Right lower arm	3	3	3	3	3			
Left lower arm	3	3	3	3	3			
Right hand	2½	2½	2½	2½	2½			
Left hand	2½	2½	2½	2½	2½			
Right thigh	5½	6½	8	8½	9			
Left thigh	5½	6½	8	8½	9			
Right leg	5	5	5½	6	6½			
Left leg	5	5	5½	6	6½			
Right foot	3½	3½	3½	3½	3½			
Left foot	3½	3½	3½	3½	3½			

G. American Burn Association (ABA) grading system
 1. The ABA uses extent, depth, age, and associated injuries to grade burns as minor, moderate, or major.
 2. A major or severe burn injury has the following characteristics:
  a. >10% TBSA in a child
  b. >5% full thickness
  c. Burn to face, eyes, ears, genitalia, or joints
  d. Known inhalation injury
  e. Known high-voltage injury
  f. Significant associated injuries
V. Primary survey and triage
 A. Overview
  1. As with all trauma patients, a field assessment of airway, breathing, and circulation must be performed rapidly (see Chapter 1).
  2. A quick assessment of the extent of the burn, as part of the primary survey, determines the need for intravenous (IV) access, fluid resuscitation, and possible transfer to a burn center.
  3. Signs and symptoms of inhalation injury should prompt early intubation.

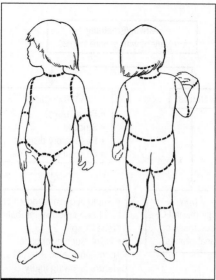

FIGURE 30-1

Total body surface area (TBSA). The areas demarcated in the figure correspond to the areas listed in Table 30-2. The surface area of a given body part varies by age, as noted in the table. TBSA is estimated by adding the percentages of all the burned areas found in the appropriate column based on the child's age.

4. Associated injuries influence field stabilization and transport to an appropriate first hospital.
5. Prior communication with the regional trauma or burn center will help facilitate prehospital care and triage.

B. Stop the burning process

General guidelines for prehospital care are as follows:

1. All patient clothing must be removed to prevent further burn injury and to allow completion of the primary survey.
   a. Intertriginous areas, such as axilla, groin, and perineum must be inspected for residual clothing.
   b. Local cooling is thought to improve perfusion if performed within the first 30 minutes.
   c. Care should be taken to prevent hypothermia.
2. In the case of a chemical burn, all contaminated clothing should be removed.
3. Electrical burn patients must not be touched by paramedics until the source of electricity has been deactivated or

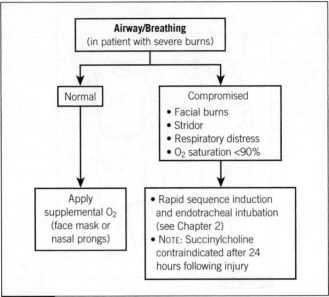

Airway/Breathing
(in patient with severe burns)

Normal

Compromised
- Facial burns
- Stridor
- Respiratory distress
- O_2 saturation <90%

Apply
supplemental O_2
(face mask or
nasal prongs)

- Rapid sequence induction
  and endotracheal intubation
  (see Chapter 2)
- NOTE: Succinylcholine
  contraindicated after 24
  hours following injury

FIGURE 30-2

Primary survey and emergency management of the airway and breathing in the child with a severe burn.

O_2, Oxygen.

    removed from the patient by means of a nonconducting
    material.
  C. Airway and breathing
    See **Figure 30-2.**
      1. Indications for immediate endotracheal intubation:
        a. Facial burns
        b. Singed eyebrows and nasal hairs
        c. Carbon deposits and inflammatory changes of the pharynx
           and nasal alae
        d. Carbonaceous sputum
        e. Stridor or hoarseness
        f. Retractions or respiratory distress
        g. Altered level of consciousness
        h. Restrictive ventilation secondary to circumferential
           full-thickness injury of the chest
      2. Patients with signs of inhalation injuries will require
         intubation, and delay will make intubation progressively more
         difficult.

3. Seek immediate surgical consultation for possible escharotomy if there is a full-thickness circumferential burn around the neck, chest, or extremities.
4. See Section XVI for treatment of inhalation injury including CO and cyanide (CN) poisoning.
   a. Suspect CO poisoning in comatose patient after house fires.
   b. CO poisoning may make mucous membranes cherry red.
5. Suspect CN poisoning in a comatose patient when a fire has been built with large amounts of burned plastics, polyurethane (insulation), synthetic rubber, or wool, silk, or nylon fibers.
6. Anticipate the need for frequent suctioning of the endotracheal tube (ETT).
   a. After the initial phase, burn tissue will begin to separate from the airway.
   b. This debris can occlude the airway.
   c. Frequent suctioning, humidification, and positioning of the ETT are crucial.
7. Inhalational injury can result in small airway disease (bronchospasm and bronchorrhea).
   a. β-Agonists and anticholinergics may improve symptoms.
   b. Steroids are usually reserved for patients with severe obstructive airway disease unresponsive to β-agonists or patients with a history of steroid-responsive asthma.

D. Circulation
   See **Figure 30-3.**
   1. Secure large-bore venous access, preferably in an unburned area.
   2. If unable to obtain IV access, intraosseous infusion should be used.
   3. Quickly estimate the TBSA involved in partial- and full-thickness burns.
   4. Initiate fluid therapy for thermal burns of >10% BSA in infants or >15% BSA in older children.
      a. Use the Parkland formula (see later).
      b. No first-degree burn should be included in the formula.
      c. Give half the calculated fluid volume in the first 8 hours and the remainder in the next 16 hours.
   5. Inhalational injury increases fluid requirements by approximately 6%.
   6. Catheterize the urinary bladder; urine output goal ≅ 1 mL/kg/hr
   7. Shock:
      a. Use Ringer's lactate solution
      b. Infuse 20 mL/kg aliquots rapidly until adequate circulation is restored.

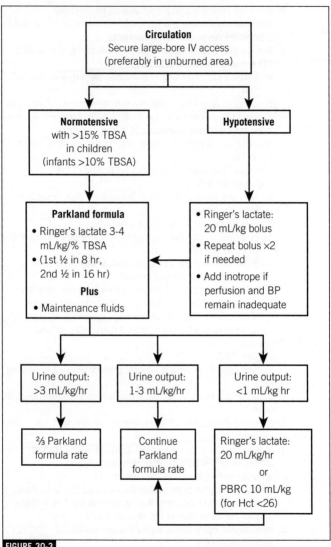

FIGURE 30-3

Primary survey and emergency management of the circulation and fluid administration based on the Parkland formula in the child with a severe burn. *BP*, Blood pressure; *Hct*, hematocrit; *IV*, intravenous; *PBRC*, packed red blood cells; *TBSA*, total body surface area.

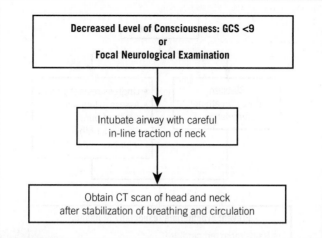

FIGURE 30-4

Primary survey and emergency management of (neurologic) disability in the child with a severe burn.

CT, Computed tomography; *GCS,* Glasgow Coma Scale.

8. Add inotropic support and initiate careful search for additional traumatic injuries if >60 cc/kg IV fluids via bolus has not restored adequate perfusion.
9. Communication with a burn center is helpful in guiding prehospital fluid resuscitation (see Fig. 30-3).

E. Disability and exposure
   1. Assess level of consciousness.
      a. For Glasgow Coma Scale (GCS) score <9: Intubate airway and obtain computed tomography scan of head and neck after patient has been stabilized (**Figure 30-4**).
   2. With large BSA–to–body weight ratio
      a. Additional evaporative heat loss is common through disruption of the cutaneous barrier.
      b. Patients can quickly become hypothermic.
   3. Warmed IV fluids and a heated room can help prevent hypothermia (**Figure 30-5**).
   4. Dry sterile or clean dressings should be used during transport to a burn center to prevent evaporative heat loss that occurs with damp dressings.
   5. Blankets or heating devices can maintain normal body temperature.

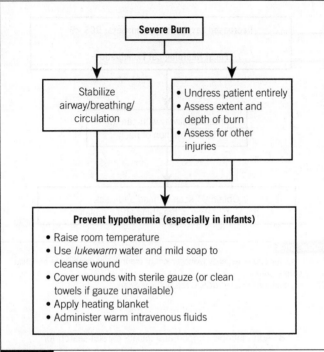

Severe Burn

Stabilize airway/breathing/circulation

- Undress patient entirely
- Assess extent and depth of burn
- Assess for other injuries

Prevent hypothermia (especially in infants)

- Raise room temperature
- Use *lukewarm* water and mild soap to cleanse wound
- Cover wounds with sterile gauze (or clean towels if gauze unavailable)
- Apply heating blanket
- Administer warm intravenous fluids

FIGURE 30-5

Primary survey and emergency management of exposure and prevention of hypothermia in the child with a severe burn.

F. Pain control
  1. Appropriate doses of opioids such as fentanyl (0.5 to 1 mcg/kg titrated every 5 minutes until effective) may be administered IV in the initial stages of resuscitation but only after the airway, breathing, and hemodynamic stability have been secured.
  2. See **Table 30-3.**
  3. See Section XIII for more details.
G. Tetanus immunization
  1. No tetanus immunization needed if patient is known to have received more than three tetanus immunizations, with the last dose given within 5 years.
  2. Give tetanus toxoid intramuscularly if patient is known to have received more than three tetanus immunizations, but time since last dose is more than 5 years.

TABLE 30-3

FENTANYL DOSING

Age (yr)	Dosage
1-3	2-3 mcg/kg IV q1-4h PRN
	Alt: 1-2 mcg/kg IV ×1, then 0.5-1 mcg/kg/hr infusion; titrate upward
3-12	1-2 mcg/kg IV q1-4h PRN
	Alt: 1-2 mcg/kg IV ×1, then 0.5-1 mcg/kg/hr infusion; titrate upward
>12	0.5-1 mcg/kg IV q1h

IV, Intravenous; *PRN,* as needed.

       a. Age younger than 7 years: DTaP (diphtheria–tetanus–acellular pertussis)
       b. Age 7 to 11 years: Td (adult tetanus)
       c. Age older than 11 years: Tdap (booster tetanus toxoid–reduced diphtheria toxoid–acellular pertussis)
   3. If tetanus immunization status unknown or patient has less than three tetanus immunizations:
       a. Give tetanus toxoid (as described earlier) *and*
       b. Give tetanus immune globulin, 250 international units intramuscularly, at a site different from the tetanus toxoid administration site.
  H. Wound dressing prior to transport
   1. If directed by burn center or if transport is delayed: Gently clean wounds with sterile gauze and the following:
       a. Tap water and mild soap *or*
       b. Sterile saline
   2. Cover burns with dry sterile gauze.
   3. Do not rupture blisters (decision to be made by burn center).
   4. Do not apply antibacterial ointments unless instructed to do so by the burn center.
  I. Criteria for transport to a burn center
   See **Box 30-1.**
VI. Secondary survey
  A. Reassess primary survey
  B. Circumstances of burn injury
   1. Type of burn: Flame, scald, electrical, chemical
   2. Possibility of inhalation injury
   3. Consider the possibility of child abuse.
  C. Complete systems examination noting any associated injuries such as the following:
   1. Thoracoabdominal injuries (see Chapters 21 and 22)
       a. Tension pneumothorax
       b. Flail chest, pulmonary contusion
       c. Solid organ injury with hemorrhage

30

BOX 30-1

CRITERIA FOR TRANSFER TO A BURN CENTER

BURN FEATURES

- Partial-thickness burn >10% total body surface area
- Any full-thickness burn
- Burns of face, neck, hands, feet, genitalia, or major joint
- Electrical burns (including lightening)
- Chemical burns (including caustic ingestion)

COMORBIDITY

- Any comorbidity that might complicate management, prolong recovery, or affect mortality
- Concomitant trauma—if the concomitant trauma is more severe than the burn, the patient should be referred to a trauma center first.

FACILITY

- A facility that lacks either personnel or equipment for the care of a child with a burn

---

    2. Orthopedic injuries
       a. Long bone or pelvic injuries
       b. Spinal injury
       c. Compartment syndrome
  D. Medical history
    Use the mnemonic AMPLE.
    1. **A:** Allergies
    2. **M:** Medications and immunizations
    3. **P:** Prior history of medical/respiratory problems
    4. **L:** Last meal
    5. **E:** Events related to the injury
  E. Pain assessment
    Age-appropriate drugs are discussed in Chapter 20.
  F. Gastric decompression
    1. Insert nasogastric tube to decompress the stomach in the patient with severe burns.
       a. Ileus is common in 15% to 20% BSA and will usually resolve within 72 hours.
       b. Prolonged ileus can be expected in larger burns and parenteral nutrition is often necessary.
    2. Begin enteral feedings via nasogastric tube as soon as hemodynamic stability and bowel motility have returned (see Section XI).
  G. Radiographs
    1. Chest (lung injury may take 24 to 36 hours to develop)
    2. Evaluation of associated injuries

H. Laboratory studies
   1. Complete blood count
   2. Electrolyte, blood urea nitrogen, creatinine levels
   3. Glucose: Early treatment of hyperglycemia with insulin may improve outcome.
   4. Type and crossmatch
   5. Arterial blood gas, co-oximetry, carboxyhemoglobin
I. Fluid resuscitation (see Fig. 30-3)
   1. Massive fluid, electrolyte and protein losses can be expected in the acute setting of a major burn.
   2. Early and adequate fluid resuscitation (see Fig. 30-3)
      a. Can reduce organ failure and mortality in pediatric burn patients
      b. Goal of the resuscitation is to restore hemodynamic stability and maintain organ perfusion and cell function while minimizing edema formation.
   3. Initiation of fluid resuscitation within 2 hours of thermal burn injury reduces the risk of sepsis, multiorgan failure, and mortality.
   4. Parkland formula
      a. Frequently used as a guide for calculating total isotonic fluid resuscitation volume during the first 24 hours
      b. Resuscitation volumes are based on the weight of the child and the extent of the partial- and full-thickness burn.
   5. Parkland formula: 4 mL/kg/TBSA burn (%) + maintenance fluid
      a. Half of total volume should be given during the first 8 hours after the burn.
         (1) This is when most of the fluid shifts occur.
         (2) If there is a delay in resuscitation, the missed volume of fluid should be given over the remaining time.
      b. The second half of the volume is infused over the following 16 hours.
      c. During the second 24 hours, postburn capillary wall integrity is usually restored and colloids can be given, if indicated.
   6. It is important to administer only the volume of fluid required to maintain an adequate urine output of 1 to 2 mL/kg/hr.
   7. Burned extremities are elevated to limit peripheral edema.
VII. Principles of burn wound management
   After the initial resuscitation and stabilization, wound care management becomes the priority to do the following:
   A. **Prevent** infection
   B. **Remove** necrotic tissue
   C. **Close** the wound

VIII. Burn wound management for superficial burns
  A. Wound care
    1. Clean the wound daily with lukewarm water and bland, nonperfumed soap.
    2. Pat with gauze or air-dry.
    3. Cover wounds with sterile, dry, nonadherent, porous gauze; if possible, secure with gauze rather than tape.
    4. Evaluate wound daily for redness, swelling, drainage, odor.
    5. An oral narcotic may be given 30 to 45 minutes before dressing change for patients with severe pain and anxiety (see Section XIII and Chapter 20 for guidelines).
    6. Encourage active patient and family participation in the dressing process.
    7. Wound healing is anticipated in 2 weeks for partial-thickness burns.
  B. Medications
    1. No antibiotic prophylaxis
    2. Steroids are not routinely used because of possible increased risk of pulmonary infection and death.
    3. However, there may be some demonstrable benefit to lung healing or pulmonary function with steroid use.
IX. Burn wound management for severe burns
  A. General comments
    1. Superficial partial-thickness burns can spontaneously reepithelialize in 2 to 3 weeks.
      a. Usually managed nonoperatively with topical therapy and dressing changes
      b. Any open blisters undergo superficial débridement.
    2. Indeterminate partial-thickness scald burns may be observed for up to 2 weeks to assess the need for operative intervention.
    3. Deeper burns require excision and grafting.
  B. Cleansing
    1. Maintain sterile technique during dressing changes
    2. Cleanse wounds once or twice daily (see Section VIII).
    3. Dressing changes for severe burn wounds usually require deep sedation with ketamine or propofol in addition to baseline narcotic analgesia.
    4. Protect against hypothermia by increasing room temperature, applying a heating blanket, and warming IV fluids.
    5. Topical antibiotic agents and dressings are dependent on the depth of the burn wound (see Section X).
    6. Elevate burned extremities.
  C. Escharotomy
    1. Indicated for full-thickness circumferential burns of the neck, chest, or extremities

2. More superficial circumferential burns should be monitored closely for signs of the following:
   a. Decreased distal perfusion
   b. Delayed capillary perfusion
   c. Diminishing pulses
   d. Worsening pain
   e. Sensory, vibratory loss
3. Compartment pressures >30 mm Hg are often the result of edema and fluid resuscitation and require escharatomy.
4. Escharotomies may need to be performed in noncircumferentially but badly burned extremities if tissue perfusion is threatened.
5. The escharotomy should be performed through the entire depth of the eschar and dermis.
6. Fasciotomy is rarely needed in routine thermal burns but may be indicated for the following:
   a. Very deep thermal burns
   b. High-voltage electrical injuries
   c. Patients with associated trauma if there is concern for vascular compromise

X. Topical antimicrobial wound care
   Properties of topical wound care agents are summarized here. Topical antimicrobials are designed to penetrate the wound surface and limit microbial proliferation in the wound.
   A. Silicone membrane-nylon fabric composite (biobrane) and fibronectin-coated skin substitute (TransCyte)
      1. Used for the management of clean, partial-thickness burns
      2. Should be applied during the first 24 hours
      3. Provides no antibacterial activity
      4. Promotes epithelialization
   B. Silver sulfadiazine 1%
      This is most commonly used.
      1. May be painful
      2. Apply daily in children (after cleansing and débridement).
      3. Cover with dry sterile dressing.
      4. Some gram-negative organisms may be resistant.
      5. Fair eschar penetration
      6. Contraindications
         a. Sulfa allergy (may substitute polymyxin-bacitracin)
         b. Infants younger than 2 months
      7. Adverse effects: Transient neutropenia
   C. Polymyxin-bacitracin
      1. Painless
      2. Limited antimicrobial activity
      3. Poor eschar penetration

4. Apply to small, partial-thickness flame burns or larger, partial-thickness scald burns.
5. Typically used for facial burns
6. Can cause conjunctivitis; ophthalmologic bacitracin should be used around the eyes.

D. Mafenide acetate

   5% solution = 50 g powder in 1 L saline or water

   1. Painful
   2. Broad antimicrobial activity
   3. Excellent eschar penetration
   4. Apply daily in children.
   5. Cover with dry sterile dressing.
   6. Contraindicated in patients with a sulfa allergy
   7. Adverse effects
      a. Myelosuppression
      b. Excoriation of new skin
      c. Metabolic acidosis secondary to carbonic anhydrase inhibition

E. Silver-coated wound dressing (acticoat)
   1. Can be painful with initial application; usually resolves quickly
   2. Broad antimicrobial activity
   3. Poor eschar penetration
   4. Apply every 3 to 5 days; primary advantage is reduced pain and cost of frequent dressing changes.
   5. Requires frequent wetting of the dressing; can cause hypothermia

XI. Nutritional support
   A. Overview
      1. Burn patients have very large caloric needs because of the hypermetabolic response to the burn injury.
      2. For patients with major burns, enteral supplementation or total parenteral support is often required.
      3. Enteral alimentation is much preferred.
         a. Helps maintain the integrity of the intestinal mucosa
         b. This in turn helps reduce translocation of bacteria across the intestinal wall and reduces the risk of gastric stress ulcers.
      4. Estimation of daily caloric requirement (**Table 30-4**)
      5. Place a nasoduodenal tube to begin feeding within 24 hours of the burn injury.
         a. Despite absent bowel sounds, the small bowel may maintain motility.
         b. Burn patients may continue transpyloric feedings before, during, and after surgery.

TABLE 30-4

FORMULA FOR CALORIC REQUIREMENTS IN CHILDREN WITH SEVERE BURNS*

Age (yr)	Daily Caloric Requirement
0-1	2100 kcal/m^2 BSA + 1000 kcal/m^2 burned surface area
1-11	1800 kcal/m^2 BSA + 1300 kcal/m^2 burned surface area
12-18	1500 kcal/m^2 BSA + 1500 kcal/m^2 burned surface area

BSA, Body surface area.
*Shriners Hospital for Children, Galveston, Tex.

6. Administer 5% or 25% albumin IV to prevent hypoalbuminemia if aggressive nutritional support fails to prevent hypoalbuminemia.
   a. Anticipate hypoalbuminemia when TBSA >40%.
   b. Hypoalbuminemia is common in severe burn victims because of capillary leak, protein catabolism, and decreased albumin production (secondary to the inflammatory response and malnutrition).
   c. Although controversial, albumin administration is at least not harmful and may decrease edema as well as improve survival.
7. Administer insulin infusion to maintain normoglycemia; although controversial, the preponderance of the evidence suggests that insulin therapy and normoglycemia do the following:
   a. Retard protein catabolism
   b. Decrease infections
   c. Decrease mortality in burned patients
8. Monitor nutritional progress with indirect calorimetry, urinary nitrogen excretion and nitrogen balance, and patient weight.
9. For burns >40% TBSA, a combination Oxandrolone (1 mg/kg once to twice a day) and beta blocker therapy (propranolol titrated to decrease tachycardia by 20% to 25%)
   a. Decreases the hypermetabolic response
   b. Increases lean body mass
   c. May improve outcome
10. Administer histamine receptor blockers (e.g., ranitidine) to reduce the risk of gastric stress ulcers.
11. Ileus is common with larger burns but usually resolves within 72 hours.
    a. Gastric decompression should be started presumptively after the airway has been secured.
    b. Parenteral nutrition should be converted to enteral feeding as soon as possible after ileus has improved.

30

XII. Burn wound infection and sepsis
  A. Overview
    1. Infection can be a major cause of morbidity and mortality in burn patients.
    2. The most common type of infection in pediatric burn patients is pneumonia (50% of all infections), followed by burn wound sepsis and urinary tract infections.
    3. Immediately after a burn, cutaneous bacterial growth is sparse.
    4. Gram-positive organisms soon predominate but are replaced by gram-negative bacteria from the gut within the first week following the burn.
    5. Burn wound excision and the appropriate use of topical and systemic antibiotics significantly reduce the risk of burn wound infections.
  B. Factors that contribute to infection in burn patients
    1. Generalized immunosuppression
    2. Reduced blood flow to the zone of stasis results in a decrease in the number of white blood cells and humoral immune factors available to fight infection.
    3. Nonviable tissue in the zone of coagulation provides an excellent medium for bacterial growth.
  C. Diagnosis of burn wound infection
    1. Tissue bacterial counts
      a. Surveillance can be performed with quantitative bacterial counts of burned tissue.
      b. Patients with bacterial counts less than 105 organisms/g of tissue usually have low risk of burn wound sepsis or graft loss.
      c. In contrast, bacterial counts greater than 105 organisms/g of tissue are associated with a 50% increased incidence of burn wound sepsis and skin graft loss.
      d. Thus, bacterial counts greater than 105 organisms/g of tissue can warrant treatment with systemic antibiotics, *if* signs of local or systemic infection are present.
    2. Signs
      a. Progression of burn wound depth from partial to full thickness
      b. Worsening erythema
      c. Dark discoloration of burn wound
      d. Systemic signs (fever, hypotension)
      e. New hyperdynamic cardiovascular state after the acute burn period
      f. Leukocytosis, thrombocytopenia, elevation of creatinine level
      g. Hypothermia or hyperthermia
      h. Diminished urine output despite adequate resuscitation

D. Treatment
   1. Antibiotic therapy should initially be broad spectrum and later tailored, based on culture results.
   2. Although the role of systemic antibiotics in treating pneumonia and urinary tract infections is uncontested, burn eschar excision is the most effective means of treating burn wound sepsis.
   3. **There is no proven role for prophylactic antibiotics.**

XIII. Pain control

Pain control is crucial. Comfort measures must be implemented for pain, suffering, anxiety, pruritus, and sleep disruption. The types of pain that must be treated include pain at rest, procedure-related pain, and psychic pain (e.g., suffering, loss of body image).

A. Pain at rest
   1. Nonpharmacologic comfort measures
      a. These include distraction with music, TV, and toys; positive reinforcement needs to be implemented from the onset.
      b. The use of child life resources with parental and patient's active involvement is crucial.
   2. Severe burns
      a. IV patient-controlled anesthesia with morphine or fentanyl is often required during the first 24 to 48 hours.
      b. A basal infusion is appropriate (see Chapter 20).
   3. Extended relief
      a. Enterally administered opioids (e.g., MS Contin, OxyContin, methadone) for moderate to severe ongoing pain
      b. Liquid methadone may be given via a feeding tube.
      c. Sustained-release tablets cannot be given by the feeding tube route.
   4. Oxycodone (0.1 mg/kg/dose every 4 to 6 hours) for mild to moderate pain (i.e., healing of a partial-thickness burn wound)
   5. Weak analgesics with antipyretic activity every 4 to 6 hours for fever or mild pain
      a. Ibuprofen (6 to 10 mg/kg)
      b. Acetaminophen (15 mg/kg)

B. Procedure-related pain

Moderate to deep sedation is the rule; occasionally, general anesthesia will be required. Sedation, analgesia, amnesia, and immobility are the essential components needed for both the patient and staff to ensure success. There is never a need to induce more suffering in these patients. Monitoring, particularly for efficacy of sedation and pain control and for adequacy of ventilation, is vital. All the drugs listed here are titrated to effect.

1. IV opioids, usually fentanyl (0.5 to 1 mcg/kg), are the mainstay analgesic drugs.
   a. Given every 3 to 5 minutes and titrated to patient comfort, respiratory function, and O_2 saturation (SaO_2)
   b. Opioids are administered using the patient-controlled analgesia demand function or bolus dosing.
2. IV benzodiazepines, usually midazolam (0.05 to 0.1 mg/kg), are the mainstay sedative, anxiolytic, and amnestic drugs and are given every 3 to 5 minutes and titrated similarly. (**WARNING: There is an increased incidence of apnea when opioids are combined with benzodiazepines. Be prepared to administer naloxone. Monitor the patient's vital signs and O_2 saturation. Be prepared to provide respiratory support.**
3. IV ketamine, a dissociative general anesthetic agent
   a. May be used by practitioners skilled in its use or for patients who are already intubated
   b. Dose, 0.5 mg/kg every 3 to 5 minutes as needed
4. Oral opioids and/or amnestics (midazolam, diazepam) should be given 30 to 45 minutes before the procedure to allow the drug to reach its peak action during the procedure.
5. Oral transmucosal fentanyl (10 to 15 mcg/kg) is very effective and is given 10 to 15 minutes before the procedure.

XIV. Burn wound excision and skin grafting
  A. Overview
    1. Early excision and grafting (less than 24 to 48 hours from the time of injury) should be considered the treatment of choice for all burns that will not heal spontaneously in 2 to 3 weeks.
    2. Burn eschar bacterial colonization occurs within 24 hours following the burn.
    3. Early excision is advocated to reduce the incidence of burn sepsis and graft loss.
    4. Burn wound excision can be performed as soon as the patient is assessed and stabilized.
    5. The resuscitation can safely be continued during surgery.
  B. Types of excision
    1. Tangential excision, down to healthy bleeding tissue, with a Goulian or Humby dermatome, is performed for most burns.
    2. Fascial excision is required for burns that are very deep.
      a. This can be performed with electrocautery.
      b. Blood loss is considerably less with fascial excision.
  C. Grafting
    1. Split-thickness skin grafts can be harvested from the back, legs, buttocks, abdomen, and scalp.
    2. The scalp is an excellent donor site for facial burns.
    3. Care must be taken to preserve the hair follicles.

4. Skin can be reharvested from healed donor sites, which is particularly helpful in large burns.
5. Grafts can be meshed at a ratio of 1.5:1 or 3:1 to increase their surface area and allow for efflux of effluent; unmeshed sheet grafts are used in smaller burns or in areas where cosmesis is of major concern (e.g., the face).
6. Cultured epithelial autografts (CEAs) are useful for massively burned children in whom donor sites are limited.
   a. An area of skin is biopsied on admission and grown in culture.
   b. Although a CEA can provide large quantities of skin, it is generally expensive, fragile, and less resistant to infection.
7. Human cadaveric allograft can be used while waiting for donor sites to reepithelialize for future use.
8. Blood loss is estimated at 0.5 mL/cm^2 of tissue to be excised.
   a. Blood loss is replaced during the operative procedure.
   b. Blood loss can be minimized with the use of the following:
      (1) Extremity tourniquets
      (2) Subcutaneous epinephrine clysis
      (3) Maintenance of normal body temperature

XV. Skin graft management by percentage of burn
   A. Burns <30% TBSA
      1. Excision and autografting: Meshed 1.5:1 or sheet grafts
      2. Unmeshed sheet grafts should be placed on all vital areas—face, neck, and hands.
   B. Burns = 30% to 40% TBSA
      1. Excision and grafting: Sufficient donor sites are usually available to graft the excised areas despite the fact that about 20% to 30% TBSA is unavailable for donor site (face, neck, hands, feet).
      2. Grafts should be meshed 1.5:1 or 3:1, or temporary allografts should be used while donor sites are healing.
   C. Burns >40% TBSA
      1. Excision and grafting donor sites are limited.
         a. It is impossible to cover all the excised wounds with an autograft.
         b. We typically excise 20% to 30% TBSA/day and mesh the autograft 1.5:1, 2:1, or 3:1.
         c. If the autograft is meshed 3:1, an allograft should be used as overlay to close the wide interstices.
         d. Cultured epidermis can also be used.

XVI. Inhalation injury
   A. Overview
      1. Occurs in 30% of patients with major burns
      2. More common in enclosed spaces

3. Most deaths caused by smoke inhalation are from asphyxia; fire consumes O_2 and can reduce the fraction of inspired O_2 to 10% in an enclosed space.
4. Inhalation of superheated gases causes direct injury to the tracheobronchial tree.
5. The noxious byproducts of combustion, including hydrogen cyanide, injure respiratory mucosa and cause hemorrhage.

B. Carbon monoxide
   1. CO (**Fig. 30-6**) has a high affinity for hemoglobin-binding sites (200 times that of O_2), causing tissue hypoxia and direct cytotoxic effects.
   2. Half-life of carboxyhemoglobin
      a. 4 hours in room air
      b. Reduced to 40 minutes on 100% O_2 and 25 minutes with O_2 delivered at 3 atmospheres of pressure
   3. Patients become symptomatic with carboxyhemoglobin levels of >20%.
   4. Carboxyhemoglobin levels of >60% are fatal.
   5. Management includes the following:
      a. Measurement of arterial blood gas carboxyhemoglobin levels
      b. Prompt administration of 100% O_2.

C. Signs and symptoms of smoke inhalation
   1. Hoarseness, stridor, and wheezing
   2. Hypoxia, hypercapnia
   3. Facial burns
   4. Singed facial hairs
   5. Carbonaceous sputum or soot in the oropharynx
   6. History of a burn in a closed-space area, such as a burning room, car, or tent
   7. Altered level of consciousness

D. Diagnostic studies
   1. SaO_2
   2. Arterial blood gas
   3. Carboxyhemoglobin level
   4. Chest radiographic changes may take 24 to 36 hours to become apparent.
   5. Bronchoscopy

E. Treatment
   1. Endotracheal intubation when signs and symptoms of significant inhalation injury are present
   2. Delayed intubation can be difficult secondary to airway swelling and secretions.
   3. Intensive care unit observation for smoke inhalation injuries
   4. Warm humidified O_2
   5. Bronchodilators, postural drainage, chest physiotherapy, and suctioning

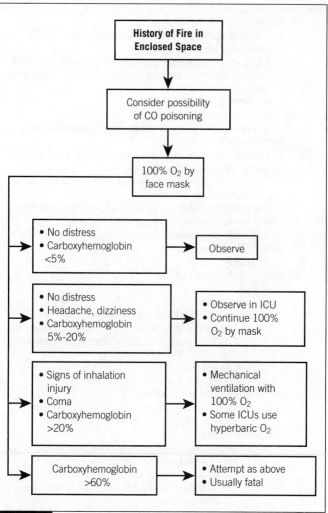

FIGURE 30-6

Recognition and management of carbon monoxide poisoning in the child with smoke inhalation.

CO, Carbon monoxide; *ICU;* intensive care unit; *O₂,* oxygen.

XVII. Electrical injuries
  A. Epidemiology
    1. Electrical injuries account for 1000 deaths and 20,000 emergency room visits/year.
    2. 5% of all burn admissions are caused by electrical injuries.
    3. Common causes of electrical injuries in children include the following:
      a. Chewing on electrical cords
      b. Placement of objects into household outlets
      c. Contact with overhead power lines during play activity
  B. Pathophysiology
    1. Electrical burns result from the conversion of electrical energy into heat.
    2. Injury also occurs from the disruption of the body's normal electrical activity.
    3. High-voltage current can cause depolarization of the heart and nervous system, resulting in the following:
      a. Cardiac arrhythmias
      b. Unconsciousness
      c. Apnea
  C. Determinants of extent of injury
    1. Voltage
      a. Low voltage
        (1) Household current (110 to 440 V)
        (2) Most household current is 110 V (United States) or 220 V (Europe, Asia); some larger appliances require 110 to 240 V
      b. High voltage: >1000 V
        (1) Overhead power lines and transformers
        (2) High tension: >1000 V
        (3) Lightning: May involve a single blast of current equivalent to 2000 to 2 billion V of electricity.
    2. Type of current
      a. Alternating current (AC) versus direct current (DC)
        (1) Most low-voltage and high-voltage current is AC.
          (a) AC current produces sustained muscle contraction (tetany), causing the nonrelease phenomenon.
          (b) AC injuries are associated with higher morbidity and mortality than DC injuries.
        (2) DC current (e.g., lightening bolt)
          (a) Produces a single muscle contraction and large release, often causing the victim to be thrown from the source
          (b) Hence, blunt trauma often accompanies DC injuries.

    3. Resistance of body tissue to the path of current
        a. Skin (especially when dry) > bone > blood vessels
           > nerves
    4. Duration of contact
    5. Arc burns
        a. The result of current hitting the skin but not penetrating
           the body
        b. The ionization of air particles between conductors (e.g.,
           body parts) generates massive amounts of heat that can
           produce flame (arc) burns.
 D. Primary survey and cardiopulmonary resuscitation (CPR)
    See Chapters 1 and 5.
    1. Along with the thermal burn, high-voltage electrical injuries
       can result in numerous cardiac abnormalities, necessitating
       securing the airway and commencing CPR.
    2. If the patient is found in cardiac arrest after an electrical
       injury, asystole is the common dysrhythmia after a lightening
       strike; ventricular fibrillation is the more common
       dysrhythmia after injury from household current or high-
       voltage power lines.
    3. Tetanic contraction of respiratory muscles presents as a
       respiratory arrest.
    4. Ensure that the patient has been separated from the power
       source before attempting CPR.
    5. Sustained resuscitative efforts are indicated despite a GCS of
       3 and/or fixed pupils; paralysis and/or autonomic dysfunction
       may cause these neurologic abnormalities.
 E. Secondary survey
    See Chapter 1.
    1. Identify entrance and exit wounds.
    2. Beware of associated injuries, such as bony injuries and
       compartment syndrome.
    3. Superficial wounds often markedly underestimate the extent
       of deep tissue injury.
    4. Organ-specific considerations
        a. Cardiovascular
           (1) As many as 25% of patients have cardiac arrhythmias
               (usually occur with high-voltage injuries).
           (2) Sudden death from asystole or ventricular fibrillation
               can result from massive depolarization of the heart
               after high-tension injuries.
           (3) Cardiac injuries are more common when current
               crosses from hand to hand.
        b. Gastrointestinal
           (1) Possible intraperitoneal damage because of the
               low-resistance mesenteric vascular system

30

      c. Renal (rhabdomyolysis management)
         (1) Rhabdomyolysis and myoglobinuria may result from severe electrical burns.
         (2) Fluid (at 1.5 to 2 times maintenance rates) should be administered to maintain urine output of 3 to 5 mL/kg/hr.
         (3) Mannitol (250 to 500 mg/kg IV) can be administered as a bolus to improve urine output.
         (4) Urine should be alkalinized with the addition of sodium bicarbonate to IV fluids.
   F. Laboratory studies
     1. Full laboratory workup as described for thermal injuries; in addition, urine should be checked for myoglobin.
     2. Cardiac enzyme levels (creatine kinase MB fraction or troponin) do not reliably predict the extent of myocardial injury.
     3. Monitor for hyperkalemia.
   G. Imaging studies
     1. Chest radiograph
     2. Bone radiographs if high suspicion for related orthopedic injury

XVIII. Chemical burns
   A. Epidemiology
     1. Most chemical burns in adults are a result of industrial accidents.
     2. National prevention initiatives have made them much less common.
     3. However, because of the higher ratio of BSA to weight, these injuries can be lethal in children.
     4. Most chemical burns in children result from inadvertent exposure to common household products.
   B. Pathophysiology
   The extent of tissue damage is dependent on a number of factors as follows:
     1. Nature of the chemical
     2. Quantity of the chemical
     3. Concentration of the chemical
     4. Length of the exposure
     5. Delay in treatment
     6. Mechanism of action
     7. Chemical agents injure tissue through corrosion, dehydration, oxidation, dessication, and denaturation.
   C. Treatment
     1. Primary and secondary surveys
     2. General treatment involves the following:
       a. Removing the contaminated clothing
       b. Instituting copious irrigation of the burned area

      c. Irrigation should be started as soon as possible and should continue for at least 30 minutes initially.

      d. Irrigation may be required for up to 12 hours.

XIX. Treatment considerations for specific chemical agents

  A. Hydrofluoric acid

    1. Injury through denaturation

    2. Irrigate with water to remove hydrogen ions.

    3. Inject 10% calcium gluconate (0.5 mL/cm^2) subcutaneously into multiple sites in and around the burn.

    4. Fumes have toxic effects on the lungs and can cause pulmonary edema.

  B. Gasoline

    1. Injury through dessication

    2. Irrigate with water.

    3. Excreted by the lungs; inhibits surfactant, causing atelectasis and pulmonary infiltrates

    4. Progressive liver and kidney failure with large exposures

  C. Phenol

    1. Injury through corrosion

    2. Aromatic hydrocarbon derived from coal tar

    3. Apply polyethylene glycol or vegetable oil to burns.

    4. Skin appears grey and may turn black.

    5. Monitor electrocardiogram (ECG)—significant risk of cardiac arrhythmias

  D. Phosphorus

    1. Injury through corrosion

    2. Can ignite if allowed to desiccate

    3. Mechanically remove individual phosphorus particles.

    4. Irrigate with 2% copper sulfate.

    5. Monitor ECG—T wave and ST changes

    6. Can cause renal failure

30

Chapter 31

Child Abuse
Allen R. Walker, MD, MBA

I. Background
   A. Epidemiology
      1. Incidence: Maltreatment of children, including physical, sexual, and emotional abuse and neglect, is based on the number of report-based counts of child victims; reporting is not uniform throughout the United States.
         a. The U.S. National Child Abuse and Neglect Data System (NCANDS) reported a maltreatment rate of 11 per 1000 children in 2007.
         b. Young children are the most common victims; in 2007, NCANDS reported the following rates per 1000 children:
            (1) 22, younger than 1 year
            (2) 13, ages 1-3 years
            (3) 12, ages 4-7 years
            (4) 9, ages 8-11 years
            (5) 9, ages 12-15 years
            (6) 5, ages 16-17 years
         c. Neglect is the most common type of maltreatment reported in the United States; highest in the 0- to 3-year age group.
            (1) The type of maltreatment varies by age.
            (2) Among NCANDS-reported cases, physical and sexual abuse was highest in the 16- to 17-year age range.
      2. Increased risk
         a. Abused children are at risk for repeated episodes of abuse, including escalating severity of injury.
         b. Such events, including lethal insults, can even happen during hospitalization.
      3. Mortality rate and profile
         a. The Child Welfare Information Getaway, published by the Administration on Children, Youth and Families, reported an estimated 1760 child fatalities (ages 0 to 17 years) in 2007, which corresponds to a rate of 2.35/100,000 children (http://www.childwelfare.gov/pubs/factsheets/fatality.cfm). See **Box 31-1.**
         b. Over 5 years (2002-2006), this number steadily increased.
         c. Almost half of these nonaccidental deaths are children younger than 1 year of age, and children younger than 4 years make up 75% of total fatalities.

BOX 31-1

CAUSES OF FATAL CHILD ABUSE

- Asphyxiation
- Blunt thoraco-abdominal injury
- Burn injuries
- Drowning, aspiration
- Exposure to temperature extremes
- Gunshot wound
- Head injury
- Poisoning
- Sepsis, inadequately treated infection
- Stab wound
- Starvation, dehydration

   d. In 75% of cases reported in 2007, the perpetrator was an individual (or individuals) responsible for the care and supervision of the child.
   e. Although there is no single profile for perpetrators of fatal abuse cases, reappearing characteristics include the following:
   (1) Young adult (male or female) in the mid-20s
   (2) No high school diploma
   (3) Living at or below the poverty level
   (4) Depressed
   (5) Experienced violence firsthand
   (6) Has difficulty coping with stress
4. Chronic morbidity: Long-term sequelae of childhood maltreatment include the following:
   a. Low-level scholastic performance
   b. Juvenile delinquency
   c. Substance abuse
   d. Mental health disorders
5. Global perspective
   The International Society for the Prevention of Child Abuse and Neglect, in its *World Perspective on Child Abuse* (8th ed., 2008), reported emerging agreement that sexual and physical abuse, children living on the streets, and childhood prostitution are the worldwide behaviors constituting abuse and neglect.
B. Role of medical personnel
1. Roles
   Medical personnel suspect, diagnose, treat, report, and document nonaccidental trauma and child maltreatment. They are also concerned with prevention.
2. Child protective teams
   a. The approach to child abuse is a team effort, involving hospital personnel (social work, nursing, and medicine) and community agencies (police, social services, prosecutors) concerned with the welfare of children and families.

b. Many hospitals now have child protective service teams, and their interaction with state agencies such as the Department of Children and Families is invaluable.

3. Suspicion of child maltreatment is based on the following:
   a. Inadequate, inconsistent, or changing history of injury
   b. Discrepancy between severity of injury and history of injury
   c. Suspicious patterns of injury
   d. History of delay in seeking medical attention
   e. Parental substance abuse
   f. Inappropriate parental response to medical professionals

4. Differential diagnosis
   a. Child abuse may be difficult to differentiate from sudden infant death syndrome (SIDS) or other diseases at the first encounter.
   b. Therefore, a nonaccusatory manner works best.

5. Reporting requirements
   a. All health care providers in the United States are obligated by law to report cases of suspected maltreatment to either the local police and/or child welfare agencies.
   b. All states are required to have a toll-free reporting hotline.
      (1) Verbal reports should be made within 24 hours of presentation.
      (2) Health care workers are protected from prosecution when they report suspected cases.
      (3) Reports should not wait until maltreatment can be proven.
      (4) Suspicions should be based on objective evidence.
         (a) Failure to diagnose and/or report renders the professional liable.
   c. The likelihood of adverse parental responses may be lessened by the following:
      (1) Telling the family about the nature of the concern and the obligation to report on behalf of the patient
      (2) Carefully documenting the basis for concern, including verifying information given by other providers
      (3) Having the health care team reach consensus on the need for a report and letting the family know that the decision is supported by all members of the team

6. Documentation
   a. Document the caretaker's explanation in writing and verbatim when possible.
   b. Obtain labeled photographs of relevant injuries when possible.
      (1) Include a measurement scale in photographs.

   (2) Include the patient's name and date of birth, and date
    photo was taken as a label on digital or hardcopy
    photos.
  c. Draw pictures of body surfaces and describe injuries in
   terms of length, width, texture, and color.
  d. Admission orders should state the facts, such as the
   following:
   (1) Physical findings and history are not compatible.
   (2) Admitting diagnosis can be "Rule out nonaccidental
    trauma."
 7. Focus on the child's needs, not the parent's shortcomings.
  a. If in doubt, give the benefit of the doubt to the child,
   because children cannot protect themselves.
  b. Nevertheless, do not alienate the parents, if possible,
   because the social service system will need to work with
   them extensively.

II. Shaken baby syndrome
 A. Definition
  1. A constellation of intracranial injuries, including the
   following:
   a. Subdural hematoma, other central nervous system (CNS)
    hemorrhages, fractured skull, retinal hemorrhages, and
    bone fractures in young infants
   b. Not all findings are present in all victims.
  2. Subdural hemorrhage with or without a skull fracture is not
   usually associated with a minor fall (<4 feet).
  3. Median age: 6 months
  4. Survivors often have long-term neurologic sequelae such as
   mental retardation, cerebral palsy, or paralysis.
 B. Cause
  1. Reflects violent shaking with acceleration-deceleration CNS
   injury
  2. May involve striking the head against an object
  3. Diffuse axonal injury and more extensive shear injury deep in
   white matter may be found.
 C. Symptoms
  Shaken baby syndrome usually presents with symptoms
  suggesting acute neurologic injury.
  1. Seizures
  2. Apnea
  3. Lethargy
  4. Irritability
  5. Vomiting
 D. Physical examination
  1. May be unrevealing
  2. Vital signs often abnormal

31

3. Ophthalmology examination
   a. May show retinal hemorrhages and occasionally optic atrophy, retinal detachment, and macular schisis
   b. Retinal hemorrhage is rarely associated with the following:
      (1) Severe head trauma
      (2) Birth trauma
      (3) Cardiopulmonary resuscitation (CPR)
      (4) Hematologic disease
      (5) Vascular malformation
   c. Recognition of retinal hemorrhages mandates consideration of abuse.

E. Diagnostic testing
   1. Computed tomography (CT) brain scan may reveal subdural hematoma, atrophy, hygroma, or other pattern of cerebral hemorrhage. Atrophy and hygroma are consistent with chronic abuse.
   2. None of these CT findings are specific to abuse, although mixed-density (as opposed to homogeneous) subdural hematoma is more frequent in abused infants (because it likely represents hematomas of different ages).
   3. Radiographs of all long bones and the ribs ("skeletal survey") should be obtained whenever the diagnosis of shaken baby syndrome is entertained.

III. Patterned or suspicious cutaneous lesions
   A. Bites
      Human (versus animal) bites usually crush more than lacerate.
      1. Circular or oval, with an obvious impression from the canines (adult human intercanine distance is generally >3 cm).
      2. Forensic odontologists may help identify the perpetrator.
      3. Photographs and deoxyribonucleic acid (DNA) testing of the skin surface are helpful if done immediately.
   B. Burns
      These include scalds, patterned burns, electrical burns, and chemical burns. Consider abuse if burn injury from fire is caused by neglect.
      1. Scalds: Most frequent burn injury
         a. Usually associated with tap water
         b. Quick, forced immersion in hot water usually leaves no splash or run marks and a sharp demarcation between burned and normal skin, often with trunk burn injury and sparing of the following:
            (1) Central buttocks (caused by the cooler porcelain)
            (2) Inguinal and abdominal wall creases (caused by flexion)
            (3) Soles of the feet (because of thicker skin)
         c. Accidental immersion is often characterized by splash and run marks as the child struggles to get away.

    d. Clothing worn at the time of forced immersion may alter the pattern by retaining hot liquids close to the skin, leaving an outline of elastic or fold of clothing.

    e. Observation over several hours or débridement may be required before a pattern emerges.

  2. Patterned burns may be caused by the following:

    a. Cigarettes (7 to 10 mm in diameter with deeper central ulcer)

    b. Irons, curling irons, or other appliances

    c. Usually well-demarcated and deeper than accidental burn injuries

C. Contusions

  1. Epidemiology

    a. Progression of colors confirms lesion as a contusion or bruise (as opposed to a Mongolian spot)

    b. Color changes may not be helpful for purposes of dating the injury.

  2. Contusions and abrasions are rare in infants younger than 6 months who are not yet mobile.

  3. Definitions

    a. Ecchymosis: Hemorrhage in subcutaneous tissue

    b. Hematoma: Any collection of extravasated blood

    c. Petechiae: Hemorrhages in the dermis <3 mm in diameter, which may be associated with the following:

      (1) Asphyxia, strangulation (neck)

      (2) Binding (wrists, ankles)

      (3) Gagging (oral commissures)

      (4) Foreign objects (oral mucosa)

  4. Location

    a. Hematomas over relatively protected areas (upper arms, thighs, hands, trunk, neck, ears, abdominal wall, and genitalia) are suggestive of nonaccidental trauma in the absence of a consistent history.

    b. Abdominal wall ecchymosis in this context mandates a search for internal injury, because significant blunt trauma is usually required to produce the injury.

    c. Small abrasions over the eyes or face may be self-inflicted in young infants with long fingernails.

  5. Appearance: The shape of an ecchymosis may become more distinct with time, suggesting the responsible object (whereas petechiae are characterized by sharp borders).

  6. Hematoma pattern or extent

    a. May suggest a hemorrhagic diathesis

    b. Coagulation workup, including complete blood count (CBC), international normalized ratio, partial thromboplastin time, and fibrinogen, at a minimum, is indicated in selected patients.

IV. Physical examination
  A. General considerations
    1. The often misleading history does not typically provide the correct diagnosis in cases of child abuse.
    2. Most diagnoses are made from physical and/or laboratory examinations.
    3. The physical examination of acutely injured, ill victims of abuse includes the elements of any standard trauma evaluation.
  B. Primary survey
    Perform the primary survey as in any general trauma case (see Chapter 1).
  C. Secondary survey
    Complete physical examination.
    1. Should proceed concurrently with ongoing resuscitation efforts by a multidisciplinary team
    2. Specific findings
      a. Evidence of neglect or poor hygiene may suggest nonaccidental trauma.
      b. The examination may change markedly over the first few hours following injury.
      c. As with any trauma patient, pay strict attention to avoid secondary injury caused by persistent or recurrent hypoxemia or hypoperfusion.
V. Laboratory studies
  A. General considerations
    1. Laboratory tests
      a. CBC
      b. Electrolyte levels with renal function tests
      c. Liver function tests
      d. Amylase, lipase levels
      e. Urinalysis to screen for occult blood
      f. Toxicology screen
    2. Radiology
      a. CT scans of head, chest, abdomen, and pelvis
      b. Skeletal survey
    3. Ophthalmology examination
  B. Laboratory examinations for children with specific presentations
    1. Sudden and unexplained infant death
      a. Blood, urine, and other secretions should be sent for metabolic and infectious disease workup.
      b. Skin biopsy (2-4 mm wide sample) for fibroblasts and workup of metabolic disease
        (1) Requirements include:
          (a) Signed consent by the parent/guardian
          (b) Strict aseptic technique
          (c) Prior notification of the receiving lab

      c. An autopsy, which may include postmortem imaging (i.e., a skeletal survey), is essential.

      d. A multidisciplinary mortality review by a specialized team is helpful when risk factors suggest the possibility of intentional asphyxia.

2. Infants or young children with possible abuse and bone fracture(s)

    a. Skeletal survey

      (1) Neither a skeletal survey nor bone scans are 100% sensitive or specific for fractures.

      (2) Skeletal survey is less costly, more readily available, more sensitive at detecting bilateral lesions and fractures that may be obscured by areas of rapid bone growth, and uses less radiation.

    b. Workup for bone fragility

      (1) CBC, calcium, phosphorus, and alkaline phosphatase levels

      (2) If hypocalcemia and hyperphosphatemia are present or rickets is suspected, check vitamin D levels.

      (3) Other tests for selected patients

        (a) Serum copper level

        (b) DNA sequencing

        (c) Skin biopsy (for osteogenesis imperfecta) **Box 31-2**

3. Infants or children with possible abuse and acute neurologic injury

    a. CT scans of head, chest, abdomen, and pelvis

      (1) Head CT identifies all lesions requiring immediate surgical intervention, but may miss subtle manifestations of abuse.

      (2) CT scan does not delineate the age of a lesion as well as magnetic resonance imaging (MRI).

    b. MRI may identify traumatic lesions not identified by CT. Spinal imaging may be needed in selected cases.

    c. Lumbar puncture, depending on imaging results and clinical assessment

      (1) Bloody fluid may not represent a *traumatic* tap.

      (2) Xanthochromic supernatant after centrifugation of cerebrospinal fluid suggests CNS hemorrhage.

BOX 31-2

SKELETAL DISORDERS WITH FRAGILITY AND INCREASED TENDENCY TO FRACTURE

- Congenital syphilis
- Copper deficiency—Menkes syndrome
- Myelophthisis
- Osteogenesis imperfecta
- Osteomalacia (e.g., rickets)
- Osteomyelitis
- Osteopenia of prematurity

VI. Skeletal injuries
   A. General considerations
      1. Bone fractures are the second most common clinical manifestation of child abuse (after skin findings), although the fracture pattern is generally nonspecific.
      2. Cause
         a. Twisting of extremity
         b. Direct compression or force
         c. Firmly holding extremities while shaking
      3. The frequency of cervical spine injury associated with child abuse is unknown; it may present as spinal cord injury without radiologic abnormality.
      4. There are no fractures pathognomonic of child abuse, although the following fractures should suggest the possibility of nonaccidental injury:
         a. Metaphyseal fractures in infants: Tufts, chips, arcs of bone ("bucket handles"); these occur with shearing injury perpendicular to the long axis of the bone as the infant is held firmly and shaken.
         b. Multiple fractures of various ages: Abuse is more common than diseases characterized by bone fragility or increased tendency to fracture.
         c. Differential diagnosis in selected patients
            (1) Osteogenesis imperfecta—characterized by the following:
               (a) Abnormal dentition
               (b) Blue sclera
               (c) Easy bruisability
               (d) Limb deformities, scoliosis, and/or kyphosis
               (e) Hyperextensible joints
               (f) Hearing impairment
               (g) Demineralized bones: Diagnosis made with skin biopsy and DNA sequencing
            (2) Osteopenia of prematurity
               (a) Bone density may normalize only after the first year.
               (b) Cause is multifactorial but usually involves infants with a history of critical illness (i.e., hyperalimentation, multiple medications, and limited mobility).
            (3) Other disorders of bone fragility (see Box 31-2)
   B. Posterior rib fractures
      1. Likely related to thoracic compression during violent shaking in infants. Fingerprint ecchymoses may not develop until hours after injury.
      2. Typically unrelated to CPR

3. Usually nondisplaced; may not be visible on radiograph until callus formation seen at 10 to 14 days
4. Location
    a. Posterior—near attachment to spine as well as laterally
    b. May be obscured on standard chest films
C. Long bone fractures in infants
    1. Most common in distal femur and proximal tibia, but also seen in upper extremity
    2. Spiral or transverse fractures are not unique to abuse
        a. Spiral fractures can occur whenever there is sufficient rotational force.
        b. Transverse fractures occur with significant direct trauma.

VII. Skull fractures
A. Diagnosis
    1. Conventional radiographs are preferred to CT scans.
    2. Short falls (<4 feet, such as from a bed) at home are very unlikely to result in serious injury.
        a. With skull fracture resulting in only 1% to 3% of these children, assuming the impact is spread over a relatively large area of the skull
        b. Usually simple, nondisplaced linear (usually parietal) fractures
        c. Features suggestive of greater force associated with minor trauma (and thus raising the possibility of intentional injury) include the following:
            (1) Complex skull fractures (branching lines, multiple fractures, fractures crossing suture lines)
            (2) Bilateral skull fractures

VIII. Blunt thoraco-abdominal trauma (see also Chapters 21 and 22)
A. Victims
    1. Older infants or young children, often presenting with multiple injuries
    2. Injuries may be a marker for later stages of abuse in families with multiple children already known to the social service system.
    3. Mortality rate is high (25% to 50%).
B. Rib fractures, hemo-pneumothorax, and pulmonary contusions
    1. Cause: Posterior rib fractures are associated with physical abuse.
    2. Manifestations
        a. Hemo-pneumothorax may be seen on chest radiograph.
        b. Ecchymoses over the chest wall may be delayed in appearance or masked by monitoring devices.
    3. Diagnosis: Chest CT scan is more sensitive than chest radiograph for pulmonary contusions.

C. Small bowel hematoma and perforation
1. Cause
    a. Blunt force compresses small bowel against thoracolumbar spine, usually producing intramural bleeding in the duodenum (much of it in a retroperitoneal location)
    b. Pancreatitis—also a retroperitoneal injury—may coexist.
    c. External evidence of injury may be lacking.
2. Diagnosis: Chest CT scan with intravenous contrast (oral contrast may be poorly tolerated in these patients) is best for accurate diagnosis.
3. Associated injuries
    a. Obstruction often develops slowly (1 to 5 days) and may progress to perforation, especially if unsuspected.
    b. Alternatively, acute perforation with severe compressive injury may occur early.
    c. Associated injuries include mesenteric laceration and solid organ injury.
D. Solid organ injury
1. Most common types
    a. Hematoma
    b. Laceration
    c. Vascular injury of the liver and spleen
2. Symptoms
    a. Often nonspecific (abdominal discomfort, nausea, vomiting)
    b. Hemodynamic changes occur with worsening injury and thus may be attributed to other injuries, possibly resulting in delayed diagnosis.
3. Diagnosis: Abdominal CT scan for diagnosis and grading of injury
4. Management: Expectant and typically nonsurgical
E. Retroperitoneal injury
1. Types of injury: Retroperitoneal portion of the duodenum, pancreas, kidneys, upper urinary tract, and part of the colon
2. These injuries require significant severe blunt force; multiple injuries are the rule, including:
    a. Acute traumatic pancreatitis
    b. Renal hematoma and laceration
    c. Delayed complication: Pancreatic pseudocyst (caused by traumatic duct disruption)
IX. Asphyxiation
A. Causes
    Fingers, hands, clothing, bedding, and other foreign bodies have been used to suffocate infants.
B. Physical examination
1. May be normal

BOX 31-3

POSSIBLE RISK FACTORS FOR INTENTIONAL ASPHYXIA IN VICTIMS OF PRESUMED SUDDEN INFANT DEATH SYNDROME

- Recurrent cyanosis, apnea, or acute life-threatening event occurring only while in the care of the same person
- Age at death older than 6 months
- Previous unexpected or unexplained death of one or more siblings
- Simultaneous or nearly simultaneous death of twins
- Previous death of infants under the care of the same unrelated person, or
- Evidence of previous pulmonary hemorrhage (such as marked siderophages in the lung)

(Modified from AAP Hymel KP. Distinguishing sudden infant death syndrome from child abuse fatalities. Pediatrics 2006;118:421-7)

2. May reveal the following:
   a. Bleeding from nose or mouth
   b. Petechiae on the face, scalp, conjunctivae, lips, neck, chest
   c. Signs of neurologic injury in survivors
C. Acute life-threatening event episodes or SIDS
   Intentional asphyxiation in the form of Munchausen syndrome by proxy should be considered (**Box 31-3**).
X. Sexual abuse
   See **Tables 31-1** and **31-2.**
   A. Definition
      1. Sexual abuse is a spectrum.
         a. Includes noncontact activities (e.g., exhibitionism, voyeurism, pornography) as well as genital, anal, or oral-genital contact.
         b. Sexual play between young children and age-appropriate sexual activity in adolescence are differentiated from abuse.
      2. History
         a. Do not ask leading questions.
         b. Instead, ask "Has anyone touched you?"
         c. Behavioral abnormalities are common.
         d. Specific complaints may be suggestive (e.g., prepubertal vaginal bleeding suggests trauma or foreign body).
      3. Physical examination
         a. Forensic evidence (e.g., body swabs, sampling of hair, saliva, clothing, photographs, drawings) may be helpful when performed and labeled properly within 72 hours of alleged abuse.
            (1) The examination and forensic evidence are frequently normal in victims of sexual abuse.

31

TABLE 31-1

IMPLICATIONS OF COMMONLY ENCOUNTERED STDS FOR THE DIAGNOSIS AND REPORTING OF SEXUAL ABUSE OF INFANTS AND PREPUBERTAL CHILDREN

STD Confirmed	Sexual Abuse	Suggested Action
Gonorrhea*	Diagnostic[†]	Report[‡]
Syphilis*	Diagnostic	Report
HIV infection[§]	Diagnostic	Report
*Chlamydia trachomatis**	Diagnostic[†]	Report
Trichomonas vaginalis	Highly suspicious	Report
Condylomata acuminata (anogenital warts)*	Suspicious	Report
Herpes simplex (genital location)	Suspicious	Report[¶]
Bacterial	Inconclusive	Medical follow-up

Modified from Kellogg N, American Academy of Pediatrics Committee on Child Abuse and Neglect: The evaluation of sexual abuse in children. Pediatrics 2005;116:506-512.

HIV, Human immunodeficiency virus; *STD*, sexually transmitted disease.

*If not perinatally acquired and rare nonsexual vertical transmission is excluded.

[†]Although the culture technique is the "gold standard," current studies are investigating the use of nucleic acid-amplification tests as an alternative diagnostic method in children.

[‡]To the agency mandated in the community to receive reports of unsuspected sexual abuse.

[§]If not acquired perinatally or by transfusion.

[¶]Unless there is a clear history of autoinoculation.

TABLE 31-2

GUIDELINES FOR MAKING THE DECISION TO REPORT SEXUAL ABUSE OF CHILDREN

Data Available				Response	
History	Behavioral Symptoms	Physical Examination	Diagnostic Tests	Level of Concern	Report Decision
Clear statement	Present or absent	Normal or abnormal	Positive or negative	High	Report
None or vague	Present or absent	Normal or nonspecific	Positive test for *C. trachomatis*, gonorrhea, *T. vaginalis*, HIV, syphilis, or herpes*	High	Report
None or vague	Present or absent	Concerning or diagnostic findings	Negative or positive	High[†]	Report
Vague, or history by parent only	Present or absent	Normal or nonspecific	Negative	Indeterminate	Refer when possible
None	Present	Normal or nonspecific	Negative	Intermediate	Possible report,[‡] refer, or follow

HIV, Human immunodeficiency virus.

*If nonsexual transmission is unlikely or excluded.

[†]Confirmed with various examination techniques and/or peer review with expert consultant.

[‡]If behaviors are rare or unusual in normal children.

        (2) Caution is indicated in the interpretation of tests for sexually transmitted disease (STD).

        (3) Positive results, within the context of sexual abuse, mandate reporting of sexual abuse.

        (4) Reporting is also mandated for children whenever the level of concern about sexual abuse is high, despite a normal history, physical examination, or diagnostic tests.

    b. Physical examination should include thorough identification of all findings (particularly contusions, abrasions, scars) in the following:

        (1) Males: Anus, mouth, penis, perineum, scrotum, thighs

        (2) Females: Anus, clitoris, hymen, labia majora, minora, mouth, perineum, thighs, urethra

        (3) A speculum or digital examination should be performed only under general anesthesia in prepubertal victims.

           (a) Injuries to posterior parts of external genitalia are more suggestive of penetrating trauma.

           (b) Anterior injuries are compatible with crush and straddle trauma.

    c. Laboratory testing

        (1) Universal STD screening for postpubertal victims

        (2) Selective STD testing in prepubertal victims

        (3) Pregnancy testing for postpubertal female victims is mandatory.

    d. Victims should be referred to a physician and a mental health professional with expertise in pediatric sexual abuse; some states require a pediatric forensics interview.

XI. Munchausen syndrome by proxy

  A. Definition

    Caretaker simulates, falsely reports, or induces illness in the child

  B. Features

    1. Extensive but vague history of difficult-to-document complaints without an obvious cause

    2. Often overlooked as a diagnostic possibility

    3. Parental level of denial is high.

    4. Responsible caretakers

      a. More commonly involves the mother

      b. Suspected perpetrator often skilled at hiding evidence

      c. May change physicians when diagnosis is suspected

    5. Victims

      a. May have underlying systemic disease

      b. The presence of a medical device (e.g., feeding tube, venous catheter) may allow the caretaker to induce illness by using the device to introduce toxin, infection, or medication.

BOX 31-4

ABUSIVE MANEUVERS EMPLOYED BY CARETAKERS IN MUNCHAUSEN SYNDROME BY PROXY

- Altered or adulterated laboratory tests
- Asphyxiation, suffocation
- Fabricated history of previous illness
- Inflicted injury

- Injection into intravenous catheters
- Poisoning
- Starvation

    C. Abusive maneuvers in Munchausen syndrome by proxy (See **Box 31-4**)

    D. Approach to diagnosis
       1. Laboratory tests to show that blood specimens are not from the patient or that specimens have been adulterated
       2. Isolation of patient with documentation that symptoms do not occur when suspected caretaker not present
       3. Occult video surveillance
       4. Referral to experienced specialists

Chapter 32

Neonatal Emergencies
S. Lee Woods, MD, PhD

I. Overview
  A. Definition
     A neonate or newborn is defined as an infant younger than 1 month of age.
  B. General considerations
     1. Many medical and surgical emergencies in this population are similar in diagnosis and treatment to those in older infants and children.
     2. Some situations are unique, however, especially in the *newly born* infant, defined as the first minutes to hours after birth.
     3. At birth, the neonate undergoes a dramatic transition from intrauterine to extrauterine life.
     4. The "Golden Hour" may be reduced to "Golden Minutes" when resuscitation is needed.
     5. Timely and effective resuscitation may make a lifetime of difference.
     6. Birth is associated with unique causes of hemorrhage that can be life-threatening for the newborn.
     7. At or shortly after birth, many congenital anomalies and metabolic disorders become apparent and may represent an emergency situation.
     8. Intestinal obstruction, infection, and jaundice may also present as neonatal emergencies.
II. Neonatal resuscitation
  A. Transitional physiology
     1. Exposure to air or fall in temperature: Provides a stimulus to begin spontaneous respirations
     2. Lung expansion
        a. Fluid-filled fetal lungs must be expanded with air to establish gas exchange.
        b. Fetal lung fluid is absorbed through the lymphatics.
           (1) Process that begins during labor
           (2) Lung fluid cannot be suctioned out, and little is *squeezed* out during the birth process.
        c. With the first few breaths, the neonate establishes a functional residual capacity (FRC).

3. First breaths
   a. High end-expiratory pressure is generated by expiration against a closed glottis.
   b. This maneuver assists the lungs in expanding evenly and establishing FRC.
4. Umbilical cord clamping
   a. Accompanied by a rapid rise in central blood pressure (BP)
   b. Sympathetic stimulation results in *shocked* appearance of the neonate and blue hands and feet (acrocyanosis).
5. Pulmonary vascular resistance (PVR)
   a. In utero, high PVR results in shunting blood away from the lungs toward the placenta through fetal shunts (ductus arteriosus and foramen ovale).
   b. Rapid fall in PVR occurs with lung inflation after birth, followed by a more gradual decrease over hours and days, with transition from fetal to adult circulation.

B. Abnormal events
1. In utero or perinatal compromise (asphyxia)
   a. Respirations are the first vital sign to cease in a fetus or newborn deprived of oxygen (O_2).
   b. After initial period of rapid gasping
      (1) The fetus or newborn enters a period of *primary apnea*.
      (2) Spontaneous respirations can be induced in this period by vigorous stimulation (see Section III).
   c. If O_2 deprivation continues, the infant will make several irregular gasps and then enter a period of *secondary apnea*.
      (1) Spontaneous respirations **cannot** be induced by stimulation in this period.
      (2) Positive-pressure ventilation is required.
   d. If an infant is not breathing at birth, it may be in primary *or* secondary apnea.
      (1) A brief period of stimulation should be tried, but
      (2) Positive-pressure ventilation **MUST** be initiated quickly (no more than 30 seconds after birth) if spontaneous respirations do not begin.
2. Effects of prematurity
   a. Poor respiratory effort and lung expansion initially, as well as poor lung compliance caused by surfactant deficiency
   b. Rapid heat loss caused by lack of subcutaneous tissue and immature skin with larger than normal evaporative heat loss

C. Assessment of need for resuscitation
1. Approximately 10% of newborns will require some help in establishing breathing at birth; 1% will need extensive resuscitation.

BOX 32-1

EQUIPMENT FOR NEWBORN RESUSCITATION

STANDARD EQUIPMENT SETUP

Radiant warmer
Stethoscope
Oxygen source with heated humidifier
Suction source, suction catheter, and bulb suction
Nasogastric tubes (5 Fr, 8 Fr, Replogle)
Apparatus for bag and mask ventilation
Ventilation masks (small sizes)
Laryngoscope (handles, blades, and batteries)
Endotracheal tubes (2.5, 3.0, and 3.5 mm)
Intravenous fluids (10% dextrose, Ringer's lactate solution)

DRUGS

Epinephrine (1:10,000 solution)
Naloxone hydrochloride (0.2, 0.4, or 1.0 mg/mL)
Sodium bicarbonate (0.5 mEq/mL)
Volume expanders (5% albumin, Plasmanate, normal saline)

OTHER

Plastic wrap or bags
Equipment for umbilical vessel catheterization
Micro blood gas analysis availability
Warm blankets

32

2. A rapid assessment using four questions is used to determine if resuscitation is needed:
   a. Was the infant born after a full-term gestation (≥37 weeks)?
   b. Is the amniotic fluid clear of meconium and evidence of infection?
   c. Is the infant breathing or crying?
   d. Does the infant have good muscle tone?
3. If the answer to any of the questions is "no," resuscitation should be initiated immediately.
4. If the answer to all four questions is "yes"
   a. The infant does *not* need resuscitation.
   b. The infant should be dried and wrapped, with ongoing observation.
5. The equipment necessary to carry out a neonatal resuscitation is listed in **Box 32-1.**
   a. This equipment should be available in any location in which a delivery might occur.
   b. It should be available to teams responding to deliveries in the field.
   c. **Figure 32-1** provides an overview of neonatal resuscitation.

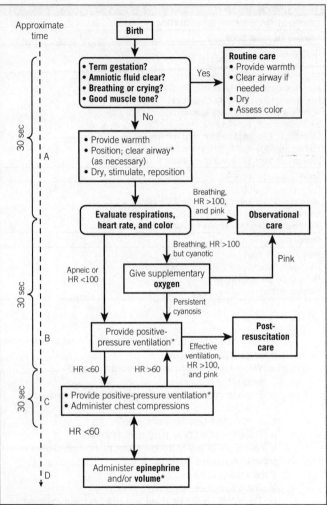

FIGURE 32-1

Overview of neonatal resuscitation. (Redrawn from American Heart Association. Part 13: neonatal resuscitation guidelines. Circulation 2005;112:IV188-IV195.) HR, Heart rate.

*Endotracheal intubation may be considered at several steps.

III. Resuscitation techniques
    A. Initial steps of resuscitation
        1. Provide warmth.
            a. Place the infant on a radiant warmer.
            b. Dry quickly to prevent evaporative heat loss.
            c. Outside of a delivery room setting, chemically activated heat packs can be used. Do not use hot water bags because the temperature is poorly controlled and can cause burns (especially in preterm infants).
            d. Preterm infants of very low birth weight (<1500 g) require additional measures.
                (1) Cover the body with plastic wrap or a bag (food-grade heat-resistant plastic).
                (2) Cover the scalp with a small sandwich bag using a standard stocking cap to hold it in place.
                (3) All subsequent resuscitative procedures can be done with these coverings in place.
        2. Position the infant's head in a *sniffing* position to open the airway.
            a. Avoid flexion or overextension of the neck.
            b. Either of these can cause airway obstruction in the newborn.
        3. Suction
            a. Clear the airway with a bulb syringe or suction catheter.
            b. Avoid prolonged or deep suctioning, which may cause a profound vagal response, resulting in apnea and bradycardia.
            c. To avoid deep suctioning, turn the infant's head to the side, allowing secretions to pool in the dependent cheek; suction only to the angle of the jaw.
        4. Stimulate: Breathing can be safely stimulated by firmly rubbing the infant's back or slapping or flicking the soles of the feet.
    B. Assessment
        1. The decision to progress from each step to the next in resuscitation is based on the *simultaneous* evaluation of three vital signs:
            a. Respiration
            b. Heart rate (HR)
            c. Color
            This assessment is repeated **every 30 seconds**.
        2. Respirations are evaluated by observing chest rise or auscultating breath sounds.
        3. HR is best determined by listening to the apical beat or by feeling the pulse by lightly grasping the base of the umbilical cord.

TABLE 32-1

APGAR SCORES*

	Score		
Sign	0	1	2
Heart rate	Absent	Slow (<100 beats/min)	≥100 beats/min
Respirations	Absent	Slow, irregular	Good, crying
Muscle tone	Limp	Some flexion	Active movements
Reflex irritability (catheter in nares)	No response	Grimace	Cough or sneeze
Color	Blue or pale	Pink body, blue extremities	Completely pink

*Apgar scores are an objective numerical expression of the newborn's condition on a scale of 0 to 10. The scores are recorded at 1 and 5 minutes after delivery. If the 5-minute score is <7, additional scores should be assigned every 5 minutes, up to 20 minutes. Apgar scores are not used to direct resuscitation. They have clinical usefulness later, when clinical status at delivery may have a bearing on diagnostic assessments. The system was originally described in 1953 by Dr. Virginia Apgar, an anesthesiologist.

    4. Color is best assessed by looking at the tongue and mucous membranes.
       a. The catecholamine surge at birth often causes the hands and feet to stay blue (acrocyanosis) and appear poorly perfused; the average fetal partial pressure of arterial oxygen (PaO_2) is 25 mm Hg, so all infants appear blue at birth.
       b. It can take several minutes for circulatory transition to occur and central cyanosis to disappear.
       c. *Provide supplemental O_2 if the infant is breathing but has central cyanosis 30 seconds after the initial steps of resuscitation.*
    5. Note that Apgar scores (**Table 32-1**) are not used to determine if resuscitation is needed or what resuscitative steps are necessary; resuscitation **must begin before** these scores are assigned.
  C. Positive-pressure ventilation
    Lung inflation is the single most important resuscitative maneuver and is the key to a successful resuscitation.
    1. Begin bag and mask ventilation if the infant is apneic or gasping or if HR is <100 beats/min after the initial steps of resuscitation, approximately 30 seconds after birth.
    2. A neonatal-sized bag with a pressure manometer and pressure release valve (set at 30 to 40 cm H_2O) should be used, if possible, to avoid delivering excess pressure.
    3. Supplemental O_2 should be used whenever positive-pressure ventilation is needed—use 100% O_2 if there is no equipment available to monitor O_2 saturation (SaO_2) or vary O_2 concentration.
    4. If O_2 is not immediately available, begin bag and mask ventilation with room air; lung inflation is the most immediate goal.

TABLE 32-2

ENDOTRACHEAL TUBE SIZE

Tube Size (mm internal diameter)	Birth Weight (g)	Gestational Age (wk)
2.5	<1000	<28
3.0	1000-2000	28-34
3.5	2000-3000	34-38
3.5-4.0	>3000	>38

5. To inflate the lungs successfully
   a. The first few breaths require higher pressure (up to 30 to 40 cm H_2O) and longer inspiratory time.
   b. Subsequent breaths usually require less pressure (15 to 20 cm H_2O with normal lungs, 20 to 40 cm H_2O with diseased or immature lungs).
6. The best measure of adequate ventilation is a prompt improvement in the HR.
   a. Also watch for a **gentle** rise and fall of the chest.
   b. Avoid overinflation.
7. Provide breaths at a rate of 40 to 60/min. Count it out (one-one thousand, two-one thousand, three-one thousand…) to avoid hyperventilation.
8. Place an orogastric tube to decompress the stomach if bag and mask ventilation is continued for more than several minutes.

D. Endotracheal (ET) intubation
   1. Indicated for the following:
      a. Tracheal suctioning of meconium
      b. If bag and mask ventilation is ineffective or prolonged
      c. When chest compressions are performed
      d. ET delivery of medication
      e. In special circumstances (such as diaphragmatic hernia or extremely low birth weight, <1000 g)
   2. The tube size is determined by birth weight or gestational age (**Table 32-2**).
   3. Follow the general guidelines for ET intubation (see Chapter 2).
      a. Avoid hyperextension of the neck during intubation.
         (1) The neonatal airway is very anterior.
         (2) Gentle cricoid pressure may assist visualization.
      b. The ET tube is inserted until the vocal cord guide (dark line) is at the level of the vocal cords.
         (1) The depth of insertion can also be estimated by the birth weight.

32

(2) As a rule of thumb:

Length of insertion (cm from upper lip) = weight (kg) + 6

(3) Correct position in the trachea should be confirmed by auscultating equal breath sounds in both lung fields.

  c. The best indicator of correct tube placement and effective ventilation is a prompt improvement in HR.

  d. Use of an exhaled carbon dioxide (CO_2) detection device or end-tidal CO_2 monitor to confirm tube placement is recommended; other indicators of correct tube placement include the following:

(1) Condensation in the tube during exhalation

(2) Presence of chest movement

E. Chest compressions

  1. Make certain ventilation is being delivered effectively before starting chest compressions.

    a. Ventilation is the most effective action in successful neonatal resuscitation.

    b. Compressions may compete with optimal ventilation.

  2. Chest compressions are indicated if HR is ≤60 beats/min after 30 seconds of **effective** ventilation with supplemental O_2.

    a. The lower third of the sternum should be compressed to a depth of one third of the anterior-posterior diameter.

    b. The two-thumb encircling hands technique is recommended (**Fig. 32-2**).

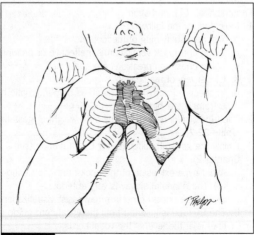

FIGURE 32-2

Technique for chest compressions in the neonate.

      c. The two-finger technique may be necessary if access to the umbilicus is needed for line insertion.

      d. Compressions and ventilation should be coordinated with a 3 : 1 compression-to-ventilation ratio at a rate to provide 90 compressions and 30 breaths/min (approximately 120 events/min).

      e. It is helpful to have someone count out the events to maintain coordination and set the rate ("one and two and three and breathe and …").

      f. Respirations, HR, and color are assessed every 30 seconds.

      g. Compressions should be stopped when HR is >60 beats/min.

F. Medications

   1. Medications are rarely indicated in neonatal resuscitation.

      a. Bradycardia is usually the result of inadequate lung inflation and hypoxemia.

      b. The most effective treatment is establishing adequate ventilation.

   2. Epinephrine or a volume expander is indicated if HR remains <60 beats/min in spite of 30 seconds of effective ventilation with 100% O_2 and chest compressions.

   3. Epinephrine

      a. Dose: 0.01 to 0.03 mg/kg intravenous (IV) (0.1 to 0.3 mL/kg of 1 : 10,000 concentration [0.1 mg/mL] epinephrine)

      b. High-dose IV epinephrine (0.1 mg/kg) is **not** recommended for the neonate.

      c. ET administration may be used, but requires a higher dose (up to 0.1 mg/kg) to be effective.

   4. Volume expanders

      a. Volume expansion should be considered when there is blood loss or the infant appears to be in shock (e.g., poor perfusion, weak pulses, pallor) and has not responded to other resuscitative efforts.

      b. Isotonic crystalloid (normal saline, Ringer's lactate) should be given IV at a dose of 10 mL/kg.

      c. In preterm infants, volume expanders should be given slowly (over 5 to 10 minutes).

      d. Rapid volume expansion has been associated with intraventricular hemorrhage.

   5. Other medications

      a. These are **not** indicated in neonatal resuscitation.

      b. Vasopressors, sodium bicarbonate, or narcotic antagonist may be indicated after resuscitation, when BP, arterial blood gases, HR, and respirations can be monitored.

32

BOX 32-2

PROCEDURE FOR UMBILICAL VEIN CATHETERIZATION

- Restrain the infant's arms and legs.
- Use sterile technique.
- Prepare and drape the area (if emergent, drape may consist of 4-inch-square gauze pads placed at the base of the umbilical cord).
- Attach a three-way stopcock on umbilical vessel catheter and flush with sterile saline. Close stopcock to catheter; **avoid air embolisms**.
- Tie the umbilical tape to the base of the cord, snug enough to prevent bleeding but loose enough to permit the catheter to pass.
- Cut the umbilical cord with a scalpel blade so that 2 to 3 cm remain.
- Identify the umbilical vein (see Fig. 32-3, *B*) and, if necessary, dilate the vessel with the curved eye dressing forceps. This is usually not necessary.
- Insert the **fully flushed** umbilical catheter (3.5 or 5 Fr) into the vein, aiming up toward the head. Advance the catheter just until blood return is obtained (usually 3 to 5 cm).
- **At all times prior to any infusion, the stopcock should be turned off** to the infant.

    G. Emergency vascular access
       1. The umbilical vein
          a. Easiest vessel in the neonate in which to establish venous access.
          b. May be accessible for up to 1 week after birth, even if the cord has dried or has been painted with triple dye.
       2. The procedure is outlined in **Box 32-2** and shown in **Figure 32-3.**
    H. Special situations
       1. Meconium-stained amniotic fluid
          a. With fetal distress, infants >34 weeks' gestation may pass meconium in utero.
          b. Aspiration of this meconium before, during, or after delivery can lead to severe aspiration pneumonia.
          c. Suctioning of the nose and mouth at the perineum as the fetal head is delivered is of no value in preventing aspiration and is no longer recommended.
          d. ET intubation and direct suctioning of the airway after delivery is also of no value if the infant is vigorous; *vigorous* is defined as having strong respiratory effort, HR >100 beats/min, and good muscle tone.
          e. ET suctioning should be performed immediately at birth (prior to the initial steps of resuscitation) in an infant with meconium staining who is not vigorous.
       2. Preterm infants
          a. Special attention should be paid to minimizing heat loss (see Section III).

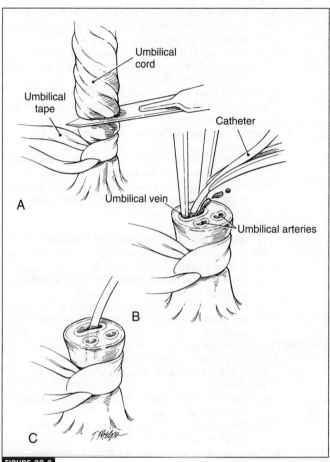

FIGURE 32-3

Umbilical vein catheterization (see Box 32-2 for complete procedure). **A,** Cut the umbilical cord. **B,** Identify the umbilical vein. **C,** Insert the umbilical catheter into the vein.

b. Premature skin can be very fragile; care should be taken in drying and handling very preterm infants to avoid bruising or sloughing.

c. Very preterm infants (<27 weeks or <1000 g) should be intubated early in resuscitation, since support with ventilation may be required.

(1) If positive end-expiratory pressure can be provided, it may help protect the immature lungs from injury and improve lung compliance.

(2) If a means to provide continuous positive airway pressure (CPAP) is available, it is reasonable to try this modality prior to intubation.

d. Surfactant is **not** a resuscitative drug; it should only be given when ongoing ventilatory management and blood gas analysis can be done.

3. Congenital diaphragmatic hernia

a. Diagnosis

(1) Decreased breath sounds on the affected side (usually the left) and a scaphoid abdomen

(2) Respiratory distress is usually evident at birth, but the diagnosis may not be obvious until a chest radiograph is obtained.

b. Therapeutic implications

(1) Bag and mask ventilation should be avoided.

(2) This is one situation in which bag and mask ventilation worsens distress.

(3) If respiratory support is needed, the infant should be immediately intubated.

(4) If a diaphragmatic hernia is suspected, the stomach should be decompressed with an orogastric tube.

4. Congenital anomalies

a. An unexpected congenital anomaly, such as spina bifida, cleft lip and palate, or gastroschisis, should be noted.

(1) It is difficult in a delivery setting to evaluate the severity or extent of an anomaly.

(2) After the infant has been stabilized, the necessary evaluation can be done.

b. Resuscitation should proceed in the usual manner, following the steps outlined earlier.

c. Open defects (e.g., spina bifida, gastroschisis)

(1) Should be covered to protect the tissue and minimize fluid loss

(2) Sterile saline-soaked gauze covered by plastic wrap is adequate.

5. Ambiguous genitalia

a. The birth of an infant with ambiguous genitalia is a very traumatic event for a family; the delivery setting is not the appropriate place for extensive discussion of this emotional issue.

b. **Do not assign a gender.**

   c. It is better to say, "The baby's genitalia have not completed
      their development. We will need a few days to perform
      some studies to determine the sex of your baby."
6. Withholding or discontinuing resuscitation
   a. Certain conditions have very high mortality and poor
      outcome
      (1) It may be reasonable to withhold resuscitation,
          especially if there is parental agreement.
      (2) Ideally, the care team should discuss possible
          scenarios in advance.
   b. From an ethical perspective, withholding resuscitation and
      discontinuing life support (during or after resuscitation) are
      equivalent.
      (1) Initiating resuscitation does not imply that all supportive
          measures must be used.
      (2) Decisions about the appropriateness of support can be
          made as more information becomes available.
   c. For conditions in which early death is almost certain and
      unacceptably high morbidity in survivors is likely,
      resuscitation is not indicated; such conditions include the
      following:
      (1) Extreme prematurity (gestation age <23 weeks or birth
          weight <400 g)
      (2) Anencephaly
      (3) Major chromosomal abnormalities incompatible
          with life
   d. In conditions with a high survival rate and acceptable
      morbidity, resuscitation is indicated.
      (1) Includes infants of gestational age ≥24 weeks and
          infants with most congenital anomalies
      (2) However, evidence of serious fetal compromise, such
          as intrauterine infection or hypoxia-ischemia, must be
          considered in such decisions.
   e. In conditions with uncertain prognosis, parental wishes
      concerning resuscitation should be supported.
I. Physical assessment
   1. Assess cardiorespiratory adaptation and reassess the following:
      a. HR and murmurs
      b. Respirations
      c. Color
      d. Work of breathing
   2. Look for the presence of congenital anomalies and examine
      the following:
      a. Face and ears
      b. Palate for cleft
      c. Spine for neural tube defects

32

       d. Extremities and digits
       e. Genitalia and anus
       f. Cord stump for three vessels
    3. Evaluate for evidence of birth injury.
       a. Skull, scalp for cephalohematoma or subgaleal hemorrhage
       b. Face for asymmetrical movement (facial nerve injury)
       c. Movement of upper extremities (brachial plexus injury)
       d. Bruising or laceration, especially with instrumented or surgical delivery
       e. Inspiratory stridor (possible vocal cord paralysis from injury to the recurrent laryngeal nerve)

IV. Ongoing supportive measures
  A. Blood sugar
    1. Blood sugar should be checked within 30 minutes of birth with the following conditions:
       a. Prematurity
       b. Small for gestational age
       c. Large for gestational age
       d. Infant of a diabetic mother
       e. Prolonged resuscitation or asphyxia
    2. If the blood sugar is <25 mg/dL, give an IV bolus of 2 mL/kg 10% dextrose in water (D10W) and start an IV infusion of dextrose.
    3. Maintain a plasma glucose concentration of 40 mg/dL or higher.
       a. This can be maintained by enteral feedings in stable term infants or by parenteral glucose at a 5 to 6 mg/kg/min glucose infusion rate.
  B. Maintenance fluids
    1. Infants requiring transport or ongoing evaluation and care should have IV access established.
    2. Suggested maintenance fluids and infusion rates based on birth weight are shown in **Table 32-3**.
    3. For a quick calculation of infusion rates:

$$3 \, mL/kg/hr \cong 75 \, mL/kg/day$$

$$4 \, mL/kg/hr \cong 100 \, mL/kg/day$$

$$6 \, mL/kg/hr \cong 150 \, mL/kg/day$$

TABLE 32-3

MAINTENANCE FLUIDS ON THE FIRST DAY OF LIFE

Weight (kg)	Fluid	Infusion Rate
<1 g	D5W	120-150 mL/kg/day
1-1.5 kg	D10W	90 mL/kg/day
>1.5 kg	D10W	80 mL/kg/day

D5W, 5% dextrose in water; *D10W*, 10% dextrose in water.

C. Thermoregulation
   1. Infants should be kept in a neutral thermal environment (NTE).
      a. The NTE is that environmental temperature at which O_2 and caloric consumption are at their lowest.
      b. This temperature is higher for infants of lower gestational age.
   2. Hypothermia
      a. Causes
         (1) Environmental cooling
         (2) Sepsis (low temperature is more common than fever in neonates)
         (3) Hypothyroidism
         (4) Hypothalamic dysfunction
      b. Consequences
         (1) Increased O_2 consumption
         (2) Tissue hypoxia caused by left shift in O_2 dissociation curve
         (3) Hypoglycemia secondary to increased anaerobic metabolism and increased metabolic rate
         (4) Apnea
         (5) Pulmonary hemorrhage
         (6) Intraventricular hemorrhage
   3. Mechanisms of heat loss
      a. Evaporation: Wet infant at the time of delivery or after preparation for procedures
      b. Conduction: Infant being placed on a cold radiograph plate or treatment table
      c. Convection: Infant being placed in a draft or under an air-conditioning duct.
      d. Radiation: Infant lying close to but not in contact with a cold wall or window
   4. Treatment and prevention of hypothermia
      a. A hypothermic infant should be rewarmed slowly at a rate of 1° C/hr.
      b. Healthy infants >2.5 kg usually do not require additional thermal support beyond blankets, a hat, and a crib.
      c. Preterm, low birth weight, or ill infants may require thermal support. The goal is an axillary temperature of 36.3° to 36.8° C.
      d. A double-walled incubator provides the best mode of thermal support.
         (1) A radiant warmer that provides thermal support and access for procedures or care of unstable infants is recommended in the acute care setting.

32

   (2) A skin probe is necessary to prevent overheating and should be set at 36.5° C.
   e. Extremely low birth weight infants (<1000 gm) may require increased environmental humidity or a blanket of plastic or bubble wrap to prevent evaporative heat loss.
5. Hyperthermia
   a. Causes
      (1) High environmental temperature or overbundling
      (2) Sepsis: Bacterial or viral
      (3) Dehydration: More common in breast-fed infants
      (4) Drug withdrawal
      (5) Hyperthyroidism
      (6) Maternal fever (in newly born infant)
   b. Consequences
      (1) Increased metabolic rate
      (2) Increased fluid requirement
      (3) Apnea
      (4) Tachycardia and tachypnea
      (5) Central nervous system (CNS) damage
6. Treatment of hyperthermia
   a. Correct underlying cause (e.g., sepsis, overbundling)
   b. Acetaminophen, orally (PO) or by rectum (PR)
      (1) PO: Loading dose, 20 to 25 mg/kg; maintenance, 12 to 15 mg/kg/dose
      (2) PR: Loading dose, 30 mg/kg; maintenance, 12 to 18 mg/kg/dose
      (3) Dosing interval
         (a) Term infant, q6h
         (b) Preterm, ≥32 weeks q8h
         (c) Preterm, <32 weeks q12h
7. Vitamin K: All neonates should receive vitamin K prophylaxis within 1 hour of birth.
   a. Term or near-term infants: 1 mg intramuscularly (IM)
   b. Preterm, <32 weeks: Birth weight >1000 g, 0.5 mg IM; birth weight <1000 g, 0.3 mg IM
8. Gonococcal eye prophylaxis: All infants should receive prophylaxis against gonococcal ophthalmia neonatorum with a 1 to 2 cm ribbon of sterile ophthalmic ointment containing 0.5% erythromycin to each eye within 1 hour of birth.
9. Parental support
   a. Inform the parents as soon as possible about the infant's condition.
   b. Let them see or hold the infant, if at all possible.
V. Neonatal respiratory distress
   A. Signs and symptoms of respiratory distress
      1. Tachypnea

    2. Grunting

    3. Nasal flaring

    4. Intercostal, suprasternal retractions

    5. Cyanosis

    6. Apnea

B. Causes of respiratory distress

    1. Respiratory distress syndrome (RDS)

      a. More common in preterm infants and infants of diabetic mothers

      b. Respiratory distress presents at birth or shortly thereafter.

      c. Diffuse *ground glass* pattern on chest radiograph

      d. Treatment includes the following:

        (1) Ventilatory support

          (a) Supplemental O_2

          (b) CPAP

          (c) Intubation with mechanical ventilation

        (2) Surfactant replacement

    2. Pneumothorax

      a. The greatest risk of spontaneous pneumothorax occurs in the immediate postnatal period (1% of all deliveries).

      b. Pneumothorax also occurs after positive-pressure ventilation (including during resuscitation).

      c. Asymptomatic pneumothoraces generally resolve spontaneously and require no treatment.

      d. Symptomatic pneumothorax—poor respiratory compliance, hypotension, progressive hypoxemia, increased work of breathing—requires the following:

        (1) Needle aspiration

        (2) Followed by thoracostomy tube if there is continued air leak (see Chapter 21)

        (3) Respiratory support should be provided as needed.

    3. Airway obstruction

      a. Nasal obstruction caused by *choanal atresia*

        (1) Presents with respiratory distress when the infant is not crying but resolves with crying

        (2) Initial treatment is establishing an oral airway.

      b. Obstruction in the larynx and trachea often presents with inspiratory stridor.

      c. Causes of lower obstruction include the following:

        (1) Congenital malformations of the airway

        (2) Paralysis of the vocal cords

        (3) Masses

        (4) Vascular rings

        (5) Laryngomalacia

        (6) Tracheomalacia

        (7) Presence of a foreign body

32

4. Congenital malformations of the lungs include the following:
    a. Diaphragmatic hernia
    b. Pulmonary sequestration
    c. Congenital lobar emphysema
    d. Cystic adenomatoid malformation
    e. Diagnosis
        (1) Chest radiograph
        (2) Chest computed tomography (CT) scan
        (3) Magnetic resonance imaging (MRI)
5. Infection
    a. Pneumonia
        (1) Radiograph may be diagnostic with persistent localized or diffuse infiltrate.
        (2) Congenital group B β-hemolytic streptococcal pneumonia can mimic RDS on chest radiograph.
    b. Sepsis
        (1) Signs and symptoms are nonspecific.
        (2) Sepsis should always be considered in an infant presenting with respiratory distress (see later, Section VI).
    c. Neonatal tetanus
        (1) Although rare in the United States, up to a 10% mortality rate exists in underdeveloped countries.
        (2) It should be considered in cases with a history of home birth or omphalitis.
        (3) Treatment
            (a) Respiratory support
            (b) Tetanus immune globulin
            (c) Penicillin G
            (d) Sedation
            (e) Neuromuscular blockade in severe disease
6. Congestive heart failure
    a. Signs and symptoms
        (1) Respiratory distress
        (2) Tachycardia
        (3) Poor perfusion
        (4) Hypotension
        (5) Cardiomegaly
        (6) Hepatomegaly
        (7) Pulmonary edema
    b. Causes
        (1) Congenital heart disease
        (2) Cardiomyopathy
        (3) Asphyxia
        (4) Hydrops fetalis
        (5) Arteriovenous malformation

   7. Polycythemia
      a. Hyperviscosity caused by the following:
         (1) Venous hematocrit (Hct) >65% *or*
         (2) Venous hemoglobin ≥22 g/dL
      b. Causes
         (1) Transfusion (twin to twin, placental)
         (2) Intrauterine growth retardation
         (3) Asphyxia
         (4) Infant of a diabetic mother
   8. Inborn error of metabolism
      a. Presents with the following:
         (1) Poor feeding
         (2) Vomiting
         (3) Lethargy
         (4) Seizures
         (5) Coma
      b. Metabolic findings
         (1) Hypoglycemia
         (2) Metabolic acidosis and/or hyperammonemia (see Chapter 8)
VI. Neonatal sepsis
   A. Signs and symptoms
      1. Temperature instability—hypothermia is more common than fever.
      2. Irritability or lethargy
      3. Poor feeding or feeding intolerance
      4. Respiratory distress
      5. Poor perfusion, hypotension, shock
      6. Disseminated intravascular coagulation (DIC)
      7. Seizures
      8. Hypoglycemia
   B. Risk factors
      1. Prematurity
      2. Prolonged rupture of membranes (>18 hours)
      3. Intrapartum signs of infection, including the following:
         a. Maternal fever (≥38° C).
         b. Uterine tenderness
         c. Fetal tachycardia
      4. Mother cultures positive for group B β-hemolytic streptococci, especially with a history of group B streptococcus (GBS) urinary tract infection during pregnancy, or history of GBS sepsis in a previous child
      5. Any infant, even if asymptomatic, born to a mother with chorioamnionitis should be cultured, started on antibiotics, and observed closely for at least 48 hours.

32

TABLE 32-4

AMPICILLIN DOSING INTERVAL CHART*

Postmenstrual Age (wk)	Postnatal Age (days)	Interval (hr)
≤29	0-28	12
	>28	8
30-36	0-14	12
	>14	8
37-44	0-7	12
	>7	8
≥45	All	6

*100 mg/kg/dose.

    C. Common organisms
        1. Early neonatal sepsis (<1 week old)
            a. Group B β-hemolytic streptococci
            b. *Escherichia coli*
            c. *Listeria monocytogenes*
            d. Herpes simplex virus
        2. Late neonatal sepsis (>1 week old)
            a. Group B β-hemolytic streptococci
            b. *E. coli*
            c. *Staphylococcus aureus*
            d. *Enterobacter* spp.
            e. Herpes simplex virus
    D. Management
        1. Supportive measures
            a. Respiratory support
            b. BP support
            c. Treat coagulopathy
            d. Treat seizures
        2. Obtain culture of the following:
            a. Blood
            b. Urine
            c. Cerebrospinal fluid (CSF)
            d. ET secretions (if intubated)
        3. Parenteral antibiotics
        Ampicillin, *plus* an aminoglycoside or cephalosporin, should be started according to the following dosing schedule:
            a. Ampicillin, 100 mg/kg/dose IV (meningitis dose) (**Table 32-4**)
            b. Gentamicin, IV infusion over 30 minutes (**Table 32-5**)
            c. Cefotaxime, 50 mg/kg/dose IV over 30 minutes (**Table 32-6**)
        4. Herpes simplex virus infection
            a. Should be suspected in any infant presenting with fever or vesicular rash in the first week of life, regardless of the maternal history

TABLE 32-5

GENTAMICIN* DOSING INTERVAL CHART

Postmenstrual Age (wk)	Postnatal Age (days)	Dose (mg/kg)	Interval (hr)
≤29[†]	0-7	5	48
	8-28	4	36
	≥29	4	24
30-34	0-7	4.5	36
	≥8	4	24
≥35	All	4	24

*NOTE: There is a risk of ototoxicity in the presence of renal insufficiency, concomitant diuretic usage, or prolonged gentamicin usage. Gentamicin administration should be guided by measurement of peak and trough levels.
[†]Or significant asphyxia, patent ductus arteriosus (PDA), or treatment with indomethacin.

TABLE 32-6

CEFOTAXIME DOSING INTERVAL CHART*

Postmenstrual Age (wk)	Postnatal Age (days)	Interval (hr)
≤29	0-28	12
	>28	8
30-36	0-14	12
	>14	8
37-44	0-7	12
	>7	8
≥45	All	6

*50 mg/kg/dose over 30 minutes.

32

   b. Because the diagnosis of herpes sepsis may be subtle, there is a low threshold for starting acyclovir in any critically ill newborn pending diagnosis.
   c. If suspected
      (1) Obtain cultures (nasopharynx, eye, rectum, skin vesicles, CSF)
      (2) Add acyclovir, 20 mg/kg/dose q8h IV over 1 hour.
      (3) Increase dosing interval to q12h in infants younger than 34 weeks postmenstrual age.
   d. Maintain contact isolation.
VII. Congenital heart disease
   A. Presentation
      Timing of presentation depends on the lesion and how rapidly pulmonary vascular resistance falls, particularly with ductal-dependent lesions (birth to 1 week).
   B. Signs and symptoms
      1. Murmur (not always present)
      2. Click or gallop
      3. Hyperdynamic precordium

TABLE 32-7

COMMON RADIOGRAPHIC FINDINGS ASSOCIATED WITH CONGENITAL HEART DISEASE

	Cardiomegaly	Pulmonary Vascularity	LV	RV	Atrium	Comments
CHF	Yes	↑				Can have pleural effusions
PDA	Yes	↑				Pulmonary edema
VSD	Yes	↑	↑		Left, ↑	
Coarctation of the aorta*	Yes	Normal	↑		Left, ↑	↑ Pulmonary artery ↑ Ascending aorta
Tetralogy of Fallot	No	↓		↑	Right, ↑ Left, normal	Small pulmonary artery
Transposition of the great arteries	Yes, ±	±		↑	Right, ↑	Narrow mediastinum; *most* are normal
Total anomalous pulmonary venous return	Minimal or none	↑				Congestive failure or pulmonary edema
Hypoplastic left heart*	Yes, initially normal	↑		↑	Right, ↑	
Tricuspid atresia*	Yes	↓	↑			Small pulmonary arteries
Truncus arteriosus	Yes	↑	↑	↑		Straightening of left cardiac border
Ebstein anomaly	Yes	↓			↑	
Pulmonary stenosis*	No	↓		No		

CHF, Congestive heart failure; *LV*, left ventricle; *PDA*, patent ductus arteriosus; *RV*, right ventricle; *VSD*, ventricular septal defect.

*May be ductal-dependent lesions.

4. Tachypnea without distress
5. Diminished pulses or BP in lower extremities (BP gradient >10 mm Hg)
6. Shock with metabolic acidosis
7. Difference between preductal and postductal SaO_2 (right upper extremity vs. lower extremity)
8. Arterial blood gas
   a. Normal or near-normal partial pressure of arterial CO_2
   b. Hypoxia in cyanotic lesions
C. Diagnosis
   1. Chest radiograph (**Table 32-7**).
      a. Cardiomegaly
      b. Absent or significant pulmonary vascular markings
      c. Right aortic arch
   2. Hyperoxia test
      a. Measure arterial blood gas in room air.
      b. Administer supplemental O_2 with fraction of inspired oxygen (FIO_2) of 1.0 for 10 to 20 minutes and repeat measurement.

        c. Infants without cyanotic congenital heart disease will generally have PaO_2 >150 mm Hg.

        d. Infants with cyanotic heart disease will not have a significant elevation in PaO_2.

    3. Echocardiogram is diagnostic.

  D. Management

    1. Prostaglandin E_1 (PGE$_1$), 0.01 to 0.4 mcg/kg/min IV infusion.

      a. Indications: Any newborn with refractory shock or hypoxemia should receive PGE_1 until a ductal-dependent lesion can be ruled out with echocardiogram.

      b. Dose

        (1) Usual starting dose is 0.05 mcg/kg/min.

        (2) Side effects include the following:

          (a) Apnea

          (b) Fever

          (c) Hypotension

          (d) Cutaneous vasodilation

          (e) Seizures (CNS irritability).

    2. Supportive care

      a. Support ventilation.

      b. Support BP.

      c. Correct acidosis.

      d. Correct hypoglycemia.

VIII. Gastrointestinal (GI) emergencies

  A. Bowel obstruction (**Fig. 32-4**)

    1. Neonatal intestinal obstruction

      a. Surgical emergency

      b. Malrotation with volvulus

        (1) First diagnostic consideration

        (2) Initial management should be directed to this possibility.

    2. Causes

      a. Malrotation with volvulus

      b. Esophageal atresia

      c. Pyloric stenosis

      d. Duodenal atresia

      e. Other small bowel atresias and stenoses

      f. Meconium ileus

      g. Intussusception

      h. Colonic atresia or stenosis

      i. Hirschsprung disease

      j. Imperforate anus

      k. Adhesions (past history of abdominal surgery or necrotizing enterocolitis [NEC])

Text continued on p. 544.

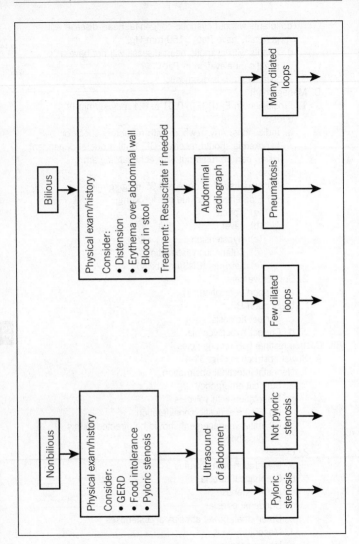

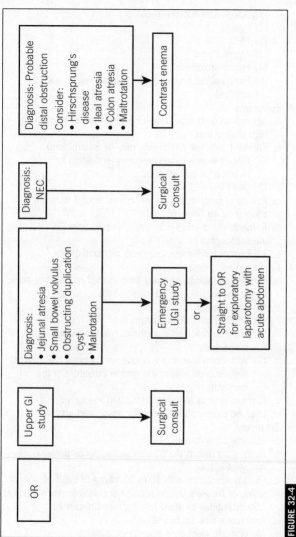

FIGURE 32-4

Diagnostic and management algorithm for vomiting in the newborn.

GERD, Gastroesophageal reflux disease; *GI,* gastrointestinal; *NEC,* necrotizing enterocolitis; *OR,* operating room; *UGI,* upper gastrointestinal.

    l. Physiologic obstruction (ileus)
      (1) Sepsis
      (2) NEC
      (3) Hypokalemia
      (4) Hypothyroidism
      (5) Perinatal drug exposure (e.g., magnesium sulfate, opiates)

3. Symptoms
  a. Abdominal distention (may be intermittent or minimal in high obstruction)
  b. Emesis (bilious or nonbilious, may be intermittent)
    (1) Bilious emesis always requires evaluation for malrotation and volvulus.
    (2) See Figure 32-4.
  c. Failure to pass stool (first meconium stool is normally passed by 48 hours of age)
  d. Palpable mass (olive in pyloric stenosis, bowel in intussusception)
  e. Abdominal tenderness (suggests peritonitis)

4. Evaluation
  a. Abdominal radiograph (may show dilated stomach or bowel loops; **cannot** rule out malrotation with volvulus)
  b. Upper GI series
    (1) If upper obstruction suspected
    (2) Must be obtained if malrotation with volvulus is suspected.
    (3) With normal anatomy, duodenum crosses the midline and ascends toward the greater curvature of the stomach.
  c. Contrast enema (if lower obstruction suspected)
  d. Detailed examination looking for associated anomalies

5. Treatment
  a. Surgical consultation
  b. Nothing by mouth (NPO) with gastric decompression via nasogastric tube
  c. Fluid resuscitation with 10 to 20 mL/kg IV bolus of normal saline or Ringer's lactate solution and maintenance fluids at 150 mL/kg/day for *third spacing* (see Chapter 6)
  d. Antibiotics (see Section VI)
  e. Monitor BP, electrolyte levels, Hct, platelets.

B. Incarcerated hernia
  1. Generally evident on physical examination
  2. Attempt manual reduction
    a. Sedation may be helpful or necessary.
    b. Hold infant in frog-leg position to relax abdominal wall.
    c. Fix the hernia with one hand while the other hand presses the incarcerated mass upward toward the inguinal canal.

        d. Apply steady pressure; several minutes may be required.

        e. Immediate surgery is necessary if not reducible.

C. NEC

  1. Presentation

     a. Generally occurs within first 2 weeks of life but may occur as late as 3 months after birth

     b. The overwhelming majority of cases involve preterm infants.

     c. Term infants with intrauterine cocaine exposure, hyperviscosity syndrome, or cyanotic congenital heart disease are at increased risk.

  2. Signs and symptoms

     a. Feeding intolerance, vomiting (bilious or nonbilious)

     b. Abdominal distention and tenderness

     c. Bloody stools

     d. Hypotension/shock

     e. Nonspecific signs of sepsis (e.g., lethargy, respiratory distress, apnea)

     f. DIC

     g. Abdominal mass (usually right lower quadrant)

     h. Abdominal wall erythema

  3. Laboratory findings

     a. Leukopenia (<5,000 white blood cells [WBCs]) or leukocytosis (>25,000 WBCs)

     b. Increased immature neutrophils on complete blood count (CBC)

     c. Thrombocytopenia

     d. Metabolic acidosis

     e. Hyperkalemia

  4. Radiographic findings

     a. Pneumatosis intestinalis (air in bowel wall)

     b. Dilated bowel loops

     c. Thickened bowel wall

     d. Portal venous air

     e. Peritoneal free air (most easily detected on left lateral decubitus view)

  5. Management

     a. Ventilatory support

     b. Fluid resuscitation with 10 to 20 mL/kg IV bolus of normal saline or Ringer's lactate solution and maintenance fluids at 150 mL/kg/day for *third spacing* (see Chapter 6).

     c. BP support with vasopressors as needed

     d. Consider sodium bicarbonate for correction of metabolic acidosis

     e. Provide blood products (packed red blood cells, platelets) as needed

     f. NPO with gastric decompression via nasogastric tube

BOX 32-3

POTENTIAL CAUSES OF SEIZURE ACTIVITY IN NEONATES

AT BIRTH

- Acute drug effects (maternal anesthetic agents or cocaine)
- Hypoxic-ischemic brain injury

DAY 1

- Hypoglycemia
- Hypocalcemia
- Hypoxic-ischemic brain injury
- Infection
- Intracranial hemorrhage
- Hyperviscosity syndrome
- Drug withdrawal

DAYS 2-3

- Infection (meningitis)
- Drug withdrawal

DAYS 3-7

- Infection (prenatal and neonatal)
- Hypocalcemia
- Drug withdrawal
- Developmental defects, inborn errors of metabolism

>1 WEEK

- Infection
- Drug withdrawal (methadone)
- Trauma
- Intracranial hemorrhage (suspect vitamin K deficiency)

---

      g. Sepsis evaluation and initiation of broad-spectrum antibiotic therapy

      h. Surgical consultation

IX. Seizures

   A. Overview

      1. The management of neonatal seizures does not differ from that in the older child.

      2. The cause and initial presentation may be different.

      3. Seizures in the neonatal period can present as apnea (**Box 32-3**).

   B. Evaluation

      1. History should include birth history and characteristics of seizure activity.

      2. Physical examination should include the following:

         a. Neurologic and retinal examination

         b. Assessment of the fontanelles

   3. Laboratory evaluation
      a. Serum **glucose** and electrolyte levels (include Na^+, Ca^{2+}, Mg)
      b. Sepsis evaluation (include CBC, blood, urine, and CSF cultures)
      c. Metabolic evaluation
         (1) Ammonia
         (2) Lactic acid
         (3) Plasma amino acids
         (4) Urine organic acids
         (5) Pyruvate
      d. Arterial blood gases
      e. Urine toxicology screen
   4. Neuroimaging (head CT or MRI)
 C. Treatment
   1. Assure adequate oxygenation and ventilation.
   2. Treat the underlying cause.
   3. Pharmacologic intervention does not differ from that in the older child, except for a trial of pyridoxine, 50 to 100 mg IV push, if the seizures are refractory to other interventions.
X. Coma
 A. Overview
   1. Many of the causes of coma or unresponsiveness in the neonate are the same as in older infants and children (see Chapter 16).
   2. Intracranial hemorrhage, drugs transmitted from the mother, and inborn errors of metabolism must be considered.
 B. Causes
   1. CNS abnormalities
      a. Intracranial hemorrhage
         (1) Intraventricular most likely in preterm; subarachnoid or subdural in term infants
         (2) Vascular abnormality should be considered in all patients.
      b. Hypoxic-ischemic encephalopathy
      c. Meningitis
      d. Maternal drugs of abuse
         (1) CNS depression from opiates
         (2) Cerebral infarctions from cocaine
      e. Trauma, physical abuse
      f. Seizures, postictal state
      g. Kernicterus (see Section XI)
   2. Metabolic abnormality
      a. Hypoglycemia
      b. Electrolyte imbalance
      c. Uremia

d. Diabetic ketoacidosis
e. Hypercapnia
3. Inborn errors of metabolism
   a. Symptoms generally occur after a period of well-being.
   b. CNS symptoms
      (1) Hypotonia
      (2) Coma
      (3) Seizures
   c. GI symptoms
      (1) Poor feeding
      (2) Vomiting
      (3) Hepatomegaly
      (4) Hyperbilirubinemia
   d. Metabolic findings
      (1) Acidosis
      (2) Hyperammonemia
      (3) Hypoglycemia
      (4) Ketosis
   e. Other findings
      (1) Abnormal hair
      (2) Abnormal odor
   f. Evaluation includes the following:
      (1) Serum glucose level
      (2) Electrolyte levels
      (3) Blood gas (to evaluate acid-base status)
      (4) Ammonia, lactate and pyruvate levels,
      (5) Urinalysis (ketones)
      (6) Plasma amino acid levels
      (7) Urine organic acid levels
   g. Initial management:
      (1) ABCs of resuscitation as needed
      (2) **Stop feedings containing protein** (pending diagnosis)
      (3) **Start infusion with D10W** (and maintain euglycemia).
      (4) Metabolic disease consultation and diagnostic workup
4. Toxins (see Chapter 17): Consider toxins or medications, including herbal remedies, that can be transmitted through breast milk.
XI. Hyperbilirubinemia
   A. Indirect hyperbilirubinemia
      1. Signs and symptoms
         a. Jaundice
         b. Dark-colored urine
         c. Lethargy or irritability
         d. Poor feeding
         e. Signs of dehydration

2. Initial laboratory evaluation (rule out hemolytic process)
   a. Total and direct serum bilirubin levels
   b. CBC with reticulocyte count and smear
   c. Blood type and direct Coombs' test
3. Nonhemolytic causes
   a. Physiologic jaundice
   b. Dehydration
   c. Breast milk jaundice
   d. Extravasation of blood (cephalohematoma, bruising)
   e. Infant of diabetic mother
   f. Prematurity
   g. Polycythemia
   h. Urinary tract infection
   i. Sepsis
4. Hemolytic causes
   a. Isoimmunization (ABO or Rh incompatibility)
   b. Glucose-6-phosphate dehydrogenase deficiency (or other red cell enzyme defects)
   c. Red blood cell membrane defects
   d. Hemoglobinopathies
5. Infants with hemolysis:
   a. Often present with jaundice before 24 hours of age
   b. May have pallor, anemia, and hepatosplenomegaly
6. Bilirubin toxicity (kernicterus)
   a. Risk factors
      (1) Prematurity
      (2) Hemolytic disease
      (3) Acidosis
      (4) Sepsis
      (5) Asphyxia
      (6) Hypoalbuminemia
   b. Initial symptoms
      (1) Lethargy
      (2) Hypotonia
      (3) Poor suck
   c. Subsequent symptoms
      (1) Hypertonia (arching of the neck and opisthotonus)
      (2) Fever
      (3) High-pitched cry
      (4) Hypotonia returns after about 1 week.
   d. Symptoms in survivors
      (1) Choreoathetoid cerebral palsy
      (2) Sensorineural hearing loss
      (3) Paralysis of upward gaze
      (4) Dental enamel hypoplasia

32

7. Treatment
   a. Hydration
   b. Intensive phototherapy
   c. Exchange transfusion
8. Indications for phototherapy
   a. Phototherapy converts bilirubin in the skin to less toxic and more soluble metabolites that are excreted in the urine, thereby lowering the serum bilirubin level.
   b. Phototherapy is initiated when the total serum bilirubin level exceeds a threshold value that poses a risk for kernicterus.
   c. See **Figure 32-5.**
9. Indications for exchange transfusion: The total serum bilirubin values at which exchange transfusion is recommended are given in **Figure 32-6.**

B. Direct hyperbilirubinemia
   1. Defined as direct serum bilirubin >2 mg/dL
   2. Usually accompanied by a history of the following:
      a. Prolonged hyperbilirubinemia
      b. Acholic stool, and/or
      c. Dark-colored urine
   3. Requires evaluation for possible biliary atresia, hepatitis, or choledochal cyst.

XII. Polycythemia-hyperviscosity syndrome
   A. Definition
      1. Polycythemia is defined as a central venous Hct >65%.
      2. May be associated with hyperviscosity syndrome, which can lead to CNS infarctions and poor circulation to a variety of organs.
      3. Blood viscosity increases almost linearly when Hct >65%.
   B. Associated conditions
      1. Infants with intrauterine hypoxia
      2. Placental insufficiency
      3. Delayed cord clamping
      4. Pregnancy at high altitude
      5. Maternal diabetes mellitus
      6. Trisomy 21
   C. Signs and symptoms
      1. Asymptomatic
      2. Tachypnea
      3. Cyanosis (especially acrocyanosis)
      4. Lethargy, hypotonia
      5. Poor feeding
      6. Irritability, seizures
      7. Hypoglycemia
      8. Hematuria

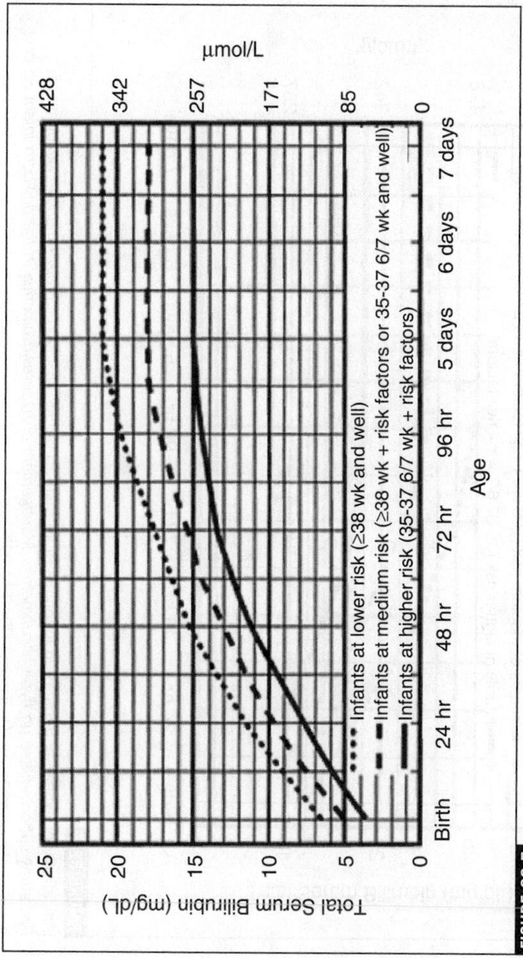
Total Serum Bilirubin (mg/dL)
25
20
15
10
5
0
µmol/L
428
342
257
171
85
0
Infants at lower risk (≥38 wk and well)
Infants at medium risk (≥38 wk + risk factors or 35-37 6/7 wk and well)
Infants at higher risk (35-37 6/7 wk + risk factors)
Birth
24 hr
48 hr
72 hr
96 hr
5 days
6 days
7 days
Age

FIGURE 32-5 Indications for phototherapy in infants more than 35 weeks' gestation. *(From American Academy of Pediatrics subcommittee on hyperbilirubinemia. Management of hyperbilirubinemia in the newborn infant 35 or more weeks of gestation. Pediatrics 2004;114:297-316.)*

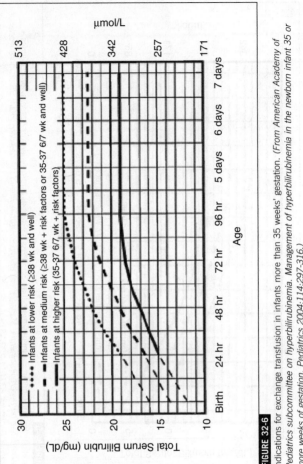

FIGURE 32-6

Indications for exchange transfusion in infants more than 35 weeks' gestation. *(From American Academy of Pediatrics subcommittee on hyperbilirubinemia. Management of hyperbilirubinemia in the newborn infant 35 or more weeks of gestation. Pediatrics 2004;114:297-316.)*

9. Jaundice
10. Thrombocytopenia
11. Cerebral infarction
12. NEC
13. Cardiomegaly
14. Pulmonary hypertension

D. Treatment
1. Rehydration alone may reduce the Hct if the newborn is dehydrated.
2. Symptomatic
   a. Partial exchange transfusion, replacing blood with a plasma substitute
   b. Isotonic saline is as effective as plasma or saline plus albumin.
   c. The volume to be exchanged is determined by the following equation:

$$\text{Volume (mL)} = \frac{(\text{Initial Hct} - \text{desired Hct}) \times \text{weight (kg)} \times 90 \text{ mL/kg}}{\text{Initial Hct}}$$

   d. 50% is generally used as the desired Hct.
3. Asymptomatic
   a. Prophylactic treatment of asymptomatic infants is controversial.
   b. Hydration may be tried as an initial step.

XIII. Neonatal transport checklist
A. Thermal stability
1. External heat source to maintain skin temperature at 36.5° C and rectal temperature at 36.5° to 37.5° C.
2. Infant should be kept warm, dry, and away from drafts.
B. Vital signs
1. Respiratory rate: 30 to 60 breaths/min (rates in the upper range seen in younger infants)
2. HR: 100 to 160 beats/min (rates in the upper range seen in younger infants)
3. BP (**Table 32-8**): If the need for vasopressor support is anticipated, initiate prior to transport or have vasopressor drip available on transport.

TABLE 32-8

BLOOD PRESSURE MEASUREMENTS (mm Hg)

Weight (kg)	Systolic	Diastolic	MAP
1	35-60	18-35	25-45
2	45-65	20-40	30-50
3	50-70	25-45	35-55
4	58-80	30-50	42-62

MAP, Mean arterial pressure.

C. Respiratory support
   1. Ensure adequate airway and oxygenation.
      a. SaO_2 in preterm infants, 88% to 94%
      b. SaO_2 in term infants, 95% to 100%
   2. Assume that respiratory distress will worsen during transport.
   3. Consider prophylactic intubation if there is evidence of increasing respiratory distress or compromised airway.
   4. Secure ET tube well with tape applied to skin.
   5. Sedation may be helpful, if not medically contraindicated.
D. Intravenous access
   1. Ensure functioning IV line with sufficient fluid for transport.
   2. Have backup line in place if critical infusion (e.g., PGE_1, dopamine) is required.
E. Documentation
   1. Copies of all records (maternal records if available), radiographs, and laboratory results
   2. Transport permit signed
   3. Phone numbers of referring hospital and parents obtained

Chapter 33

Transportation of the Critically Ill and Injured Child

Lynn D. Martin, MD, MBA,
Susan Ziegfeld, MSN, CRNP-Pediatric,
and Charles N. Paidas, MD, MBA

I. Overview

   A. Reducing further harm to child

   1. Effective stabilization and timely safe transport, from the scene or interhospital, are vital to reduce further harm to an injured child.

   2. Regardless of the scene of origin, life-threatening illnesses and injuries need to be cared for immediately.

   3. For severely ill or injured children, optimal care is ultimately provided at specialized centers.

   4. Physicians caring for children in other designations must be knowledgeable of who in their community is best prepared to treat the severely ill or injured child and when a transfer to a specialized pediatric center is necessary.

   B. Why a pediatric center?

   1. Patient outcome is directly related to time from injury to proper definitive care.

   2. The outcome of pediatric trauma is enhanced if injured children are cared for in pediatric centers.

   3. No longer should the child be transferred to the closest hospital, but instead to the closest pediatric center.

   4. Prehospital providers are trained to *scoop and swoop*, transporting the child to an appropriate center as quickly as possible.

   5. Whether critically ill or injured, children can deteriorate rapidly and develop severe complications.

   6. The unique anatomic characteristics of children require specialized attention to assessment and management, which is better provided by pediatric specialists.

   7. Furthermore, psychological needs and child development considerations warrant a specialized team accustomed to caring for the ill or injured child.

33

II. Public education and prevention
   Injury and illness can be prevented or controlled on three levels.
   A. Primary prevention
      1. This is twofold, involving both the public health and legislative systems.
      2. The public health system addresses access to health care and appropriate immunization of children, whereas the legislative system can influence traffic laws and gun control.
   B. Secondary prevention
      1. This involves minimizing the severity of an illness or injury.
      2. *Damage control* is considered secondary prevention.
   C. Tertiary prevention
   This involves optimizing the child's outcome through treatment and eventual rehabilitation.
III. Emergency medical services (EMS) for children
   A formal curriculum for prehospital providers is imperative to ensure that a high standard of care is consistently provided to patients (**Table 33-1**). Those who provide transport services must ensure that the staff has an adequate baseline level of training and/or licensure, an ongoing system of educational review, and the frequency of activity necessary to maintain skills.
   Established in 1984, the Emergency Medical Services for Children (http://bolivia.hrsa.gov/emsc) addresses the unique needs of children within the EMS system, and serves as a resource for statewide

TABLE 33-1

PREHOSPITAL PROVIDER DESCRIPTIONS AND SKILLS

Provider	Description
Emergency medical dispatch	Call intake, call allocator, medical interrogation, medical prearrival and postdispatch instructions, medical call prioritization, EMS allocation and management
First responder	Patient assessment, bleeding control and bandaging, fracture management, medical emergency management, CPR, optional O_2 administration, optional automated external defibrillator use
Basic EMT (BLS)	Patient assessment, bleeding control and bandaging, shock management, fracture management, CPR, O_2 administration, medical emergency management, patient assisted medication, spinal immobilization, patient movement and transport.
CRT (ALS)	Intravenous fluid administration, medication administration, monitoring of the ECG and defibrillation-cardioversion, endotracheal intubation, external jugular cannulation, intraosseous cannulation, decompression thoracostomy, external transcutaneous pacing
Paramedic (ALS) CPR	All skills listed above plus additional medication administration, nasotracheal intubation, external transcutaneous pacing

ALS, Advanced life support; *BLS*, basic life support; *CPR*, cardiopulmonary resuscitation; *CRT*, cardiac rescue technician; *ECG*, electrocardiogram; *EMS*, emergency medical services; *EMT*, emergency medical technician; O_2, oxygen.

guidelines, resources, and networking on emergency care for
children and their families.

IV. Primary transport

Defined as the prehospital care phase of treatment

The child may be transported by a layperson or by the EMS
system. This type of transport can be divided into three phases.

A. Entry phase

1. This is the time from when the *system* is activated until the
arrival of EMS personnel.

2. This is often accomplished by dialing 911; however, access to
this system may not be available in all cities.

B. Response phase

Defined as the period of time from the arrival of EMS providers
until transport to a medical center

This phase can be further divided into several task-oriented
time periods.

1. Scene assessment

a. On arrival, EMS providers must perform a brief scene
assessment for personal safety hazards and an assessment
of the environmental needs for clues regarding mechanism
of injury.

b. Moreover, it is important to document clues that could
suggest signs of possible neglect or abuse.

c. Crash scene information, such as intrusion space into a
vehicle, may help determine the severity of injury as well as
help with future injury prevention initiatives and research.

2. Patient assessment, treatment, and triage

a. Life-threatening illnesses and injuries need to be cared for
immediately. Emphasis in the prehospital phase should be
based on the ABCDE (airway, breathing, circulation,
disability, exposure) priorities.

b. Treatment decisions can be made with the help of protocols
and online medical direction, which can vary by city or state.

3. Transport

a. Priorities, resources, and environmental condition decisions
should be driven by the EMS system.

b. The field provider must determine the level of hospital
appropriate to care for the child, resources available, and
transport time.

c. As a general rule, once the field provider has performed a
primary survey, the child should be transported as soon as
possible to the most appropriate facility.

C. Hospital phase

Defined as the period of time when the hospital is first notified of
the child's arrival and assumes medical direction until ultimate
discharge of the child post injury

This phase can further be divided into three phases.

1. Anticipatory preparation
   a. A designated area for pediatric emergency care should be preestablished within the medical facility.
   b. Pediatric-specific equipment and reference materials should be well visualized and contained in this area.
2. Patient care
   a. This phase begins with the arrival and report of the EMS personnel to the receiving staff (**Table 33-2**).
   b. Optimal care requires mobilization of resources and personnel into an organized team.
   c. Protocols should be developed that assign responsibility to each member of the team.
   d. Team composition may vary from facility to facility, but intervention priorities should remain consistent with attention to the ABCDE evaluation and treatment.
3. Receiving staff: Becomes medicolegally responsible for the child as soon as the child is in their care, whether at their own institution or an outside institution (in the case of a transport team)

V. Secondary transport

After initial resuscitation and stabilization, severely ill or injured children may require definitive care at a specialized trauma or pediatric center. Awareness of each institution's capability and areas of expertise is essential prior to transporting a critically ill or injured child. Early consideration of transportation is of equal importance.

A. Advanced preparation

A list of pediatric tertiary care centers and transport systems with pediatric capabilities, including phone numbers and administrative and treatment protocols, should be readily available.

B. Transport telephone information
   1. Organization of information by the referring institution prior to the initial request for transport can improve communication and the overall transport process.
   2. Preprinted forms can expedite this procedure (see Table 33-2).
   3. It is imperative that direct verbal communication between hospitals occurs prior to the transportation of the child.

C. Mode of transportation: Ground versus air

It is very important for each center to evaluate its resources and capabilities of its local transport services. Considerations should include but are not limited to the following:
   1. Maintaining optimal level of care
   2. Safety (weather conditions)
   3. Cost considerations of ground versus air transport

TABLE 33-2

CHECKLIST: COMMUNICATION WITH HOSPITAL PERSONNEL

☐ Date/time:
☐ Name:
☐ Age:
☐ Date of birth:
☐ Sex:
☐ Weight:
☐ Chief complaint: _____
☐ Medic name, phone number, or
☐ Referring physician, referring hospital phone number
☐ Insurance information if available (verify in state versus out of state)
☐ Consent (if necessary)
☐ Patient information:
☐ AMPLE history
   A: Allergies
   M: Medication
   P: Past medical history
   L: Last meal
   E: Events leading to illness or injury
☐ Interventions thus far:
☐ Physical findings:

	Symptom	Y	N	Comments
Airway	Noisy breathing			
	Retractions			
	Drooling			
	Tripoding			
	Intubated			Size, position
	Risk factors for difficult airway			
Breathing	O₂ requirement			
	Increased WOB			
	Altered LOC			
Circulation	Dysrhythmias			
	Poor perfusion, delayed CR			CR = _____ seconds
	Vascular access			
Disability	GCS			
	E:___			
	V:___			
	M:___ = ___			
	Increased ICP (pupils, posturing)			
	Seizure activity			
Exposure	Rash			

☐ *Laboratory findings
☐ *Radiologic findings (copies of films when possible)
☐ *Mode of transportation
☐ Air versus land
☐ Scene versus interhospital
☐ Approximate time of arrival

CR, Capillary refill; *E*, eye opening; *GCS*, Glasgow Coma Scale; *ICP*, intracranial pressure; *LOC*, level of consciousness; *M*, motor; *V*, verbal; *WOB*, work of breathing.
*Denotes additional information if being transported from another facility.

33

VI. Transport team

A dedicated interhospital transport team is required in addition to statewide resources. Prehospital providers, referring hospital, and regional center must cooperate closely in assigning a priority for transport of the patient (**Table 33-3**). A well-equipped transport vehicle is essential for optimal care, and the equipment should be checked on a regular schedule and before each transport (**Table 33-4**).

VII. Concerns of air transport

During the period of transfer, a critically ill child is at risk from the pathology, treatment, and the transfer itself. Air medical transportation is an important component of the prehospital EMS system because out of hospital time can be minimized and specialized in-flight delivery of care can be offered. Air transportation cannot only be costly but can also contribute some risks and restrictions based on the nature of the disease or injury itself, as well as changes in the environment (e.g., temperatures, positioning, transportation equipment).

Communication, careful evaluation and management, anticipation of complications, and a well-equipped, well-trained transport team can minimize associated risks of transport. While maintaining a level of care as close as possible to that available at the receiving critical care unit, team members should always be prepared for worst case scenarios and develop a method for problem resolution as troublesome issues arise.

A. Physiologic considerations

1. Dalton's law of partial pressure

a. This law states that the total *pressure* exerted by a *gaseous* mixture is equal to the sum of the *partial pressures* of each individual component in a gas mixture.

b. At sea level, the air mixture is approximately 78% nitrogen and 21% oxygen (O_2), with the remaining 1% being a mix of argon, carbon dioxide, neon, helium, and other rare gases.

2. Barometric pressure

a. Barometric pressure (PB) is the sum of the partial pressures of individual gases in the atmosphere.

b. PB is defined as atmospheric pressure—that is, the force exerted on a surface of unit area caused by the weight of the air column above, normally between 950 and 1050 kilopascal (kPa) at sea level.

c. It indicates the presence and movement of weather patterns and affects many physical measurements.

d. The partial pressure of O_2 in the atmosphere (PO_2) is equal to the concentration of O_2 in the atmosphere (21%) times the PB (**Table 33-5**).

TABLE 33-3

INTERHOSPITAL TRANSPORTATION PRIORITY SCALE

	Priority 1: MD/NP, RN/RT (NICU)	Priority 2: RN/Paramedic Routine, RN/RN	Priority 3: Paramedic Only	Priority 4: EMT Only
Airway	S/S of acute upper airway obstruction H/O difficult airway with S/S of respiratory failure Intubated with H/O difficult airway or <8 years by ground	Intubated with normal airway by air or >8 year by ground Tracheostomy	No S/S of upper airway obstruction No artificial airway	Normal airway
Breathing	Impending respiratory failure Mechanical ventilation with hypoxemia FiO₂ ≥60% or PEEP >5 cm Higher level supplemental O₂ (progressive)	High level supplemental O₂ (stable) Mechanical ventilation with FiO₂ <60% or PEEP ≤5 cm	Low level supplemental O₂	No acute O₂ requirement
Circulation	Poor perfusion and/or dysrhythmia despite support No vascular access in unstable patient Stable condition on acute vasopressor or antidysrhythmic	Stable condition on chronic vasopressor or antidysrhythmic	Stable condition with no support requiring cardiac monitoring	No cardiac monitoring
Disability	GCS <10 Uncontrolled or persistent seizure activity	Acute altered mental status (GCS >10) Controlled seizure activity	Chronic altered mental status	Normal neurologic status
Medications	Multiple vasopressors or antidysrhythmics	Medication or infusions not in paramedic formulary	Morphine for pain Diazepam for unanticipated seizure	No medications
Invasive lines	ICP monitor PA catheter	Arterial line Temporary CL Chest tube	Long-term CL or PIV with IVF Gastric tube Foley catheter	Long-term CL or PIC that is capped

CL, Central line; *Fio₂*, fraction of inspired oxygen; *GSC*, Glasgow Coma Scale; *H/O*, history of; *ICP*, intracranial pressure; *IVF*, intravenous fluid; *NICU*, neonatal intensive care unit; *NP*, nurse practitioner; *O₂*, oxygen; *PA*, pulmonary artery; *PEEP*, positive end-expiratory pressure; *PIC*, percutaneous inserted central line; *PIV*, peripheral intravenous catheter; *RN*, registered nurse; *RT*, registered technician; *S/S*, signs and symptoms.

33

TABLE 33-4

TRANSPORTATION EQUIPMENT CHECKLIST

☐ Airway equipment
☐ Appropriate size nasal cannulas, masks, ETT, stylets, NP, OP airways, laryngeal mask airway
☐ Intubation kit: Blades, handles, light bulbs, Magill forceps, batteries
☐ O_2 source (full e-cylinder O_2 tank: 660 liters at 1900 psi)
☐ O_2 delivery device: Bag–valve–mask, nonrebreather mask
☐ Flowmeters
☐ Suction source
☐ Various size suction catheters, Yankauer catheters
☐ Ventilators
☐ Electrical supply system
☐ Light source
☐ Functional climate control system, (heating and cooling)
☐ Medical portable radio or other communication device
☐ Means to secure all equipment and personnel
☐ Spine immobilization equipment, splinting devices, or car seat
☐ Emergency medications
☐ Glucometer or dextrose sticks
☐ Pediatric reference guide (Broselow tape, equipment and medication doses based on age or length)
☐ Intravenous access supplies (IV, IO)
☐ IV fluids (LR or NSS with and without dextrose)
☐ Chest tubes, Heimlich valve, chest air evacuation device
Monitors include:
☐ BP
☐ ECG
☐ SpO_2
☐ $ETCO_2$
☐ Capability of synchronized cardioversion/defibrillation versus AED
☐ Sanitation equipment/biohazard items
☐ Personal protective equipment

AED, Automated external defibrillator; *BP*, blood pressure; *ECG*, electrocardiogram; *$ETco_2$*, end-tidal carbon dioxide; *ETT*, endotracheal tube; *IO*, intraosseous; *IV*, intravenous; *LR*, lactated Ringer's; *NP*, nasopharyngeal; *NSS*, normal saline solution; *O_2*, oxygen; *OP*, oropharyngeal; *SpO_2*, oxygen saturation.
NOTE: All equipment should be latex-free (when possible) and include various age-specific and weight-specific sizes.

    e. Thus, at sea level, the PO_2 in the air is 160 mm Hg (0.21 × 760), but is only 110 mm Hg at 10,000 feet (0.21 × 523).
  3. Alveolar O_2
    a. As the PO_2 in the atmosphere falls, so does alveolar O_2.
    b. The relationship between the two is not linear; alveolar O_2 is dependent on the PO_2 in the atmosphere and on the alveolar partial pressure of carbon dioxide ($PACO_2$).

TABLE 33-5

RELATIONSHIP OF BAROMETRIC PRESSURE AND ALTITUDE AND EFFECTS ON PARTIAL PRESSURE OF OXYGEN IN THE ATMOSPHERE*

Altitude (feet)	Barometric Pressure (mm Hg)	P_{O_2} in Air (mm Hg)	P_{O_2} in Alveoli* (mm Hg)
0 (sea level)	760	160	110
2000	707	149	99
4000	656	138	88
6000	609	128	78
10,000	523	110	60
16,000	412	87	57
18,000	360	76	46
20,000	349	73	43
30,000	226	48	18
36,000	170	36	6

*Assumes a partial pressure of arterial carbon dioxide (Pa_{CO_2}) of 40 mm Hg at altitudes below 10,000 feet, a Pa_{CO_2} of 24 mm Hg at an altitude above 10,000 feet, and a respiratory quotient of 0.8.

c. The alveolar gas equation is defined by the following formula:

$$P_{AO_2} = P_{IO_2} - (Pa_{CO_2}/R) = (P_B - 47) \times (F_{IO_2}) - (P_{CO_2}/0.8)$$

where

P_{AO_2} = alveolar partial pressure of O_2,

P_{IO_2} = partial pressure of inspired O_2

F_{IO_2} = fraction of inspired O_2

which = $(P_B - 47) \times (F_{IO_2})$, or the barometric pressure minus the partial pressure of water at 37° C times the inspired O_2 concentration, and

P_{ACO_2} = alveolar partial pressure of carbon dioxide

R = respiratory quotient

assumed to = 0.8.

d. As P_{O_2} in the atmosphere falls, the body compensates for the diminished atmospheric O_2 by increasing minute ventilation.

e. This lowers CO_2 and minimizes the decrease in alveolar O_2 concentration.

4. Boyle's law

a. Boyle's law states that at constant temperature, the volume of a gas varies inversely with the pressure.

    b. Thus, the volume of gas within a closed space (pneumothorax, bowel obstruction, cystic adenomatous malformation of the newborn lung, and endotracheal balloon cuff) will change with changes in P_B.

    c. As P_B is halved, the volume within a closed space will double.

  5. Cabin pressurization

    a. Cabin pressurization reduces the effects of altitude by maintaining a preset P_B within the cabin of a fixed wing aircraft.

    b. Cabin pressurization is not available in helicopters, which normally fly at altitudes well below 12,500 feet.

B. Stress of flight on transport personnel

The stresses of flight are multiple and often interrelated. Modern helicopters have specialized patient care compartments, which optimize the medical crew's access to the patient and patient comfort. The aircraft has handling characteristics that allow for a gentler ride. Furthermore, noise reduction technology and climate control has lessened noise and temperature stressors. Adverse effects of altitude and flight include the following:

  1. Night vision is impaired at cabin pressures when the aircraft is higher than 5000 feet.

  2. The ability to concentrate, stay alert, and make rapid decisions is impaired by high altitude, vibration, and noise; fatigue, drugs, and sleep deprivation potentiate these effects.

  3. P_B disturbances of the middle ear are common, particularly in the presence of an upper respiratory infection, sinus infection, or allergies.

  4. Dry eyes, lips, and mouth, chapped lips, hoarseness, and sore throat are common because the absolute amount of moisture in the environment drops with increasing altitude.

  5. Motion sickness (nausea, vomiting, pallor, headache, and lethargy) is a problem during all forms of transport.

C. Medical equipment

Transport personnel should always rely on their eyes, the color of the patient (especially a baby), and chest expansion. These three components are essential for in flight care of the critically ill or injured child.

  1. All medical equipment used in an aircraft should be evaluated for altitude changes before use. Information regarding most equipment is available from the U.S. Air Force.

  2. Expansion of gas in closed containers (Boyle's law) affects the endotracheal tube cuff, blood pressure cuff, air splints, unvented glass bottles, intravenous drip chambers, flowmeters, ventilators, and unvented mattress covers in newborn isolettes.

3. Vibration can interfere with the functioning of medical devices (cardiorespiratory monitors, pulse oximeters, pacemakers) without harming the device itself.

VIII. Legal considerations

Interhospital transport of children is fraught with liability issues. Federal and state laws, as well as society standards, have been developed to establish and coordinate a uniform interhospital transport process. It is incumbent on the local hospital to know applicable federal and state laws.

A. Medical direction

The medical director should have authority over all clinical and patient care aspects of the EMS system or service, with the specific job description dictated by local needs. Medical direction of prehospital EMS can be divided into two sections, off-line and on-line.

1. Off-line medical direction
   a. Administrative promulgation and enforcement of accepted standards of prehospital care
   b. Prospective methods include the following:
      (1) Training, testing, and certification of providers
      (2) Protocol development
      (3) Operational policy and procedures development
      (4) Legislative activities
   c. Retrospective activities include the following:
      (1) Medical audit and review of care
      (2) Direction of remedial education
      (3) Limitation of patient care functions, if needed
   d. Various aspects of prospective and retrospective medical direction can be handled by committees functioning under the medical director with representation from appropriate medical and EMS personnel.

2. On-line (concurrent) medical direction
   a. Provided directly to prehospital providers by the medical director or designee
   b. Communication provided either on scene or by direct voice communication
   c. Ultimate authority and responsibility for concurrent medical direction rest with the receiving medical director.

B. HIPAA privacy regulation

The Health Insurance Portability and Accountability Act (HIPAA) of 1996 (http://www.hipaa.org) was signed into law on August 21, 1996.

1. Requires informing individuals of their rights and how their protected health information (PHI) may be used or disclosed.

In emergency situations:

a. HIPAA defers to Emergency Medical Treatment and Labor Act (EMTALA); see later.

b. The notice is provided once the individual has been stabilized and is able to sign an acknowledgment of receipt form. If the individual refuses to sign the form or notice cannot be provided (i.e., a person voluntarily leaves the emergency department), then the provider must document the individual's refusal to sign.

2. Defines a *covered entity* as any of the following:

a. A health care provider that electronically transmits health information in one of the transactions covered by the HIPAA Standards for Electronic Transaction Regulation

b. Any health care plan

c. Health care clearinghouse, which helps transmit transactions electronically between the provider and payer

3. Requires covered entities to obtain an individual's authorization before using or disclosing PHI; exceptions to this rule include the following:

a. Use and disclosure of PHI for treatment, payment, and health care operation purposes, because these are regarded as being internal activities of the covered entity

b. Use and disclosure of PHI as required by law

c. Use and disclosure of PHI as allowed by waived research

C. Emergency Medical Treatment and Labor Act

1. In 1986, Congress enacted EMTALA to ensure public access to emergency services regardless of the ability to pay.

2. This was passed as part of the Consolidated Omnibus Budget Reconciliation Act of 1986 based on concerns of increased reports that hospitals were refusing to treat or accept patients if they did not have health insurance.

3. EMTALA requires that a hospital must provide a medical screening and, if necessary, stabilize a seriously ill or injured patient prior to transfer to a facility that has agreed to provide definitive care.

4. The hospital can transfer the child, at the family's request, following an informed discussion.

5. EMTALA requires that a transfer must meet certain requirements:

a. Medical treatment is provided within its capacity.

b. The receiving hospital must have space available, qualified personnel, and officially accept the patient.

c. The transferring hospital must send the receiving hospital the appropriate medical records.

d. The transfer must be effective through qualified personnel and transportation equipment, including the use of necessary and medically appropriate equipment.

      e. The transferring hospital is legally responsible for the patient until the patient's care is accepted by the receiving hospital, and it is responsible for the adequacy and competency of the personnel and equipment used in transfer.

      f. The physician at the sending hospital is responsible for determining the appropriate mode of transfer; necessary equipment for the transfer, and necessary attendants for transfer.

      g. Medical direction shall be in accordance with individual state guidelines.

IX. Guidelines

  A. Society for Critical Care Medicine (SCCM)

    SCCM has issued guidelines for the transfer of critically ill patients (www.sccm.org).

    1. Current law and good medical practice require that the competent patient or agent give informed consent prior to the transfer.

    2. If this is not possible, then the indications for transfer and the reason for not obtaining consent need to be documented.

  B. American College of Emergency Physicians (ACEP)

    ACEP has also published guidelines regarding interhospital transfers (www.acep.org).

33

Index

Page numbers followed by *f* indicate
figures; *t*, tables; *b*, boxes.